Insights into Medical Communication

Linguistic Insights

Studies in Language and Communication

Edited by Maurizio Gotti,
University of Bergamo

Volume 203

PETER LANG
Bern · Berlin · Bruxelles · Frankfurt am Main · New York · Oxford · Wien

Maurizio Gotti, Stefania Maci & Michele Sala (eds)

Insights into Medical Communication

PETER LANG
Bern · Berlin · Bruxelles · Frankfurt am Main · New York · Oxford · Wien

Bibliographic information published by die Deutsche Nationalbibliothek
Die Deutsche Nationalbibliothek lists this publication in the Deutsche Nationalbibliografie; detailed bibliographic data is available on the Internet at ‹http://dnb.d-nb.de›.

British Library Cataloguing-in-Publication Data: A catalogue record for this book is available from The British Library, Great Britain

Library of Congress Control Number: 2015942051

Published with the support of Dipartimento di Lingue, Letterature Straniere e Comunicazione, Università di Bergamo, Italy.

ISSN 1424-8689 pb. ISSN 2235-6371 eBook
ISBN 978-3-0343-1694-1 pb. ISBN 978-3-0351-0844-6 eBook

This publication has been peer reviewed.

Hochfeldstrasse 32, CH-3012 Bern, Switzerland
info@peterlang.com, www.peterlang.com

Contents

Communicating with Patients

Communicating Healthcare Information

Communicating Research Findings

Stefania M. Maci / Michele Sala / Maurizio Gotti

Introduction

1. Investigating medical communication

Medical knowledge is represented, conveyed and questioned through communicative practices. However, the relation between medicine and communication is complex. Despite the fact that knowledge is still commonly transferred and disseminated through language, medical knowledge implies the exploitation of other means of communication, such as formulae, graphs, images, etc. as well as other communicative modes, such as traditional academic and popular genres, in addition to newly-emerging procedures offered by information technology.

Medical discourse is not just a matter of communicating with patients, about patients, and for patients. Indeed, this specialised type of communication is a very complex phenomenon, mainly relying on the fact that practitioners and researchers need to communicate in different ways, for different aims, and to different targets. As rightly pointed out by Hyland (2004, 2011), the ways in which members of the various disciplines communicate encompass different viewpoints embracing both the issue under investigation as well as their standpoints on that issue. For this reason, specialists employ as many registers as possible according to the many different options available so as to target the various audiences they need to address. Furthermore, in order to reach their goals, they need to exploit a number of interdisciplinary and multimodal strategies, both in public and in private interactions.

This new trend, therefore, has led investigators of medical communication to take into consideration newer theoretical perspectives, and to adopt a more varied range of methodological approaches. Indeed, in communicating medical research findings, this new trend has promoted the recourse to a more 'open genre network' (Swales/Feak 2000) of academic writing, which includes – besides the well-established and visible public research genres such as research articles, abstracts, or conference proposals – more modern communicative procedures such as posters, research letters and blogs (Maci 2012a, 2012b; D'Angelo 2012) in addition to newer forms of popularization, by means of which medical science can be disseminated to laymen as well to practitioners not belonging to the same professional sector (Myers 2003; Gotti 2014).

One of the challenges in medical communication studies is the ethnographic positioning of the applied linguist when studying specialised discourse in professional domains. As Sarangi states in this volume, professional practice is not easily reducible to mere language or communication because it relies on different layers of understanding involving scientific, organizational and technological knowledge, all of them explicitly realized by different discourses and not immediately recognizable at a linguistic level. This perspective has given way to a vast literature concerning the relationship existing between medical communication and professional settings. Just to quote a few contributions, we can cite: Sarangi/Roberts (1999), who propose an interdisciplinary approach to professional talk and its role in institutional settings, while offering theoretical and methodological tools for further linguistic analysis; Candlin/Candlin (2002), who focus on the discoursal strategies employed by both professionals and laymen in the achievement of rhetorical and professional goals; Roberts/Sarangi (2005), who provide an ethnographic approach to discourse analysis in order to reveal how language constructs professional practices; Gotti/Salager-Meyer (2006), who analyse both oral and written communication in medical discourse in professional settings; Garzone/Sarangi (2007), who consider issues of ideology in specialised communication in various professional, institutional and disciplinary settings, medicine included; Sarangi/Candlin (2011), who investigate medical professional practice from a linguistic standpoint.

Medical discourse has also been examined from other angles, particularly from the perspectives of conversation-analysis, pragmatics, and sociolinguistics (Bowles 2006; Heritage/Maynard 2006; Roberts 2006; Ferguson 2013). In some cases, analyses have been carried out also from a diachronic viewpoint (Taavitsainen/Pahta 2004, 2010,

2011). In other cases, a closer intersection between health communication and applied linguistics has been sought, thus offering a multifaceted contribution in terms of methodological approach to the understanding of healthcare communication in the global context (Hamilton/ Chou 2014).

Nowadays, attention is more and more frequently paid to the way in which traditional medical interaction can be carried out in new forms of communication, such as those offered by the social media, blogs and Twitter in particular (Myers 2010; Bjerglund/Söderguist 2012; Prasad/ Kumar 2012). Although medical discourse is realized in a highly codified structure that transcends national cultures (Dahl 2004), the way in which interaction can be expressed in these new communicative modes seems to enhance a more direct access to medical information and practice. While institutional agents seem to promote health communication mainly through traditional channels (such as Doctor-Patient Communication, Patient Information Leaflets, Direct-to-Consumer Advertising), Web 2.0 has been making available medical information to an unprecedented level, sometimes revealing, unfortunately, sociolinguistic misuses of medical terminology, with serious implications. Indeed, not only are such social networks as Twitter or blogs used as new media of communication by medical professionals, these new channels are also used to present medical information to the public. Furthermore, the availability of medical information on the Net has, on the one hand, changed the relationship between doctor and patients, and, on the other, made it the place where patients look for plain explanations of complex and specialised medical concepts, for medical advice and self-medication (Eysenbach/Diepgen 1999; McMullan 2006).

Given the importance of these different perspectives – which sometimes may be perceived as divergent – in the investigation of traditional and technological interactions, this multifaceted volume tries to bridge the gap between conventional and up-to-date medical communication. Indeed, the goal of this volume is to highlight the various viewpoints and strategies that are adopted in the different ways in which medicine and healthcare are practised, communicated and understood by both professionals and non-professionals. The following section shows how the organization of this volume tries to reflect the rich complexity of this type of communication.

2. Contents of the volume

The present volume is divided into four sections, each investigating a particular issue relevant to medical communication from a different angle, namely, communication in medical practice, communication with patients, communicating healthcare information and, finally, the communication of research findings.

In the introductory chapter SRIKANT SARANGI discusses issues surrounding interdisciplinary research and interprofessional practice, specifically in the domain of healthcare. In fact, although collaboration across disciplines and professions is usually highly appreciated, it is at the same time challenging and problematic both for epistemological and ontological reasons. After discussing the notions of discourse community and community of practice, the chapter introduces the concept of community of interest, that covers long-term interprofessional collaborations which exceed the purely discursive and practical dimension of professional-client relationship yet being part of the same profession-specific system. This type of communities, though aware of the differences existing between members at the epistemological and ontological level, tend to privilege mutual interests and commitment over differences. Based on comments exchanged between a discourse analyst and a professional practitioner regarding a case instance of genetic counselling (more precisely a joint clinic session involving patients, medical experts and a genetic counsellor), the chapter illustrates the tensions and the interpretive challenges arising when discourse analysts and healthcare professionals, both part to the same community of interest, interact with the purpose of categorizing data, and discusses the strategies of negotiation which are required in the process of meaning-making.

2.1 Communication in medical practice

In the opening chapter of the first section, Greg Myers provides a corpus analysis of sample tweets from medical professionals with the aim to illustrate the range of modes which may be found in a 140-character tweet by members of the medical community. The analysis examines the most frequent keywords and strings, considering their key semantic domains and pragmatic functions in their broader communicative context, and provides a framework to investigate how experts construct their professional persona by selecting and combining a plurality of modes. While the personal mode seems to be the least relevant (occurrences of the first person are not statistically relevant, especially when compared to those found in a reference corpus of tweets), the professional mode is highly relevant and is realized through expressions whereby actors are represented through professional categories (*as consultant, as patients*), the exclusive *we* or the use of domain-specific terms. The institutional mode has to do with more abstract, general or bureaucratic aspects of the medical profession, usually instantiated by general terms (the singular *patient*, such words as *care*, *team*, *board*, etc.) as well as conventional expressions (*teaching objectives, teaching evaluation,* etc.). Finally, the public mode is expressed by those terms lying outside the strictly institutional domain and referring to political, financial or even ideological issues.

Anna Tereszkiewicz investigates how and why medical doctors (MDs) use Twitter as a medium for professional communication. The chapter analyses a corpus of tweets (and the relevant profile) of ten MDs (selected from the Doctor registry on Tweeter on the basis of their popularity in terms of followers), and groups them (according to their content and function) into three categories: updates, addressed messages and retweets. She then considers the resources writers use in order to establish a reliable persona, convey professional expertise and authority, and engage and attract their readers. Hyperlinking and multimodality (i.e. audiovisual elements) are the genre-specific resources made available by the web-based medium, and exploited to frame MDs and the meaning they communicate within a recognizable and reliable disciplinary and institutional community. At the discourse level, the chapter shows how self-representation, stance-taking, evaluation and the expression of affective and epistemic modality are used for the dissemination of information, for self-promotion and to enhance community engagement and integration.

Carol Benkenkotter, Cristina Hanganu-Bresch and Kira Dreher analyse the way and the degree to which medical terminology may influence the definition of conceptual frameworks and the interpretation of medical/psychiatric phenomena. The chapter focuses on the clinical case of John Horatio Baldwin, the first patient formally diagnosed with Manic Depressive Insanity (MDI) in terms of Emil Kraepelin's nosology, and deals with the difficulties encountered by doctors in recognizing and interpreting the patient's symptoms – namely, mania, depression and occasional 'lucid intervals', all characteristics of MDI – hence failing to cure him, until the adoption of a new nomenclature which included MDI as a diagnosis of insanity. The authors point out how the notion and the actual phenomenon of MDI became easier to deal with once it was linguistically represented in a way that allowed experts to conceptualize and frame an array of symptoms as varied as those experienced by Baldwin in a coherent way.

While current research on doctor-patient interaction focuses primarily on felicitous types of exchange, Syelle Graves, Rebecca R. Burson and Victor A. Torres-Collazo consider how the use of a non-standard variety of the language on the part of the patient may provoke miscommunication and misconceptions, and may ultimately lead to misdiagnosis. Reporting the case study of a minority English-speaking patient (speaking African America Vernacular English) suffering from Stiff Person Syndrome, whose real condition was not detected for over a decade and was instead misdiagnosed as being mental illness, the study shows how doctor-patient dialect discord and possible – even unconscious – bias towards non-standard and stigmatized language variants may alter the interpretation of the symptoms of the patient. The chapter presents the retrospective medical chart review containing the doctor reports of the patient's description, signalling how the correct interpretation was made difficult by the patient's idiosyncratic ways of describing her condition (in terms of lexical choices, syntax and pronunciation) and by the doctors' inability to disambiguate her words. This study indicates how important it is for caregivers to be aware of and understand dialectal differences and non-standard language use in order to take better care of their patients.

2.2 Communicating with patients

In the second section, CELINA FRADE examines popularization in patient information leaflets (PILs) by exploring the attempts at easification in the language of Brazilian PILs, meant to enhance clarity, consistency and domain-specific literacy. In Brazil, best practice guidance on PILs is promoted by the national health surveillance agency, and is aimed at the standardization and clarity of the genre, even though, as shown in this chapter, the practice has had to face major problems due to the very nature of PILs discourse, which looks somewhat 'unnatural', as it has to harmonize diverse and even conflicting aspects ranging from healthcare practice and policies to legal constraints, patients expectations and also genre-related requirements (i.e. its internal move structure). The chapter offers a contrastive analysis between an official PIL for a generic medicine used to cure panic and anxiety, and the 'easified' version of the same text, which illustrates how (cognitively, discursively, terminologically) the text of the original PIL suffers from lack of consistency and clarity.

ROSITA MAGLIE also analyses the genre of PILs from a contrastive angle, by comparing UK and Italian versions of the same texts, with a specific focus on those rhetorical features meant to enhance user-friendliness. Indeed, PILs, for their very nature, contain highly domain-specific contents, i.e. information about medical product provided by pharmaceutical companies but, at the same time, they have to be easily understood by the lay public; hence they need to be semantically comprehensible and cognitively clear. By investigating PILs of three different types of medical products (i.e. on-the-counter drugs, drugs requiring the supervision of an expert, and expert prescribed drugs), this chapter highlights the popularizing strategies found in the different sections of the English texts to facilitate text readability (i.e. layout and text structuring, terminological and syntactic simplification, etc.). It then compares these occurrences with those found in the Italian version of the same texts, emphasising both similarities and idiosyncrasies, the latter mainly due to different legal requirements, cultural traditions or domain-specific epistemological assumptions.

ANNA FRANCA PLASTINA offers a multimodal discourse analysis of electronic direct-to-consumer advertising (eDTCA) aimed at revealing how prescription drug ads are understood (or misunderstood) by patients. Given the proliferation of eDTCA, due both to pharmaceutical needs to promote their products and the lack of regulation on the matter in social media, the multimodal discourse found in those ads provides an interesting ground for investigation. Studying a corpus of 24 eDTCA sample videos (covering three common symptoms such as insomnia, high cholesterol and depression) and focussing both on linguistic elements and other semiotic resources (primarily audio), the chapter compares on-screen text with audio information when conveying risk/benefit – that is, negative and positive pieces of information respectively – in order to evidence parallelism and possible discrepancies between the two semiotic levels. Besides the overall (expected) tendency to emphasize positive aspects over negative ones, major differences are found between the clarity of the linguistic level when presenting risks and the inconspicuousness of other semiotic modes, which can be realized either by superimposing text on audio information or by presenting visual images not consistent with the written and spoken messages.

GIROLAMO TESSUTO presents a multimodal discourse analytic description of online self-care communication, with a particular emphasis on the possibilities that such a dynamic medium offers to empower people to self-care and engage them in matters concerning their own health. Using the UK-based Self-Care Library website as a corpus – a medic-led and evidence-based repository of patient health care information – the analysis uses an integrated framework, combining quantitative and qualitative parameters, to investigate the interplay between words and visuals and the way such resources complement each other for the benefit of effectiveness. The first part of the chapter identifies the ideational, interpersonal and textual meanings expressed in establishing identities, roles, systems of knowledge and beliefs between the participants, by emphasizing linguistic elements such as personal pronouns (inclusive and exclusive), engagement markers (imperatives and questions), active and passive voice, modal auxiliaries, adjectives, register and style. The second part focuses on visual aspects and, more specifically, the representational, interactive and compositional meanings implicit in the text on the basis of visual parameters such as framing, focus, frame size and colours.

2.3 Communicating healthcare information

The third section is introduced by a chapter where Judith Turnbull discusses the discourse of medical information for young people in websites specifically addressed to children and teenagers. Since these sites (which are usually sections of larger medical websites targeted at adult patients) are meant to provide specialised knowledge and specific contents as to how to live with diabetes in a way that is appropriate and effective, the chapter analyses the cognitive and communicative resources used to achieve this aim and compares them with those usually exploited in websites for adults. As regard the cognitive level – that is, the transfer of domain specific meanings – the main difference between young-oriented and adult sites concerns the information load, whereas at the communicative level the tendency is to emphasize the interpersonal dimension by using a more personalized tone and an emphatic and engaging style, thus combining the scientific and rational elements typical of medical communication with emotional components particularly appreciated by young audiences.

Paola Catenaccio explores the discursive construction of addiction in gambling awareness campaigns in different English-speaking countries (USA, Canada, Australia) considering how linguistic and rhetorical strategies may be exploited to represent gambling as either a pathological issue, a personal problem or a social challenge, hence by differently attributing responsibility and by presupposing different ways as to how to control and contrast it. In the course of the last decades gambling has progressively been considered as a deviant behaviour and as such dealt with: its conceptualization has been highly affected by a disease-related terminology and a medicalization-oriented interpretive framework. As the analysis of the campaigns in the corpus reveals, gambling (a term almost exclusively referred to excessive and/ or compulsive gambling, and not to responsible gambling, which is usually lexicalized through the more positively connoted term *gaming*) tends to be either fully institutionalized or co-constructed as being pathologic; hence such campaigns contribute to replicating, corroborating and, in a way, 'normalizing' the idea of gambling as illness, and by this very same act they also contribute to the de-stigmatization of this behaviour by representing it as a medical condition rather than a moral flaw.

The chapter by Miriam Bait discusses the communicative strategies adopted by government agencies in the UK and US on their websites in order to promote healthy eating for children and provide food advice, nutritional tips and dietary recommendations. Such texts have both an informative and persuasive function, and this is mirrored in their conventional two-move structure which comprises an introductory section (usually reporting scientific definitions) and a section providing guidelines for the appropriate selection of food (in terms of both quantity and quality). The investigation of the way actors and agency are differently represented in the UK and US shows how institutional websites contribute to the ideological construct of power by balancing authority and empathy.

2.4 Communicating research findings

The fourth section opens with a chapter by Ruth Breeze in which the author investigates the communication of scientific research findings in the media focussing specifically on the transformations affecting both the language and the content of a scientific research article when it is recontextualized and made to fit the generic conventions typical of media communication. The chapter compares the text of the original paper with the way laboratory findings and health implications are reformulated in an online press release issued by the Oregon State University, on the one hand, and, on the other, three news stories (published in the *Daily Telegraph,* the *Daily Express* and the *Mirror*), focusing in particular on the substitution of domain specific terms and phrases (*stilbenoids*) with more transparent expressions (*red wine* and *blueberries*). Using the Appraisal system as a methodological framework, the chapter outlines the popularizing strategies used to transform the original claims so as to make them appropriate for media communication in terms of dialogistic positioning and graduation. The analysis shows that, while the text of the press release is more mitigated – displaying neutral attribution and hedging –, the newspaper articles show a more assertive and monoglossic style, combined with intensification resources.

MARÍA JOSÉ LUZÓN's chapter examines the rhetorical phenomenon of recontextualization of specialised discourse in medical weblogs. Unlike traditional media of written expert communication, blogs, like most part of Internet-based channels, offer the possibility for a dialogic type of exchange between experts and lay public, hence between informative comments and interested requests. On the basis of this assumption, the chapter analyses the strategies exploited by experts to communicate health research to blog users, with a specific focus on how they popularize specialised contents not only through reformulation, but by recontextualizing them, that is, by adjusting them with respect to the participants, their expectation, their roles, their assumed background knowledge, the purpose of the their exchange and the channel. The study shows that the resources used to accomplish this purpose may range from the use of hyperlinks and visuals, to that of code glossing such as explanations, examples, comparisons, metaphors, etc., to the use of interactional resources like personalization, engagement markers and evaluative comments.

DAVIDE MAZZI investigates the pragmatics of the most frequent semantic sequences – i.e. co-occurring items, phrases or lexical clusters – found in medical RAs. Today doctors are required to be experts not only in carrying out research but also in communicating it, and they are expected to do so in the most effective way, that is, by respecting the domain-specific discourse conventions to shape hypotheses and discuss results on the one hand, and by framing meanings with respect to the epistemology underlying the discipline on the other. The data retrieved from a corpus of 280 medical RAs indicate that at the micro-level of the language there are indeed preferred semantic sequences occurring more frequently than others in the Introduction section, used to make topic generalizations and present new evidence to be discussed (namely the sequence *for patients with*), in the Methods section, to introduce the research criteria (*used for the*; *on the basis of*), in the Results part, to describe salient phenomenological features and cause-effect relationships (*as a potential […] for*; *in the pathogenesis/regulation of*) and, finally, in the Discussion section, where data are interpreted with respect to existing knowledge (*the finding/possibility/observation that; our hypothesis that*).

The chapter by STEFANIA MACI discusses the changes affecting medical discourse as a consequence of discipline-external factors such as globalization and, more specifically, the global crisis, on the one hand, and the urge represented by marketing or corporate concerns and competitive publishing, on the other. The ties between medicine and business are becoming more and more evident since members of the medical community engaged in clinical research are increasingly adopting a marked business-oriented approach in order to cope with the economical crisis when collecting funds, upon which medical research highly depends. This tendency also seems to be reflected in the way medical experts represent and discuss their research. Based on a corpus of 50 Research Letters published in the *Journal of American Medical Association* and *The Lancet,* the chapter points out that, beyond the traditional and conventional generic organization (replicating the IMRD structuring typical of academic genres), the micro-linguistic level of such texts displays a range of lexical elements pertaining to the corporate representation of the medical world and the financial aspects of healthcare and medical research (through words such as *management, funding, free, sponsor, cost,* etc.), thus evidencing the progressive dissemination and appropriation of marketing and corporate thinking when discussing discipline-specific contents.

Finally, the chapter by ANNA STERMIERI focuses on the dissemination of specialised knowledge in academic weblogs written by scientists working in the field of genetics, with the aim to discover how experts manage to communicate scientific contents in a way that is comprehensible and effective to audiences lacking specialised competence. Based on a corpus of posts taken from four genetics blogs, and with the aid of a reference corpus, the chapter provides an analysis of the keywords selected on the basis of their semantic category and concordances, and then focuses on the collocates of two relevant terms – namely *disease* and *risk* – in order to reveal how experts popularize the presentation of disease (i.e. by introducing and reformulating specialised concepts) and how they communicate risk or their own perspective on a medical condition (i.e. how they categorize and assess risk in terms of observation, hypothesis or investigation).

3. Closing remarks

This book analyses the subject of medical communication from a range of innovative perspectives, covering a broad spectrum of approaches and procedures that are particularly significant in this field. As the various chapters of this volume show, medical communication has been analyzed from many viewpoints: not only from a merely linguistic angle, with a focus on the description of the genres used in medical and healthcare contexts, but also from a social and cultural standpoint, with an emphasis both on the doctor-patient relationship and on the social relevance of the other types of communicative links existing between the many communities involved in this type of interaction. This richness of viewpoints is mainly due to the influence of the results of studies carried out in parallel disciplines and linguistic branches, which have promoted a more integrated approach. This interdisciplinary perspective has been favoured by the recent developments of linguistic studies, which have adopted theoretical approaches and analytical tools typical of various disciplines other than linguistics, such as sociology, anthropology and psychology.

The presentation of some of the main fields typical of medical communication has highlighted a considerable variety of themes, data and research methods which are clearly representative of the eclectic interest in this specific domain and of the wide range of approaches developed for its investigation. As the various chapters show, linguistic analysis is applicable to many types of multiparty encounters involving multiple interactions and practices, and several kinds of participants, including different healthcare professionals, trainees and patients. There are a number of reasons why linguistic studies are likely to continue to expand in medical fields. Indeed, thanks to their interdisciplinary nature, methodologically adaptable characteristics and applicability to all forms of text, they are well placed to keep up with the continuous diversification of healthcare settings and practices, thus making optimal use of the adaptive ability and linguistic creativity of the medical discourse community.

Taken together, the various chapters of this volume are indicative of the multifarious methods, resources and procedures adopted by scholars engaging in the analysis of medical and healthcare communication from a range of different backgrounds and cultures. Obviously, we do not claim to be comprehensive and offer a complete, definitive account of the way both practitioners and non-practitioners communicate in this sector. Rather, we hope that the chapters in this volume will open up new perspectives, provide subjects for fresh discussion, and stimulate debate among all those scholars and practitioners interested in medical and healthcare communication.

References

Bjerglund, Nina / Söderguist, Thomas 2012. *Social Media and Public Health Research.* <http://bjerglund.files.wordpress.com/2012/11/final-social-media-and-public-health-research1.pdf>.

Bowles, Hugo 2006. Conversation Analysis and Health Communication: Updating a Developing Relationship. In Gotti / Salager-Meyer (eds), 43–64.

Candlin, Christopher, N. / Candlin, Sally 2002. Discourse, Expertise, and the Management of Health Care Settings. *Research on Language and Social Interaction* 35, 115–137.

D'Angelo, Larissa 2012. Academic Poster Presentations: Mapping the Genre. In Gotti (ed.), 263–281.

Dahl, Trine 2004. Textual Metadiscourse in Research Articles: A Matter of National Culture or of Academic Discipline?. *Journal of Pragmatics* 36, 1807–1825.

Eysenbach, Gunter / Diepgen, Thomas 1999. Patients Looking for Information on the Internet and Seeking Teleadvice: Motivation,

Expectations, and Misconceptions as Expressed in E-mails Sent to Physicians. *Archives of Dermatology* 135/2, 151–156.

Ferguson, Gibson 2013. English for Medical Purposes. In Paltridge, Brian / Starfield, Sue (eds) *The Handbook of English for Specific Purposes*. Chichester: Wiley-Blackwell, 243–261.

Garzone, Giuliana / Sarangi, Srikant (eds) 2007. *Discourse, Ideology and Ethics in Specialised Communication*. Bern: Peter Lang.

Gotti, Maurizio 2014. Reformulation and Recontextualization in Popularization Discourse. *Ibérica* 27, 15–34.

Gotti, Maurizio (ed.) 2012. *Academic Identity Traits: A Corpus-Based Investigation*. Bern: Peter Lang.

Gotti, Maurizio / Salager-Meyer, Francoise (eds) 2006. *Advances in Medical Discourse Analysis: Oral and Written Contexts*. Bern: Peter Lang.

Hamilton, Heidi E. / Chou, Wen-ying Sylvia (eds) 2014. *The Routledge Handbook of Language and Health Communication*. London: Routledge.

Heritage, John / Maynard, Douglas (eds) 2006. *Communication in Medical Care: Interaction Between Primary Care Physicians and Patients*. Cambridge: Cambridge University Press.

Hyland, Ken 2004. *Disciplinary Discourses: Social Interactions in Academic Writing*. London: Longman.

Hyland, Ken 2011. Disciplines and Discourses: Social Interactions in the Construction of Knowledge. In Starke-Meyerring, Doreen / Paré, Anthony / Artemeva, Natalia / Horne, Miriam / Yousoubova, Larissa (eds) *Writing in the Knowledge Society*. West Lafayette: Parlor Press, 193–214.

Maci, Stefania M. 2012a. Fast-track Publications: The Genre of Medical Research Letters. In Gotti (ed.), 243–262.

Maci, Stefania M. 2012b. The Genre of Medical Conference Posters. In Gotti (ed.), 283–301.

McMullan, Miriam 2006. Patients Using the Internet to Obtain Health Information: How this Affects the Patient-health Professional Relationship. *Patient Education and Counseling* 63/1–2, 24–28.

Myers, Greg 2003. Discourse Studies of Scientific Popularization: Questioning the Boundaries. *Discourse Studies* 3, 265–279.

Myers, Greg 2010. *The Discourse of Blogs and Wikis*. London: Continuum.

Prasad, Murali / Kumar, Vijaya 2012. Specialty Medical Blogs: A Tool to Disseminate Health Information. *National Journal of Research in Community Medicine* 1/4, 178–241.

Roberts, Celia 2006. Continuities and Discontinuities in Doctor-Patient Consultations in a Multilingual Society. In Gotti / Salager-Meyer (eds), 177–196.

Roberts, Celia / Sarangi, Srikant. 2005. Theme-oriented Discourse Analysis of Medical Encounters. *Medical Education* 39, 632–640.

Sarangi, Srikant / Candlin, Christopher. N. 2011. Professional and Organisational Practice: A Discourse/Communication Perspective. In Candlin, Christopher N. / Sarangi, Srikant (eds) *Handbook of Communication in Organisations and Professions*. Berlin: De Gruyter Mouton, 3–58.

Sarangi, Srikant / Roberts, Celia (eds) 1999. *Talk, Work and Institutional Order: Discourse in Medical, Mediation and Management Settings*. Berlin: Mouton de Gruyter.

Swales, John M. / Feak, Christine B. 2000. *Academic Writing for Graduate Students: Essential Tasks and Skills: A Course for Nonnative Speakers of English (English for Specific Purposes)*. Ann Arbor: University of Michigan Press.

Taavitsainen, Irma / Pahta, Päivi (eds) 2004. *Medical and Scientific Writing in Late Medieval English*. Cambridge: Cambridge University Press.

Taavitsainen, Irma / Pahta, Päivi (eds) 2010. *Early Modern Medical Texts: Corpus and Studies*. Amsterdam: Benjamins.

Taavitsainen, Irma / Pahta, Päivi (eds) 2011. *Medical Writing in Early Modern English*. Cambridge: Cambridge University Press.

Srikant Sarangi

Experts on Experts: Sustaining 'Communities of Interest' in Professional Discourse Studies

1. Introduction

Building upon and expanding on a number of earlier publications (Sarangi 1998, 2002, 2005, 2007, 2010; Sarangi/Candlin 2011, Sarangi *et al.* 2003), this chapter is primarily a practising discourse analyst's reflections on 'interpretive repertoires' surrounding interprofessional collaborative research, with particular reference to the domain of healthcare. In a classic study of scientists' discourse, Gilbert and Mulkay (1984) draw attention to scientists' use of two distinct 'interpretive repertoires': while the 'empiricist repertoire' exemplifies impersonal accounts of scientific discovery and the rules and procedures governing the production of factual knowledge, the 'contingent repertoire' appeals to personal motives, biases and intuitions. It is the simultaneity of these two repertoires that gives rise to 'interpretive variability'. This distinction between empiricist and contingent repertoires easily maps onto the objective-subjective dialectics and also applies to discourse analysts' accounts of data-based findings. The situation becomes complex when a discourse analyst's account is subjected to further interpretation by professional practitioners on a collaborative footing.

For many of us, collaborating and partnershipping across disciplinary and professional boundaries is assumed not only to be desirable and value-added, but also as being a smooth operation without visible challenges. Indeed one's experience of collaboration can be productive, but at times one is confronted with interpretive dilemmas. My own collaboration with professional practitioners in the field of genetics and genetic counselling over the past two decades has yielded many fruits but not without interpretive challenges that underpin the long-term marriage. The aim here is not to offer an evaluative assessment of collaborative research or to set out criteria and principles that one should follow. Instead I wish to argue that collaborative interpretive practices provide a useful platform for inevitably reflecting upon one's own assumptions, especially in the context of language/discourse-oriented qualitative inquiry.

Collaboration takes many forms: with colleagues from different academic disciplines, with professional practitioners, with clients and service users, and with managers and policy makers. Collaboration with colleagues representing different disciplines can be as demanding as collaboration with professional practitioners at practical, epistemological and ontological levels (see Sarangi 2002 on a distinction between interdisciplinary and interprofessional collaboration, each posing different challenges for the communication/discourse researcher). The holy grail of interdisciplinary and interprofessional research – what I characterise here as *experts on experts* – is the subject of the present chapter.

I first briefly visit existing notions – communities of practice, communities of discourse (or discourse communities) and communities of interpretation (or interpretive communities) – and propose the notion of 'communities of interest' which characterises the lasting interprofessional collaboration of the kind I am engaged in. I then outline the key features of professional practice in relation to clients as well as interprofessional communication. I single out the notion of categorisation as 'biased' interpretation and apply this to selected data to make the point about 'analyst's paradox' (Sarangi 2002, 2007) embedded within interpretive operations. The 'interpretive variability' across the professional practitioner and the discourse analyst is cast as a tension between 'scientific-technical-specific knowledge' (knowing that) and 'discourse-analytical-specific knowledge' (knowing how).

2. Communities of practice/discourse/interpretation and communities of interest

The notion of 'community' has received critical attention within sociological and anthropological literature. Gusfield (1975) distinguishes between two meanings of community – locational/geographical vs. relational – and it is the relational dimension of community that concerns us. The relational dimension, however, should not be taken to mean primordial attachment or loyalty in an absolute sense. Following the seminal work of Lave and Wenger (1991), a community of practice is characterised by the following features: mutual engagement, a joint enterprise and a shared repertoire (Wenger 1998: 73). These features go beyond mere social categorisation, interpersonal relationship and geographical proximity. A key point is that a community of practice "does not entail homogeneity" (Wenger 1998: 75). Instead it affords diversity and partiality, similarities and differences, self and other competencies. In a nutshell, communities of practice are sustained via intelligible 'interpretive variability'.

Of the three definitional features of communities of practice, the affordance of a shared repertoire is relevant here. This idea coincides with Wuthnow's (1989) notion of community of discourse, which can also be traced to the sociolinguistic notion of 'speech community' (Gumperz 1968). Other scholars such as Swales (1990) and Porter (1992) have talked about the notion of discourse communities. Swales (1990) characterises discourse communities as socio-rhetorical networks with access to participatory mechanisms such as specific genres and communicative acts through which certain goals and purposes can be achieved. Porter (1992: 106) defines discourse communities as:

> a local and temporary constraining system, defined by a body of texts (or more generally, practices) that are unified by a common focus. A discourse community is a textual system with stated and unstated conventions, a vital history, mechanisms for wielding power, institutional hierarchies, vested interests, and so on.

At one level, notions such as community of practice and discourse community are conceived of as organic systems involving dynamic interrelationships with their environments. At another level, these notions remain abstract and normative and thus prove difficult to operationalise at an analytic level.

Shared practices – inclusive of the discursive, communicative dimension – no doubt exist, but intra-community tensions also emerge. The classic example here is Stanley Fish's (1980) notion of 'interpretive communities' (see also Bleich 1978 on 'communities of interpretation'), exemplified by different interpretations of the utterance "Is there a text in this class?". While one colleague interprets the question with the answer "Yes, it's the *Norton Anthology of Literature*", Fish would prefer to interpret the question as it was originally intended – whether a literary text can be autonomous from its contexts and readers. Can Fish and his colleague claim membership in the same interpretive community despite their differences in interpretation? As Schauber and Spolsky (1986: 146) observe:

> If, on the one hand, every variation in interpretive perspective or strategy indicates a new community, then the notion of community loses its force. If, on the other hand, major variations in perspective do not mark community boundaries, then again the notion has little use.

The community of discourse scholars – whether seen as communities of practice or discourse communities or interpretive communities – is divided on professed lines, resembling tribal warfare, each safeguarding their own territories. In systemic thinking, such demarcations can be seen as sub-systems with overlapping stakes and interests, rendering any neat classification of sub-communities nearly impossible.

Here I would like to introduce the notion of 'communities of interest' which acknowledges differences in ontologies and epistemologies across given communities of practice/discourse/interpretation, but privileges the mutual interest in the phenomena under study. This is parallel to the broader notion of 'interest groups' who organise themselves, with shared attitudes, to mobilise political action and are motivated by a purpose. The phenomenon of 'special interest groups' in academic disciplines and conferences also serves as a good example.

'Communities of interest' concern scenarios in which one crosses different communities of discourse/interpretive practice – where one may share 'interests' but not 'practices', 'discourses' and 'interpretations'. Consider, for example, multiprofessional teams in the healthcare setting who work towards a shared interest in the patient's wellbeing, independent of their belonging to different communities of discourse/ interpretive practice as manifest in different explanatory frameworks and in differential uses of acronyms/jargons. Mary Douglas' (1985: 95) definition of community foregrounds 'commitment': "The full sense of the term community is a committed group in which individuals derive their life support and which bounds their commitments". Likewise, the notion of commitment assumes utmost significance in communities of interest. One not only derives support from source but is also bound by a goal in the future. Differences in empiricist and contingent discourse/ interpretive practices do not stand as a barrier to shared membership in communities of interest.

When a particular tribe of discourse analysts studies another profession (e.g. a community of healthcare practitioners) tensions can arise during the research process, especially in relation to how data is to be interpreted and findings are to be disseminated. Categorisation of observable phenomena, or more generally the sense of meaning-making, is likely to be marked by discretions and differential inferences, leading to formulation of subjective reporting/judgements.

3. Expertise, guilty knowledge and professional practice

Notions of profession and practice are nuanced in the literature. The same is true of notions like expertise, knowledge and authority (Walton 1997). Practice, according to Bourdieu (1977), always implies a cognitive operation including perception. For him, practice is socially and discursively constructed, and is always culturally relative (both in terms of ethno-linguistic cultures and institutional ones). Whatever the manifestations of practice, or to use Bourdieu's pet notion of 'habitus', these are always historically determined and durable, although allowing for flexibility, contingency and improvisation. Over time, practice assumes theoretical significance (cf. contemporary interest in practice theory).

According to Hughes (1975: 249, cited in Walmsley *et al.* 1993: 9–10): "Professions profess. They profess to know better than others the nature of certain matters, and to know better than their clients what ails them or their affairs". This 'knowing better' is premised on theoretical knowledge as well as experience, which jointly affords authority. To this mix one can add knowledge of technology, knowledge of institutional orders, and more importantly, communicative knowledge. 'Knowing better' goes beyond the professional-client divide to capture the interprofessional division of expert labour. Again, in the context of multiprofessional teams, one specialist may know better than his/her counterpart about specific phenomena.

'Knowing better' can sometimes be equated with 'guilty knowledge'. Hughes (1993: 22–23) observes:

> The prototype of all guilty knowledge is, however, a different, potentially shocking way of looking at things. Every occupation must look relatively at some order of events, objects or ideas. These things must be classified, seen in comparative light; their behaviour must be analysed and, if possible, predicted. A suitable technical knowledge must be developed in which one may talk to one's colleagues about them. This technical, therefore relative, attitude must be adopted toward the very people whom one serves; no profession can operate without license to talk in shocking terms behind the backs of its clients.

For Kenneth Burke (1966: 52), 'knowing better' may amount to experts operating with a 'terministic screen' or on the basis of 'trained incapacities':

> Any definition of man in terms of specialised scientific nomenclatures would necessarily be 'over-socialised', or 'over-biologised', or 'over-psychologised', or 'over-physicised', or 'overpoeticised', and so on, depending upon which specialised terministic screen was being stretched to cover not just its own special field but a more comprehensive area.

We may add to this list over-linguisticised, over-discoursised and over-communicationised etc. Moreover, within these so-called disciplines, further sub-specialised terministic screens are noticeable. This tendency simultaneously leads to over- and under-interpretation of observed phenomena. For Burke (1965: 49), "every way of seeing is also a way of not seeing". With reference to the world of painting and art criticism, John Berger (2008: 1) writes:

> We only see what we look at. To look is an act of choice. As a result of this act, what we see is brought within our reach – though not necessarily within arm's reach.

Goodwin (1994) foregrounds the discursive practices underpinning what he calls 'professional vision'. Like Hughes, he draws particular attention to discursive practices of coding, highlighting and articulating material representations. Expert knowledge and professional experience both shape and are manifest in professional vision. However, from the Burkean perspective, professional vision can be seen as professional myopia – the act of seeing is also an act of not seeing. Here is an example, taken from Flint (1995: D8, cited in Walton 1997: 10):

> Biology students once learned that a sperm swims toward the passive egg of the female, pounds on the walls and breaks down the damsel's defenses. Conception was not so much a union as a vanquishing.
> Today's researchers see it differently. The egg, they say, sends out messages to guide the sperm, participating actively in the process, until sperm and egg find each other and merge.
> Yet because scientists came to the lab with preconceived labels for the microscopic players – sperm as aggressive male, egg as passive female – it has taken a long time for them to see what was really going on.

Two points emerge from the above example: professional vision is constituted in the act of 'biased' interpretation of phenomena and that professional interpretive repertoires, whether empiricist or contingent (Gilbert/Mulkay 1984), change over time, i.e. a kind of 'professional correctness' reigns periodically. As Kuhn (1962) points out, epochal changes occur even in the domain of 'normal science' to make it possible to codify phenomena with a degree of consensus.

4. Categorisation of professional practice and interpretive cleavages

Description is the basis of categorisation, which is central to both the natural sciences and the human/social sciences. According to Dunn (1978), while within the natural sciences descriptions take the form of statements and assertions which can withstand inter-observer reliability, within the human and social sciences 'reporting' is the preferred form of description which may have no corresponding inter-observer reliability.

One of the challenges is that if language and discourse are context-specific, who owns the description and interpretation of context? In other words, whose categorisation of observed phenomena should prevail: the discourse analyst's or the professional practitioner's, both in the historical sense of professionalism and in the contingent sense of the specific encounter? In relation to psychotherapy, what might appear as ordinary conversation to the outsider discourse analyst may be invested with psychotherapeutic meaning-potential. As O'Hanlon and Wilk (1987: 177) note:

> A 'fly on the wall' who did not know we were doing psychotherapy would not necessarily suspect that that was what we were doing: he would see and hear only an ordinary conversation. What defines the conversation as psychotherapy is simply our goal in conducting the conversation.

By extension, what might seem a mere repetition to the naked eye of the discourse analyst can be descriptively discriminated as echoing vs. mirroring depending on who repeats what and for what purpose, i.e., the communicative potential of repetition as a discourse device can be optimally interpreted in relation to the ensuing therapeutic intervention (Ferrara 1994).

The act of categorisation is intimately tied up with forms of knowing and seeing. In the tradition of philosophy of science, Hanson (1958: 86) distinguishes between 'seeing as' and 'seeing that': "it is a matter of logic, not merely a matter of fact, that seeing as and seeing that are indispensable to what is called in science, seeing or observing". As Hanson (1958: 10–24) remarks:

> Seeing that threads knowledge into our seeing; it saves us from re-identifying everything that meets our eye; it allows physicists to observe new data as physicists, and not as cameras. [...] Observation in physics is not an encounter with unfamiliar and unconnected flashes, sounds, bumps, but rather a calculated meeting with these as flashes, sounds and bumps of a particular kind.

This is echoed in Garfinkel's (1967: 78) formulation of what Mannheim originally conceptualised as the 'documentary method of interpretation':

> The method consists of treating an actual appearance as 'the document of', as 'pointing to', as 'standing on behalf of' a presupposed underlying pattern. Not only is the underlying pattern derived from its individual documentary evidences, but the individual documentary evidences, in their turn, are interpreted on the basis of 'what is known' about the underlying pattern. Each is used to elaborate the other.

The act of categorisation, when it leans heavily on 'seeing that', becomes indistinguishable from recontextualisation in many institutional/professional spheres (Sarangi 1998).

In my previous work (Sarangi 2002, 2007) I have suggested that attention to the notion of 'analyst's paradox' – the activity of obtaining members' insights to inform analytic practice, including collaborative interpretation – is a way of approximating 'ecological validity' (Cicourel 2007). This is more the case when our analytic gaze is method-centred (resembling communities of practice) rather than problem-centred (resembling communities of interest). An extension of Kaplan's (1964) generic concept of 'the law of the instrument' is discernible in 'Maslow's hammer': "It is tempting, if the only tool you have is a hammer, to treat everything as if it were a nail" (Maslow 1966: 15). Collaborative interpretation, involving the discourse analyst and the professional practitioner, is a useful safeguard against Maslow's 'law of the hammer'. I agree with Clarke (2005: 189) when he says:

> Interpretation of professional behaviour, and especially any attempt to evaluate professional practice, can only sensibly proceed with some input from the

> professionals. This is not to say that a professional's account of their practice must be taken at face value [...] but an attempt to make sense of practice without some input from professionals is unlikely to be productive.

This plea is recognisable as the process of triangulation, which also goes under the label 'respondent validation', while acknowledging the limitations of post-hoc accounts of action (Schön 1983). Such processes of triangulation need to be matched by inter-analytic reliability whenever possible. Following Dunn (1978: 155–156), this is a case of managing 'descriptive discretion' which underpins different, and even competing, interpretive practices:

> The prevalence of descriptive discretion is not in itself epistemologically alarming, though it does weaken the prospects of any very crisply incremental development of the social sciences. In itself it comes no closer to imperilling the reality of human performance than variations in the taste of landscape artists come to altering the physical properties of mountains. To make it epistemologically alarming and not merely methodologically troublesome, it would be necessary for it to extend to the assertion and negation of the same description (identically interpreted) of the same phenomena by two different competent, sincere and attentive observers.

The analyst's paradox is a continuum: it is at its most extreme when interpreting different professional and organisational practices such as the backstage activities, e.g., case records, peer-centred talk/text as in case presentations, case conferences, source texts, guidance notes etc. This is where collaborative interpretation by both professional practitioners and by discourse analysts belonging to a 'community of interest' may be an important means for minimising the analyst's paradox.

Sarangi *et al.* (2003) report in a discursive vein an attempt to minimise the analyst's paradox, which was achieved through recategorisation of the genetic counselling data corpus. For instance, what was first regarded as 'therapeutic frame' by discourse analysts gave way to 'reflective frame' preferred by the professional practitioners – the latter category being devoid of any negative connotation in the context of genetic counselling practice. Another analytical category – 'normalisation of experience' – was substituted by 'psychosocial coping', with the substituted category allowing for a deeper appreciation of subtle sub-categories that were hidden under the more generic label of 'normalisation'.

5. Knowing better: scientific-technical-specific knowledge (knowing that) and discourse-analytical-specific knowledge (knowing how)

The distinction between 'knowing that' and 'knowing how' owes to Ryle (1949); these are also characterised as 'declarative knowledge' and 'procedural knowledge', respectively. This distinction would apply to both genetics and genetic counselling as a discipline and as a professional practice as it would to discourse and communication studies as a discipline and as a professional practice, albeit with a range of variations. In a sense 'knowing that' aligns with our earlier discussion of 'seeing that' (Hanson 1958). For present purposes, I limit myself to characterising the position of the professional practitioner as representing 'scientific-technical-specific knowledge' (knowing that) and the discourse analyst as embodying 'discourse-analytical-specific knowledge' (knowing how).

Now I turn to some empirical data from genetic counselling. It concerns a situation where the parents wish to test their child for a genetic condition called polycystic kidney disease (PKD). The manifest symptoms are high blood pressure and urinary infection. My data is drawn from a joint clinic session involving the parents (PF and PM), the children (CF and CM), the genetic counsellor (G1), the kidney specialist (K1) and the genetic specialist nurse (N2) (see Appendix for transcription conventions). There is a division of labour between the two experts, G1 and K1 – in relation to what might be inheritance related and what might be dysfunctional about the kidney itself. As we will see, both experts display scientific-technical-specific knowledge (knowing that) of different kinds.

The selected data extracts were first analysed by SS and the written analytic commentaries then received feedback from the professional practitioner (AC). The opening data extract is contextualised by SS as follows, which receives a challenge from AC:

> SS: "It is worth noting that in conventional medicine, tests and test results are aimed at uncertainty reduction and for confirmation of diagnosis – as a precursor to medical intervention. In the context of genetics, only a few diagnostic

> tests are currently available. The other types of tests – carrier testing and predictive testing – not only involve cumbersome and costly procedure but could fail to provide definitive results."
> AC: "This does not sound correct at all – I'm puzzled… the test is likely to be the same as far as the lab and the clinician are concerned (in the mechanics of doing it) and whether it is diagnostic, predictive, carrier etc will depend upon the context."
> SS: "In what follows I focus on a particular genetic condition called polycystic kidney disease (PKD), normally associated with an enlarged kidney, which can present cysts at a later stage."
> AC: "The first sentence about large kidneys later showing cysts is what K was hoping to show in the children's PKD clinic but that study never got done. So while it may be that young children who are going to develop PKD have slightly larger kidneys, we don't know that. It'd be much more reasonable to say something about those with a PKD mutation develop cysts that become apparent on ultrasound scan over the course of 30+ years (becoming detectable at some stage from fetal life to>30 years old)."

Two relevant topics – testing (general vs. genetic) and the disease condition – are foregrounded by SS. Although the descriptions offered by SS may be sufficient for a discourse analytic audience, AC not only draws attention to the misconceptions inherent in SS's framing of both the topics but also suggests remedial action. AC's observations manifest a combination of theoretical, scientific knowledge and professional experience – which is not inhabited by SS. AC's comments above concern misunderstandings on SS's part about the nature of the disease condition as well as the scope of genetic testing and the professional practice underpinning testing, diagnosis and prognosis. These comments, I suggest, belong to the domain of scientific-technical-specific knowledge, with AC claiming expert authority. Under the circumstances, the discourse analyst has to concede to the other-expertise as a way of making their interpretation credible. Following Ryle (1949), this is evidence of 'knowing that' which is mainly non-negotiable.

In what follows, the genetic counselling data extracts are accompanied by written correspondence between SS and AC. In Data Extract 1, the kidney specialist (K1) is explaining the advantages and disadvantages of testing the child for PKD.

DATA EXTRACT 1

01 K1 but um (.) perhaps if I mention some of the (.) um (0.5) advantages of (0.5) knowing if the children have got it [PKD] for instance (0.5) obviously if you did know they've got it you'd make sure that if there was any (0.5) special (0.5) follow up or treatment that they ought to have [(0.5.)]

02 PM [mm]

03 K1 [then] you'd be able to make sure they've got it (0.5) but in fact =

04 PF [mm]

05 K1 = there is no treatment that (0.5) um (0.5) significantly alters the course of this condition (0.5) apart from treating blood pressure if it's high (.) and treating infections if they occur [(1.0)]

06 PF [*mm*]

07 K1 (*it's possible*) in future we [might]

08 PM [yeah]

09 K1 (.) have something different but that's all we can (.) recommend at the moment (0.5) and we could of course check the blood pressure and make sure urine infections are treated (0.5) even if people didn't have the scans to test for this condition so (0.5) you know if you wanted (.) the the two smaller children could have um (.) an annual check up in our clinic just for (.) blood pressure and (0.5) uh and that's the main thing we'd do (0.5) um (.) even if they hadn't had the scans to [say]

10 PM [yeah]

11 K1 they've got the cysts (0.5) ((sound of door)) um (1.0) so um (.) w- we (1.0) we're not pressing you at all (0.5) for them to have tests (0.5) um (.)>>*you know*<<specially in your in your family as (0.5) it sounds like it's quite a mild problem

12 PM yeah

13 K1 um (0.5) if of course they (.) they developed a problem that needed to be investigated we'd say (0.5) should we investigate it in its own right (1.0) uh (0.5) the the disadvantages of (.) children having tests (0.5) um (0.5) might be that (0.5) if the child was found to have a problem (0.5) they might be treated differently they might be treated as (0.5) sickly or (.) weakly (0.5) u::m (.) and um (.) it might cause extra anxieties either to yourselves or or to the child (0.5) [uh]

14 PF [mm]

15 K1 and then (.) when they're they're older (0.5) it might interfere with (.) certain careers they might want to (.) follow like um the armed forces might (0.5) not be willing to take them or um sometimes with insurances (0.5) um (0.5) they either give you a loaded premium or they won't insure you (.) if you have certain conditions (.) so there are drawbacks [to]

16 PM [mm]

17 K1 having them tested young (1.0) u:m (1.0) I don't know whether you've (.) thought at all about whether the children should have tests

18 PF *mm*

19 PM (haven't spoken ^^^)
20 K1 not really no no I mean it's not a pressing issue at all (0.5) um (.) then of course there is the question of whether the children should have the opportunity to decide for themselves (.) [and]
21 PM [yeah]
22 K1 of course if you've already done it (0.5) then they don't have that (0.5) opportunity to decide for themselves (0.5) but it is worth thinking as they get to teenage (.) um that it's probably fair that they should at least have the knowledge that this problem is going on in the family because if they don't have knowledge (0.5) they don't have any (.) choices (0.5) and uh (1.0) again they themselves can ask either for more information (0.5) (okay) from yourselves or (.) or from ourselves whichever is easy (but quite often) the GP (.) and (.) they can (0.5) consider whether they want to be tested (.) um (1.0) in their own time a::nd um (0.5) they need to know about the advantages and disadvantages obviously (.) but in addition they need to be able to (0.5) um (.) take on board the fact that it is a genetic condition and therefore they might want to (0.5) take that into account when they're planning their own families

What follows is the correspondence between SS and AC, selectively, based on SS's analytic commentary on the above data extract.

SS: "K1 provides the information about the pros and cons of childhood testing in the form of a list structure. The list begins with the positive aspects (01–09), perhaps to align with and consolidate upon what parents might already know and expect, e.g., possible treatment scenarios following a diagnosis. However, this is immediately disclaimed – keeping with the professional stance against childhood genetic testing – although concession is made about possible future intervention."
AC: "Top page 11, sentence 2 (However, this is immediately disclaimed – keeping with the professional stance against childhood testing). I disagree with this on two counts: (i) the "we're not pressing you" statement is an attempt to retain equipoise, NOT to persuade one way or the other. The next statement (about weak family history) is getting at something else – the family history is strong (no doubt about it) but the pattern of disease is less severe than usual SO (i) the risk of severe disease in the child is less, even if they inherit the PKD, and (ii) this may have implications for which particular gene locus is involved (PKD1 or PKD2).
SS: "As we can see, the list of disadvantages outweighs the advantages with K1 deferring to the child the key decision making role, which amounts to delaying the parental decision about testing. A regular check-up of blood pressure and infections, rather than a genetic test, is proffered as a justifiable solution."
AC: "At end of that same para, you interpret K1 as recommending that the child should not be tested until older. Maybe it came out that way but it was

> not her intent. K1 was trying to be 'balanced' – countering the list of reasons for testing that were given earlier. She is bearing in mind the very real limitations of testing (the difficulty of doing a linkage study in this family, the often inconclusive results from scans in childhood). She asks the parents if they have decided whether or not to request testing now and reassures them that there is no need to make a rushed decision. The limitations of testing provide part of the background – you can hardly recommend testing as the preferred option when you know that you are unlikely to be able to deliver clear results. I take this whole performance as an attempt to remain neutral, clearly willing to go with the parents' decision once they have thought it through but remaining aware of the limitations of what is likely to be feasible."

Parental decision about testing the child is neither endorsed nor objected to as part of being professionally neutral in the face of uncertainty of test results. Through his comments AC is appealing to the broader family context, including the entire consultation. As a discourse analyst, SS's interpretation attributes to K1 a preference for non-testing which may be contextually myopic and therefore misleading in terms of intentionality underpinning routine professional practice. For AC, the preference for non-testing does not count as neutral and this amounts to a divided sense of expert judgements (unlike division of expert labour between K1 and G1). As far as SS is concerned, there are no discursive cues in the local interactional environment to support a more neutral reading of K1's communicative behavior. It is worth noting that if K1, instead of G1, were to comment in this instance, she may or may not align herself with G1's interpretation. The 'knowing how' stance of a discourse analyst may seem constrained in a situation where the intentions behind communicative behaviour are not explicitly cued.

With regard to 'knowing that' and 'knowing how', what is manifest in talk and what might be the intention underpinning professional practice may constitute 'interpretive variability'. The disagreement is heightened further in this particular situation as professional neutrality remains a central tenet of genetic counselling practice. The exact communicative dimensions of neutrality may not be so easily understood or shared both within the genetic counselling profession and across disciplinary/professional boundaries.

Let us consider a further extract from the same counselling session where the parent articulates her sense of guilt about testing the child – as a precondition for proceeding with her future pregnancy.

DATA EXTRACT 2

01 PF yeah I think I just wanted um (.) a bit more knowledge about what could happen because (.) like you said I could go through life and have (.) no problems at all in (.) but I d- (2.0) uh I didn't know whether (.) would it be selfish of me to have more children and pass it on to them then they'd have to (.) deal with what [(0.5) you] know I di- =
02 N2 [mm yeah]
03 PF = you know that I'd have to pass on all what I know about all this [(.)] like mammy's had to tell me (.) what she knows about it
04 N2 [yeah]
05 K1 I mean do you understand what are (.) the <u>worst</u> [possible things]
06 PF [yeah yeah]
07 K1 that can happen so (.) [you know (^^^^^) at the best end of the situation]
08 PF [but when you look at it like that you think well (.) yeah that's it yes] ((gap))
09 G1 yeah I suppose the chance of of a young baby (0.5) uh (0.5) inheriting the PKD and being ill from it as a young child (.) is is not zero but is really rather small [(1.0)]
10 PF [yeah]
11 G1 so the vast majority of people with PKD wouldn't (.) get health problems from it (.) in pregnancy (.) I mean s- in infancy or [(.)] childhood really (1.0) s- much more likely =
12 PF [yeah]
13 G1 = if it were to be a problem for another child [(1.0) to to] yes I mean =
14 PF [it would be like the same age as I am or whatever is it]
15 G1 = to (.) not to show itself until adult life (.) as as a problem [(1.0)] =
16 PF [yeah]
17 G1 = but occasionally it will (1.0) in younger but it would be very unusual (.) not (.) I've not got a percentage in my head for [that ((K1)]

The following is the correspondence between SS and AC, selectively, based on SS's analytic commentary on the above data extract.

> SS: "The implicitly positive endorsement for a future pregnancy is facilitated by discounting the chance of a young baby inheriting PKD. This no doubt contributes to an understanding and assessment of causal responsibility. The knowledge that a genetic test procedure involves more than simple blood

> extraction from herself and that an elaborate testing protocol involving other family members can still deliver an inconclusive result contribute towards PF's decision not to go ahead with the test, which is evidenced at the close of the encounter."
> "This then forms a robust basis for safeguarding the child's autonomy and their best interests."
> AC: "So I have reservations about that sentence, which represents the professionals as always wanting to defer testing. Well – not in this disease. And I think your interpretation of the data has been distorted a bit to let you say what you want to say."
> "I hope I am not being too unfair – you will probably find lots of counter arguments – but I think you should revisit your data analysis sections. It will not alter what you say about the theoretical aspects and would actually make the paper much more interesting as exemplifying the attempt of two professionals to work for neutrality (an active non-directiveness, trying to ensure that parents get what they want – once they have understood the situation they are in)."

The divided expert accounts here directly bear on data analytic claims, especially the language of interpretation. AC's objection alludes to the negative casting of the genetic counsellor who potentially comes across as being indifferent in deferring childhood testing as opposed to displaying a form of 'active non-directiveness'. Such differential characterisation of professional practice – directiveness vs. indifference vs. active non-directiveness – is not benign and has consequences not only for the individual professional involved but also for the profession as a whole. The genetic counselling profession is premised on an ethos of non-directiveness (parallel to the principle of neutrality in mediation), so its discursive manifestation needs to be carefully categorised and safeguarded. While this professional commitment to non-directiveness (knowing that) is easy to uphold, the difficulties lie in identifying corresponding discursive evidence (knowing how).

Let us return to the earlier distinction between 'seeing as' and 'seeing that'. Both SS and AC are engaged in 'seeing that' which underpins 'interpretative variability'. Drawing on Goffman's (1974) notion of 'frame' to refer to 'schemata of interpretation to locate, perceive, identify and label' phenomena, here we have a case of both over- and under-interpretation of discourse data vis-à-vis participants' intentionality. The risks associated with non-negotiation of interpretations can be high on both sides: the professional practitioners adopting a sceptical stance to discourse analytic findings; and the discourse analyst having very little impact in trying to inform and change professional practice.

6. Conclusion

This chapter has primarily been about the bounds of interpretation across different domains of expertise and authority in the healthcare setting. Expert interpretive authority may be claimed as the basis of knowledge (knowing that) and/or experience (knowing how). Discourse analysts are more likely to appeal to what is evidenced in the data – directly or indirectly – in the spirit of Lockean empiricism, 'light arising from the nature of things themselves'. Discourse analytic interpretation is therefore indeterminate, especially in relation to intentionality underpinning participants' communicative behaviour. Such indeterminate accounts may be seen as unsatisfactory, but any 'definitive versions' are likely to be equally unsatisfactory "because they imply unjustifiably that the analyst can reconcile his version of events with all the multiple and divergent versions generated by the actors themselves" (Gilbert/Mulkay 1984: 2). The interpretive framework adopted by the discourse analyst is always underpinned by presuppositions and prior experiences. As Chisholm (1966: 56) suggests:

> *Experience*, in one or another of its various sources, is said to be the source of our knowledge; every valid claim to knowledge, it is supposed, will satisfy certain *empirical* criteria; and these criteria, it is then concluded, may be used to determine the extent of our knowledge. Empiricism thus begins paradoxically with a general premise. [Emphasis in original]

In spite of the indeterminacy of interpretive frameworks in discourse analytic research, one feels compelled to make their interpretation count. Translational research, i.e., translating research findings into practice, is becoming the order of the day. In this context we need to ask: Can discourse analytic findings impact upon the culture of everyday professional practice? What are the challenges associated with interpretation of data as well as interpretation of findings? The nuances surrounding the different interpretive stances have been the focus of my reflections in this chapter. I feel open dialogues between experts belonging to a community of interest, albeit hailing from different communities of practice/discourse/interpretation, are a necessary – but not sufficient – condition for triangulating interpretive preferences, and consequently enhancing translationality of discourse analytic findings.

References

Berger, John 2008. *Ways of Seeing*. London: BBC in association with Penguin Books.

Bleich, David 1978. *Subjective Criticism*. Baltimore, MD: Johns Hopkins University Press.

Bourdieu, Pierre 1977. *Outline of a Theory of Practice*. Cambridge: Cambridge University Press.

Burke, Kenneth 1965 [1935]. *Permanence and Change: An Anatomy of Purpose*. Indianapolis: Bobs-Merrill.

Burke, Kenneth 1966. *Language as Symbolic Action: Essays on Life, Literature and Method*. California: California University Press.

Chisholm, Roderick M. 1966. *Theory of Knowledge*. Englewood Cliffs, NJ: Prentice-Hall.

Cicourel, Aaron V. 2007. A Personal, Retrospective View of Ecological Validity. *Text & Talk* 27/5–6, 735–752.

Clarke, Angus 2005. Commentary 1: Professional Theories and Institutional Interaction. *Communication & Medicine* 2/2, 189–191.

Douglas, Mary 1985. *Risk Acceptability According to the Social Sciences*. London: Routledge & Kegan Paul.

Dunn, John 1978. Practising History and Social Science on 'Realist' Assumptions. In Hookway, Christopher / Pettit, Philip (eds)

Action and Interpretation: Studies in the Philosophy of the Social Sciences. Cambridge: Cambridge University Press, 145–175.
Ferrara, Kathleen 1994. *Therapeutic Ways with Words*. New York: Oxford University Press.
Fish, Stanley 1980. *Is There a Text in This Class?: The Authority of Interpretive Communities*. Cambridge, Mass: Harvard University Press.
Flint, Anthony 1995. The Scientists and the Radicals Square Off. *The Globe & Mail* June 3, D8.
Garfinkel, Harold 1967. *Studies in Ethnomethodology*. Englewood Cliffs, NJ: Prentice Hall.
Gilbert, Nigel / Mulkay, Michael 1984. *Opening Pandora's Box: A Sociological Analysis of Scientists' Discourse*. Cambridge: Cambridge University Press.
Goffman, Erving 1974. *Frame Analysis: An Essay on the Organisation of Experience*. New York: Harper & Row.
Goodwin, Charles 1994. Professional Vision. *American Anthropologist* 96/3, 606–633.
Gumperz, John 1968. The Speech Community. In Sills, David L. (ed.) *International Encyclopaedia of the Social Sciences* vol. 9. New York: The Macmillan Company, 381–386.
Gusfield, Joseph R. 1975. *Community: A Critical Response*. Oxford: Basil Blackwell.
Hanson, Norwood R. 1958. *Patterns of Discovery*. Cambridge: Cambridge University Press.
Hughes, Everett C. 1975. Professions. In G. Esland / G. Salaman / M. A. Speakman (eds) *People and Work*. Edinburgh/Milton Keynes: Holmes McDougall/Open University.
Hughes, Everett C. 1993. License and Mandate, abridged from The Sociological Eye (1977). In J. Walmsley / J. Reynolds / P. Shakespeare / R. Woolfe (eds) *Health, Welfare & Practice: Reflecting on Roles and Relationships*. London: Sage, 21–24.
Kaplan, Abraham 1964. *The Conduct of Inquiry: Methodology for Behavioral Science*. San Francisco: Chandler Publishing.
Kuhn, Thomas S. 1962. *The Structure of Scientific Revolutions*. Chicago: The University of Chicago Press.

Lave, Jean / Wenger, Etienne 1991. *Situated Learning: Legitimate Peripheral Participation*. Cambridge: Cambridge University Press.

Maslow, Abraham 1966. *Psychology of Science: A Reconnaissance*. London: Harper & Row.

O'Hanlon, Bill / Wilk, James 1987. *Shifting Contexts: The Generation of Effective Psychotherapy*. New York: Guilford.

Porter, James 1992. *Audience and Rhetoric: An Archaeological Composition of the Discourse Community*. Englewood, NJ: Prentice-Hall.

Ryle, Gilbert 1949. *The Concept of Mind*. London: Hutchinson & Co.

Sarangi, Srikant 1998. Rethinking Recontextualisation in Professional Discourse Studies. Special issue of *Text* 18/2, 301–318.

Sarangi, Srikant 2002. Discourse Practitioners as a Community of Interprofessional Practice: Some Insights from Health Communication Research. In Christopher N. Candlin (ed.) *Research and Practice in Professional Discourse*. Hong Kong: City University of Hong Kong Press, 95–135.

Sarangi, Srikant 2005. The Conditions and Consequences of Professional Discourse Studies. *Journal of Applied Linguistics* 2/3, 371–394. Also published in In R. Kiely / P. Rea-Dickins / H. Woodfield / G. Clibbon (eds) [2006] *Language, Culture and Identity in Applied Linguistics*. London: Equinox, 199–220.

Sarangi, Srikant 2007. The Anatomy of Interpretation: Coming to Terms with the Analyst's Paradox in Professional Discourse Studies. *Text & Talk* 27/5–6, 567–584.

Sarangi, Srikant 2010. Healthcare Interaction as an Expert Communicative System: An Activity Analysis Perspective. In J. Streeck (ed.) *New Adventures in Language and Interaction*. Amsterdam: Benjamins, 167–197.

Sarangi, Srikant / Candlin, Christopher N. 2011. Professional and Organisational Practice: A Discourse/Communication Perspective. In C. N. Candlin / S. Sarangi (eds) *Handbook of Communication in Organisations and Professions*. Berlin: De Gruyter Mouton, 3–58.

Sarangi, Srikant / Clarke, Angus / Bennert, Kristina / Howell, Lucy 2003. Categorisation Practices across Professional Boundaries: Some Analytic Insights from Genetic Counselling. In S. Sarangi / T. van Leeuwen (eds) *Applied Linguistics and Communities of Practice*. London: Continuum, 150–168.

Schauber, Ellen / Spolsky, Ellen 1986. *The Bounds of Interpretation: Linguistic Theory and Literary Text*. Stanford: Stanford University Press.

Schön, Donald 1983. *The Reflective Practitioner: How Professionals Think in Action*. New York: Basic Books.

Swales, John M. 1990. *Genre Analysis: English in Academic and Research Settings*. Cambridge: Cambridge University Press.

Walmsley, Jan / Reynolds, Jill / Shakespeare, Pam / Woolfe, Ray (eds) 1993. *Health, Welfare & Practice: Reflecting on Roles and Relationships*. London: Sage.

Walton, Douglas 1997. *Appeal to Expert Opinion: Arguments from Authority*. Pennsylvania: The Pennsylvania University Press.

Wenger, Etienne 1998. *Communities of Practice: Learning, Meaning, and Identity*. Cambridge: Cambridge University Press.

Wuthnow, Robert 1989. *Communities of Discourse*. Cambridge, Mass: Harvard University Press.

Appendix: Transcription conventions

G1	genetic counsellor
K1	kidney specialist
N	genetic nurse
PF/PM	parent female/parent male
CF/CM	child female/child male
(.) (..) (…)	micropause/pauses up to one second/pause exceeding one second
((gap))	an interval of longer length between speaker turns and an approximation of length in seconds
word	decreased volume
>> <<	accelerated pace

underlining	increase emphasis as in stress
question mark [?]	rising intonation
–	cut-off of prior word or sound
[text in square brackets]	overlapping speech
((text in double round brackets))	description or anonymised information
(text in round brackets)	transcriber's guess
(^^^^^^^)	untranscribable
=	a continuous utterance and is used when a speaker's lengthy utterance is broken up arbitrarily for purposes of presentation.

Communication in Medical Practice

Greg Myers

Social Media and Professional Practice in Medical Twitter

1. Social media and professional practice

When I have told people that I was studying the use of Twitter by medical professionals, they have usually laughed. Twitter is often treated as a non-serious topic, because it is commonly used by celebrities and used to record mundane or trivial things. But there is also considerable media anxiety about Twitter, particularly where it intersects with serious areas of life, such as the practices of people working in fields such as medicine, social work, the military or the civil service. In this chapter, I will briefly explain why Twitter and other social media can pose problems for medical practice, show how institutional codes try to anticipate and resolve some of these issues, and draw on frameworks from discourse analysis to describe some of the issues around professional roles. The core of the study is a corpus analysis of a set of tweets from six medical professionals, using examples to show the range of different modes in which they tweet. On the basis of this analysis, I will propose that tweets by medical professionals regularly cross the usually distinct personal, professional, institutional, and public modes. But it is worth noting, here at the outset, that in my small sample, they never breach professional standards as in the occasional incidents reported in news media.

An example of these reports is a story in *The Guardian* (Laja 2011), 'Trusts reveal staff abuse of social media'. A Freedom of Information query to the largest UK hospital trusts turned up a number of disciplinary cases that year involving doctors and nurses talking about patients, criticizing managers, or just spending work time on social media. Academics have some of the same tensions around their use of social media, where the more popular academic Twitter users are playful, open, and revealing, while traditions and codes require professionals to be serious, reserved, and careful about privacy. The technological characteristics that make social media such dynamic and powerful means of social change are also those that pose problems for professions:

- There are multiple and unpredictable audiences (Bernstein et al. 2013).
- The barriers between different audiences (work, family, friends, strangers) break down in what Marwick and Boyd (2011) call 'context collapse'.
- Texts are more easily reproduced and archived than with spoken or paper media.
- The texts are more easily searched, so an interested party (a patient, a student, a journalist) can find a comment intended for an audience of immediate friends or colleagues.

The basic problem is that definitions of professions assume a clear and socially practical division between the personal and professional, a division that sometimes takes a spatial form, with the walls of the office, staffroom, or hospital. Social media could lead to discourse out of place, breaching these divisions, leading to concerns for the image of the doctors, lawyers, teachers, or social workers, and the privacy of patients, clients, students, or service-users.

While news reports about social media propose a clear division between different aspects of a professional's life and communications, discourse analysts would argue that people in any walk of life move constantly between different and often hybrid roles. For instance, Celia Roberts and Srikant Sarangi see three kinds of discourse and many activity types in medical interaction:

- *Personal experience discourse* is talk [or writing] concerned with the individual's experiences and feelings [narratives, small talk, greetings, sociability];
- *Professional discourse* is the talk of doctors in practice [interviews, rounds, consultation between doctors];
- *Institutional discourse* […] is the ways in which general practitioners account for this talk […] through language that reifies and

> abstracts these practices [activity types such as records, meetings, qualifying exams, supervision]. (Adapted from Roberts/Sarangi 1999: 480, or Roberts *et al.* 2000)

Roberts and Sarangi see all three kinds of discourse employed in the activity type they are studying, the oral examinations given to those wishing to become general practitioners. They point out that a successful candidate must move seamlessly between these discourses to respond appropriately to the questions. Since I am concerned here with a medium that reaches beyond medical institutions, I might add for our purposes another category:

- *Public discourse* involves talk aimed at influencing attitudes, in the role of a citizen, celebrity, organiser, official, or author.

I am defining public discourse here not on the basis of the audience (beyond the medical profession) but the topic (such issues as awareness, voting, funding, or regulations) and purpose (informing, criticising, sharing, campaigning). I will follow Roberts and Sarangi, but will use the term *modes* rather than *discourses* for the different kinds of communication in which they engage. In this study, I will show how medical professionals employ these modes and how they move between the modes, linking the personal, professional, institutional, and public.

2. Institutional guidelines on social media

Anticipating the kinds of tensions between different roles that I have been discussing, and the kinds of news reports I have mentioned, many professional organisations and institutions have developed codes of practice for social media use (the Appendix is a short list of examples of such codes). Typically, they build on existing guidelines on professional behaviour, for instance in matters of the confidentiality of information about clients. They are often illustrated with cases of the kinds of conflicts that can occur between one's role as a professional and one's voice on social media. They are just one part of a wider issue about the many ways social media and Web 2.0 have transformed relations between professionals, lay people, and organisations. Examples would include patients researching their symptoms, diagnoses, or treatments, on the web, campaigns to get open access to medical research data, or data-mining of Google searches to predict epidemiological trends (other chapters in this volume deal with some of these issues). The guidelines show a tension between enthusiasm for a new tool for interaction, listening, sharing, and informing, and worry about confidentiality, reputations of professionals and institutions, boundaries, team conflicts, and the sheer waste of time. They are overwhelmingly negative, about what must *not* be done, rather than about what is now made possible. And perhaps inevitably, they are often contradictory in application, probably because such complex hybrid roles will always lead to tensions that are hard to handle in a general code.

An unusually good example of a professional code is the UK Royal College of General Practitioners' *Highway Code* (2013) drafted by Ben Riley and Clare Gerada, then the Chair of the RCGP. (The title refers to the book produced by the UK Department of Motor Vehicles that contains all the regulations that learner drivers need to know before qualifying for a license). It includes some suggestions that are more general in application.

1. Be aware of the **image** you present online and manage this proactively
7. Treat others with consideration, **politeness** and respect
8. Remember that **other people** may be watching you

These suggestions apply to anyone setting out in social media, since anyone needs to think about the relations between their near circle of friends and wider possible audiences, personal discourses and public. Other suggestions apply more specifically to medical professionals, showing tensions between the different discourses I have outlined:

2. Recognise that the **personal and professional** can't always be separated [Personal/Professional]
3. **Engage** with the public but be cautious of giving personal advice [Professional/Public]
4. Respect the **privacy** of all patients, especially the vulnerable [Professional/Public]

5. Show your human side, but maintain **professional boundaries** [Personal/ Professional]
6. Contribute your **expertise**, insights and experience [Professional/Public]
9. Support your **colleagues** and intervene when necessary [Professional/Institutional]
10. Test out innovative ideas, **learn from mistakes** – and have fun! [Professional/ Institutional]

The problems of being called upon to give advice out of the institutional context (3), maintaining privacy (4), and of being assessed as a member of one's profession at all times (5, 8) were common enough in medical practice before the Internet; the point made in the guidelines is that some users of social media may not recognise them as problems in this new context. Some guidelines refer to issues raised specifically by social media, such as (in 6) the possibilities or reaching out to a much wider audience (as for instance the authors @DrBenRiley and @clairercgp regularly do), and (in 9) the new imperative to intervene when a colleague is using social media inappropriately. One reason I find the RCGP guidelines unusually useful is that they were drawn up by experienced users of social media who are enthusiastic about the new possibilities, and who recognise (as in 10) that there won't always be clear-cut rules for new situations.

3. A corpus approach to Medical Twitter

In this study, I focus on Twitter, as a hybrid public / professional / private / institutional forum; it raises rather different questions from Facebook and other social media sites that encourage more control on privacy. Though each tweet is short, 140 characters, Twitter feeds are extensive, interconnected, and rapidly passing. So they are well-suited to corpus analysis, rather than intensive qualitative analysis of a few separate texts, as is done in some other areas of discourse analysis. And indeed Twitter has been extensively studied (see Bibliography). But most corpus studies of Twitter use large decontextualized datasets. Here I chose a relatively small set of 2,489 tweets (45,210 words) from six Twitter users over one month, May 2014, so that I would know their background and interactions. I chose UK professionals who tweeted regularly with between 1,000 and 25,000 followers at the time; anyone with fewer than 1,000 followers may not have a public role and may prefer to tweet relatively private matters, while anyone with more than 25,000 followers in this area is, well, famous. I excluded those who were also associated with other media (for instance, regular columnists) or those tweeting only in an institutional capacity. I tried for a range of specialisms, professional roles, and career stages. The sample I used is:

@AMCunningham
@DJNicholl
@ElinLowri
@GrangerKate
@MelloJonny
@ShazzaHudson

The retweets in these feeds vary from between 25% and 75% of the total; I kept the retweets in my corpus, even where that led to duplicates, because they were the part of the profile each user presents to the public. I should note that Kate Granger is now much more widely known in traditional media in the UK, but that was not as obvious when I began this project.

My analysis of the corpus had four stages:

- finding the keywords, the strings that were more common in my study corpus than in a reference corpus of non-medical tweets;
- finding key semantic domains, that is, those that are more common than in the reference corpus;
- concordancing these keywords and key categories to see them in context;
- categorising some of these keywords, using their context, in terms of the personal, professional, institutional, and public discourses.

I used Wmatrix corpus software (<http://ucrel.lancs.ac.uk/wmatrix/>), developed by Paul Rayson (Rayson 2008), but the same tasks (except the key semantic categories) could be done with other corpus concordance tools, such as Wordsmith or AntConc.

For those unfamiliar with corpus tools, Wmatrix (like other corpus concordancers) starts with **frequency lists** for words; so for instance we get words like *the* and *I* as frequent. But that in itself does not tell us what is distinctive about the corpus, because words like *the* and *I* are frequent in most samples of English text. So we look for the **keywords** that are relatively more frequent in this corpus than in the reference corpus of non-medical tweets, and, as one might expect, we get words like *care* and *patient*. Keywords will vary with different reference corpora; for instance, if I compared the Medical Twitter corpus to a general corpus, such as the British National Corpus (<http://www.natcorp.ox.ac.uk/>), it would highlight all the items common in Twitter, such as *retweet*, without necessarily showing what was distinctive about this particular area of twitter. The measure of how likely it is that the difference in the frequency of an item between the two corpora is due to chance, is given by a calculation of log-likelihood (LL); I looked at words with a LL of over 15. Wmatrix also assigns words a semantic category, based on a pre-determined list and the most frequent uses of that lexical item. This assignment is often wrong, since words have many multiple meanings (e.g., *labour* as a medical term and as a UK political party), but the **key semantic categories** in this case included *medicines* and *medical treatment*, so the coding is clearly on more or less the right track.

I should give some caveats for anyone unfamiliar with corpus analysis. Corpus tools do not automatically deliver an answer to the kinds of questions I have posed here; they require a great deal of interpretation. For instance, the keywords with the highest log-likelihoods are often unsurprising, in this case, the names such as @GrangerKate, and the analyst chooses relevant keywords from a much longer list. Often grammatical words and phrases (*as a*) are more interesting than the more obvious lexical words (*medical*). There are artefacts, particularly in the semantic coding, that must be disregarded. And of course my coding into the different categories around which this chapter is structured was entirely interpretive and qualitative.

4. Modes of Medical Twitter

I present my findings from the corpus analysis in terms of the four categories of mode. Under each category, I look first at the field-specific keywords that are relevant to this mode. Then I go on to look at the grammatical words that may be less obvious indications of this mode. Finally I consider semantic codes for relevant domains. At the end, I come to the hybrid uses of these modes.

4.1 The Personal Mode

I will say very little about the personal mode in the corpus, just because it is so pervasive, and so expected for Twitter. Usually analyses of the personal vs. the impersonal start with pronouns. The pronoun *I* is very frequent in the corpus, as I have mentioned, but it is a negative keyword in relation to the reference corpus – that is, the medical professionals use it less than it is used on Twitter in general. It is more interesting to note that it is variable in its distribution; it is used five times as much by @GrangerKate as by @ShazzaHudson, @DJNicholl, or @MelloJonny. This suggests that Kate Granger, who tells about her daily life as both a patient and a doctor, has more personal narrative than those who are mainly expressing general stances on health care. Another way of looking at the personal would be to compare their tweets about holidays and meetings, and especially their use of photographs, and again, they varied widely in these practices. (I will not discuss specific examples here; it seems to me this indication of the Personal Mode really is too personal to be quoted without permission). Besides these obvious markers, there are more subtle indications of the personal, which I will come back to in discussing hybrid categories.

4.2 The Professional Mode

The professional roles of some Twitter users are indicated by their names: *@wenurses*, *@IamChirurgicus*, *@docsuzy*, *@hospicedoctor*.

We also see it in the ways doctors and patients are discussed as categories. The corpus has, as we would expect, field-specific keywords such as *doctor* and *patients*. The word *patients* (almost always plural in this category) is generally modified: *older patients*, *your patients*, or the generalisation "Patients are wise". (Since the codes focus so much on the need for confidentiality, it is worth noting that there are almost no references in my corpus to specific patients). *Doctors* are not usually modified this way. They do things; they *believe*, *learn*, *choose*, *tell*, and *drink*. The word *doctor* (singular) rarely refers to an individual; we get: *a doctor with….* and *a doctor who…* (and in one case, *Dr Who*).

We find more subtle indications of professional categories in the grammatical keywords. One of these is the relatively frequent use of *as a*:

(1) as a patient
(2) as their consultant
(3) as a person with a life
(4) as healthcare assistants
(5) as a gp

The phrase is used to indicate which role is relevant at the moment, for instance in a discussion of supervision of medical staff: "I got rather a black mark *as a senior registrar* when I asked for some!" The point is that this request came at that (earlier) career stage. Or from a participant in these discussions who represents a patient support group: "*as a pt*, I want compulsory supervision [of doctors]". The point is that doctors might not like it, but she can speak with entitlement as a patient. Of course one does not need the phrase *as a* to do this self-categorisation: "Yup. And I want HCPs, support staff etc to respect the fact that *being a patient sucks* & I need them."

I noted that *I* is the most obvious indication of the Personal Mode. In the Professional Mode, we get the use of *we*. It is occasionally used to mean the author of the tweet alone: "But *we*'ve managed to have some fun". Sometimes it is used with specific plural reference to narrate a group activity: "We spent 2 days laying ourselves totally open emotionally to make this." Here *we* refers to the people in that discussion group. And in the following example, the author of the tweet is, I believe, referring to herself and her husband, looking forward to an evening of music on the television: "Four violinists? *We*'re going to need crisps. And wine." But most often the use of *we* is inclusive and refers to the medical profession or society as a whole, usually in hortatory contexts:

(6) We all need to accept it
(7) We must stop this
(8) We can have coordinated care for COPD
(9) How we communicate with patients
(10) The words we – staff, patients, families – use

In these cases, the use of *we* reinforces the identity of the tweet writer as a professional.

Some of the key semantic codes also relate to the Professional Mode. It is not surprising that such categories as 'Medicines and medical treatment', 'Disease', 'Helping' and even 'Dead' are over-represented in a corpus of medical tweets. 'Professional' is also a key category, and when we look at the concordance lines, we see that one of the most frequent words in this category is *professionalism*. The category 'Sensory: sight' is also over-represented, both in its literal senses – *seen, gaze* – and in what are probably more metaphorical uses – *watch, reflection*.

Of course the Professional Mode is not strictly bounded; it overlaps with the Personal and Institutional. For instance, I expected to find much more of this kind of tweet:

(11) Bloody hell I have had a busy day.

That he is busy is a comment on his professional life, but the complaint itself is personal, it is about his day. But there were very few tweets that commented on the immediate work; this one was setting him up to say he was now reading a *British Medical Journal* article. Being a professional permeates almost everything they tweet, even when they are also being a parent, violinist, or patient.

4.3 The Institutional Mode

Clearly the Institutional Mode, discourse in the world of hospitals, training programmes, and colleges and associations, is related to the

Professional Mode. But it is also distinct; Roberts and Sarangi say that the professional mode is the 'what' and 'how' of daily practice, while "the why of medicine, health, and illness invokes a more abstract, analytic, or bureaucratic mode" (1999: 480). It is the world of records, bureaucracies, codes. I associated most uses of *patients*, plural, with the Professional Mode, because they were in such phrases as *older patients* or *your patients*. On the other hand, *patient*, singular, tends to be used in the Institutional Mode, especially because it is usually used as a modifier: *patient-centred, patient care, patient information, patient safety, patient narratives*.

The word *care* is also commonly used in the Institutional Mode. As a verb, it would seem to be in the Professional Mode:

(12) A doctor who has time to listen, care about them, and offer hope

But I could find only two uses as a verb in my corpus, and there are 150 uses as part of a noun phrase: *patient care, patient-centred care, palliative care, care staff, end of life care, care of the dying, care audit, good care, safe care.* These phrases involve abstracting care from being a particular relation to a particular patient into a category of action or actor, part of an institution framing and monitoring professional practices. And these phrases are used so often because they are built into the vocabulary of medical professionals, the way phrases like *teaching objectives*, *teaching plan*, *teaching evaluation*, or *teaching quality assessment* are built into the vocabularies of teachers. They are a sign of bureaucratisation, indeed, but also of a necessary structure and the way that structure is incorporated into everyday talk, not treated as separate from it.

The pervasiveness of the institutional mode is clear in some of the key semantic categories. 'Belonging to a group' is key because it includes such words as *team, group, network, association,* and *together.* The semantic category 'In power' includes such words as *board meeting, director, exec, leadership, Chief, supervision, organising,* and *bossy.* The semantic code 'Participating' includes such words as *meetings, turnout, attendance, collaboration*, and *conference*. And there is 'Education' with *training* and *exams*. The category 'Success and failure' is key just because of the frequent use of the word *outcomes*.

The semantic codes are a very rough indicator of the content of a corpus, but here they do remind us of the pervasiveness of institutional vocabulary.

Of course there is a constant and perhaps necessary tension between the sense of vocation of the professional mode and the bureaucracy of the institutional mode, as in these tweets.

(13) Unfortunately the emerging speciality of the general surgery graduate is the 'on-call-ogist'.

(14) At practice meeting yesterday we discussed how to allocate our 1000> 75 years old patient amongst the 7 GPs

As I read these tweets, they are complaining about the way the institutional demands of work organisation and intensity overpower the professional vocation for development and care. There is also a recognition of the tensions between the professional and the institutional:

(15) Picking up litter in our hospital corridor, relative said you should tell bloody mngmt. I smiled, I am bloody mngmt!

The writer is recognising that she is seen here as a professional stepping out of her role to pick up the litter that should be picked up by someone else, while in fact the "mngmt" is not some faceless institution, it is made up of people like her.

4.4 Public mode

The interactions studied by Roberts and Sarangi (1999) stay within medical institutions. But the value, interest, and danger of social media are their ability to go beyond the immediate institutional setting. Even people with no immediate interest in Medical Twitter may encounter some of these tweets when they are retweeted. And the authors of the tweets express their views on both the political issues around medicine such as funding and regulation, and about other political issues. The topics for campaigns are suggested by (but not limited to) some popular hashtags. As one might expect, *#nhs* figures frequently, usually while they are talking about wider issues of policy, not particular issues at work. Some of the professionals in my sample are concerned with end-of-life care, so one often comes across the hashtag *#yodo*, for 'you only die once' (which here seems to be a plea to make that one death a good death). And my sample includes one notably successful Twitter-based campaign, *#hellomynameis*, showing support for Kate Granger's NHS-wide effort to get all medical professionals to identify themselves to patients, a campaign that received widespread coverage in mass media and took her to a meeting with the Prime Minister (although her tweet on 11 January 2015 suggests that not everyone has gotten the message – no one introduced themselves to her in her latest outpatient visit).

The political mode is suggested by keywords that refer meta-discursively to issues and debates. The keyword *about* follows such words as *telling, writing, speaking, thinking, tweeting*, and *discussion.* For example:

(16) Magisterial bollocks about the NHS by Simon Jenkins

The ubiquitous preposition *on* can, of course, be used in many constructions, but here it often links a text (*writing, article, piece*) or source (name of a journal or author) to what it or they are writing about:

(17) @bmjlatest on #SaatchiBill

So we get a picture of doctors who are not just talking about their work, but are engaged with wider discussions. In the semantic codes, the most obvious indication of the public mode is the 'Political' category, which includes words like *politician*, *election*, *Tory*, and (showing the dictionary used in USAS semantic coding is surprisingly up-to-date) *UKIP*.

4.5 Between modes

I have argued that it is useful to see that these different modes do different kinds of work for different audiences. But as the examples so far have suggested, most tweets by medical professionals can be seen as hybrid between modes. Even the most personally expressed tweets on one's work ("Bloody hell I have had a busy day") or health, family, or friends can relate to issues or policies on professional practice, organisation, or social attitudes. Even the most public tweets about political issues involve some personal stance-taking, as in this response to policies by UKIP's opposition to Eastern European immigrants (a position that @elinlowri had criticised in a previous tweet):

(18) @agnieszka_po: @elinlowri I'm one of them. EU Migrant. Nice person. Well educated. NHS physio. Shall I be sorry? Well, I'm not. :-)

The tweet by @agnieszka_po offers her own example and contribution as an implicit response to the anti-immigrant policies – with a smiley. The hybridity is related to the ambiguities of audience on Twitter; as the organisational guidelines suggest, even personal messages have multiple audiences: friends, colleagues, managers, patients, policy-makers, media – and trolls.

The need to move between modes may account for one of the key semantic categories that puzzled me, the negative. That does not, of course, mean that these medical professionals are negative in their attitudes. Negatives are more likely to be used to project an alternative view to some view or assumption that is already out there.

(19) And it **wasn't** as scary as I anticipated!
(20) One who sees my spirit & **not** just my prostate.
(21) The media is **not** helping either
(22) Although I **didn't** find this amusing
(23) GPs **aren't** leaving because of money
(24) Doctors are still **not** good at talking about dying

These phrasings project a view, held before by the author or someone else, in which this test was scary, doctors see just the prostate to be treated and not the person, the media ideally helps in its reporting, this (whatever it was) was intended to be amusing, GPs left because of the money, and doctors are already good at talking about dying. The use of the negative signals participation in a wider discussion.

Another key semantic code that suggests hybrid modes is 'Strong obligation or necessity'. Tweets with deontic modality project professional, institutional, or cultural norms that are assumed to be shared with the audience, or irresistible forces that will be recognised:

(25) GP practices have **had to** send out text messages to patients
(26) Family **need** to be reassured

(27) I really **should** get on and study
(28) We're all going to [g]o we all **need** to accept it
(29) Nursing **must** be +ve, not fearful
(30) You can decline. The care plan **should** be jointly owned by you and your GP

So, for instance, the first example does not just report the news that the GP practices have sent out these messages; it expresses the view that external circumstances forced them to do it (in response to a poorly-timed government announcement). The last example projects a situation required by the norms of the institution – both the patient and the medical staff will be involved in a care plan. By asserting that this should be the case, the tweet also reminds us that this norm may not always be followed. The tweet, one patient advising another, expresses a personal stance on institutional practices. Putting the necessity or obligation explicitly in the text makes an institutional or professional statement into one that is also personal and public.

5. Conclusion

When using concordance tools to look at a whole corpus of tweets, one loses some of the experience of social media. Twitter is usually read in little bits of 140 characters each, or in a stream of tweets that constantly flow from the top to the bottom of the monitor. A corpus approach involves taking them as one text to be coded and searched. By doing so, one finds patterns that are lost in the individual chunks and flow, for instance in the way *care* or *patient* are used, across the corpus, not just in this one tweet. I see three benefits to seeing Medical Twitter in a corpus, and to analysing the tweets into different modes of personal, professional, institutional, and public:

1) The conventional focus on issues of public and private in social media over-simplifies and moralises issues that are complex and practical for professionals moving between these different modes.
2) The analysis brings out tensions that are specific to medical discourse, for instance the tension between the demands of professional

care and the constraints of institutional practices, or the expectations of professionalism and the daily experience of individual medical staff.

3) The corpus approach can bring out patterns across the whole corpus that are missed when focusing on individual tweets.

Medical Twitter does not usually offer a diary-like insight into the everyday lives of medical professionals. But it does show the ways they enact and reflect on their tensions between their everyday lives, their roles as professionals, the institutional frames that enable and constrain their work, and the public debates that will shape how medical practice develops.

Acknowledgements

I benefitted from discussions with, among others, Erika Darics, Julia Gillen, Ruth Page, Elena Semino, and Johnny Unger.

References and introductory bibliography on Twitter

Barton, David / Lee, Carmen 2013. *Language Online: Investigating Digital Texts and Practices*. London: Routledge.

Bernstein, Michael S. / Eytan Bakshy / Moira Burke / Brian Karrer 2013. Quantifying the Invisible Audience in Social Networks. *ACM Conference on Human Factors in Computing Systems –* CHI 2013, April 27-May 2, 2013. Paris, France.

Boyd, Danah / Golder, Scott / Lotan, Gilad 2011. Tweet, Tweet, Retweet: Conversational Aspects of Retweeting on Twitter. *Proceedings of the 43rd Hawaii International Conference on System Sciences*. IEEE.

Coeckelbergh, Mark 2011. What are we Doing? Microblogging, the Ordinary Private, and the Primacy of the Present. *Journal of Information, Communication & Ethics in Society* 9, 127–136.

Gillen, Julia / Merchant, Graham 2013. Contact Calls: Twitter as a Dialogic Social and Linguistic Practice. *Language Sciences* 35, 47–58.

Hawn, Carleen 2009. Take Two Aspirin and Tweet Me in the Morning: How Twitter, Facebook, and Other Social Media are Reshaping Health Care. *Health Affairs* 28/2, 361–368.

Honeycutt, Courtenay / Herring, Susan 2009 Beyond Microblogging: Conversation and Collaboration via Twitter. *Proceedings of the 42nd Hawaii International Conference on System Sciences*. IEEE.

Jameson, Daphne A. 2014. Crossing Public-Private and Personal-Professional Boundaries: How Changes in Technology may Affect CEOs' Communication. *Business and Professional Communication Quarterly* 77/1, 7–30.

Laja, Sade 2011 Trusts Reveal Staff Abuse of Social Media. Guardian Healthcare Network <http://www.theguardian.com/healthcare-network/2011/nov/09/trusts-reveal-staff-abuse-of-social-media-facebook>.

Mansfield, Sarah J. / Morrison, Stewart G. / Stephens, Hugh O. / Bonning, Michael A. / Wang, Sheng-Hui / Withers, Aaron H.J. / Olver, Rob C. / Perry, Andrew W. 2011. Social Media and the Medical Profession *Medical Journal of Australia* 194/12. <https://www.mja.com.au/journal/2011/194/12/social-media-and-medical-profession>.

Marwick Alice E. / Boyd, Danah 2011. 'I tweet honestly, I tweet passionately': Twitter Users, Context Collapse, and the Imagined Audience. *New Media and Society* 13, 114–133.

Page, Ruth 2012. *Stories and Social Media: Identities and Interaction*. London: Routledge.

Potts, Amanda / Simm, Will / Whittle, Jon / Unger, Johann 2014. Success in Digitally Augmented Activism: A Triangulated Approach to UK Activist Twitter Use. *Discourse Context & Media* 6, 65–76.

Rayson, Paul 2008. From Key Words to Key Semantic Domains. *International Journal of Corpus Linguistics* 13, 519–549.

Roberts, Celia / Sarangi, Srikant 1999. Hybridity in Gatekeeping Discourse: Issues of Practical Relevance for the Researcher. In Sarangi, Srikant / Roberts, Celia (eds) *Talk, Work, and Institutional Order*. Berlin: Mouton de Gruyter: 473–504.

Roberts, Celia / Sarangi, Srikant / Southgate, Lesley / Wakeford, Richard / Wass, Val 2000. Oral Examinations – Equal Opportunities, Ethnicity, and Fairness in the MRCGP. *BMJ* 320/7231, 370–375.

Zappavigna, Michelle 2011. Ambient Affiliation: A Linguistic Perspective on Twitter. *New Media and Society* 13, 788–806.

Zappavigna, Michelle 2012. *The Discourse of Twitter and Social Media*. London: Continuum.

Appendix

Social media codes and guidelines for professionals

ACAS [UK Conciliation Service]: Social media and how to develop a policy: <http://www.acas.org.uk/index.aspx?articleid=3381>.

American Medical Association: <http://www.ama-assn.org/ama/pub/physician-resources/medical-ethics/code-medical-ethics/opinion9124.page?>.

Australian Health Practitioner Regulatory Agency: <http://www.ahpra.gov.au/News/2014-02-13-revised-guidelines-code-and-policy.aspx>.

Australian Medical Association: <http://www.medicalboard.gov.au/Codes-Guidelines-Policies/Social-media-policy.aspx>.

British Medical Association: Social Media Use: Practical and Ethical Guidance for Doctors and Medical Students: <http://bma.org.uk/practical-support-at-work/ethics/ethics-a-to-z>.

UK Royal College of General Practitioners: <http://www.rcgp.org.uk/~/media/Files/Policy/A-Z-policy/RCGP-Social-Media-Highway-Code.ashx>.

UK Civil Service: <http://www.civilservice.gov.uk/news/lets-get-social/how-to-use-social-media>.

Lists of policies

Chris Boudreux, Social Media Policy Database: <http://socialmediagovernance.com/policies/>.

Rachel Miller, 300 Social Media Policies: <http://www.allthingsic.com/smpolicy/>.

Anna Tereszkiewicz

Medical Doctors on Twitter: How and Why MDs Tweet

1. Introduction

Twitter, though mostly perceived as a tool of personal communication used to share daily life narratives (Page 2012, Zappavigna 2012), is increasingly common in the area of professional communication as well. Owing to the many forms of communication it offers, (e.g. one-to-one and one-to-many communication, public and private messages), Twitter has been recognized as a useful tool in various areas of professional communication, used by businessmen, lawyers and academic researchers. An increasing number of studies is being devoted to the use of social media in general and Twitter in particular in health communication as well. The research done so far underlined a widespread use of Twitter among patients, as a channel for personal narratives on illnesses, for exchanging experiences and information (McGowan *et al.* 2012, Page 2012, Scanfeld *et al.* 2010, Sugawara *et al.* 2012, Murthy 2013). A growing number of medical doctors, as well as public health departments and health care institutions resort to Twitter for branding, marketing, patient education, and dissemination of information about medical practice and health care in general (Chaudhry *et al.* 2012, Van Eperen/Marincola 2011, Thackeray *et al.* 2012, Neiger *et al.* 2013).

The studies point out both benefits and problems associated with the use of social media in health communication. Social media may be beneficial since they offer means of exchanging experiences concerning treatment and lending social and emotional support for patients (Page 2012, Sugawara *et al.* 2012, Murthy 2013), offer access to public views on health issues and to information on patients' experiences, and thus can help improve the quality of patient care (Chaudhry *et al.* 2012,

Moorhead *et al.* 2013). Among the problems, scholars and practitioners point out low reliability and accuracy of information, low security of personal data, patient privacy in particular and the risk of incorrect advice and misdiagnosis (Chaudhry *et al.* 2012, Moorhead *et al.* 2013).

2. Aims, materials and methods

This study aims at investigating the use of Twitter by medical doctors (MDs). More specifically, the study focuses on analysing MDs' profiles and content of tweets. The analysis involves a discussion of such aspects as the purpose of tweeting, the function and content of hyperlinks and audiovisual elements. With respect to the discourse properties of tweets, the analysis focuses on stance taking strategies, as one of the most important means allowing MDs to express and mark their professional expertise. It was assumed that Twitter will predominantly serve as a tool of filtering and disseminating information, as a community forming tool, allowing collaboration with other MDs, and as a tool of impression management, promoting medical practice, thus performing the functions similar to those of academic and science weblogs.

The analysis covered profiles and tweets of ten medical doctors, selected from Doctors on Twitter registry on the basis of the highest popularity measured in the number of tweets, followers and profiles followed. For the purpose of the study 1,520 tweets were collected from the analysed profiles – during seven days of a randomly constructed week over the period of three months (November 2013, March and April 2014). Due to the number of issues which were investigated, different methods were applied in the analysis. Tweets were coded for their type (update, retweet, @reply) and function, in part based on the methodology used by Lovejoy and Saxton (2012) and Neiger *et al.* (2013). Coding was designed to determine the purpose of tweeting (dissemination of information, self-promotion, interaction/engagement). The frequency, type and function of links were investigated based on the previous research on weblog linking (Kim 2000, Thelwall 2003, Ali-Hasan/Adamic 2007, Luzon 2009). The tools applied in the study of linking, supplemented by the tools of multimodal analysis proposed by Machin (2007) were adapted in the analysis of the frequency, function and content of multimedia. With respect to discourse and stance-taking strategies, the analysis involved the investigation of the patterns of evaluation, affective and epistemic attitude, performed according to Myers' (2010) approach.[1]

3. Medical doctors' profiles

Individuals maintaining a profile in social media become involved in complex practices of self-presentation and impression management. Self-presentation in social media is associated with the problem of the author's authenticity and reliability (Page 2012: 97). This aspect seems to be particularly vital considering online medical communication – creating a credible and reliable profile may help a medical practitioner establish their position in the professional community, gain credence, expand their network of relationships, both with other professionals and patient communities.

The means of impression management in Twitter comprise visual information (profile and background photographs) and textual information (personal information, updates). As far as visual information is concerned, most of the profiles included a personal photograph, with all MDs portrayed in a close shot. The pose and type of shot (all photographs featuring an MD's bust, with direct gaze, wearing a doctor's coat or a surgeon's gown) suggest that photographs serve to confirm and enhance the owner's professional identity (cf. Machin 2007). At the same time, the photographs impart a more personal, interactive and dialogical meaning to the profile (Machin 2007). In one case, a graphic image was used as a profile photograph.

1 Tweets are quoted in their original form. However, profilers' names, as well as names of other Twitter users, have not been quoted in the analysis since they may be considered sensible data.

As far as profile details are concerned, nearly all MDs provide information on professional practice, i.e. specialization (90%) and positions held (70%). Most profiles provide links to MDs' homepages or blogs (40%), to the websites of societies and institutions to which they are affiliated or at which they are employed (50%). Such information serves to confirm the tweeter's professional identity and promote the self. The data help to increase the value and reliability of the profile and of the tweets. Apart from these, selected profiles contain a disclaimer (30%) and provide personal information (20%), such as information on hobbies, which lends a more personal touch to the profile.

4. Tweet content and function

As far as the content and function of tweets are concerned, the range of uses and forms of tweets confirms their multifunctional character (Page 2012: 99). All the forms of messages available in Twitter can be found on the profiles, i.e. updates, retweets, and addressed messages, each serving a specific function. In the analyzed material, updates proved the most frequent (43%), followed by addressed messages (32%) and retweets (25%). Updates comprise tweets disseminating popular science and health-care oriented articles from mass media, science-oriented and medical research news and articles or case reports published in academic journals, as well as health tips. A small percentage of updates (6%) comprise personal life posts, not associated with health and medicine. The following updates exemplify the above-mentioned subcategories of the posts:

(1) Let's eliminate the stigma of cancer –> Don't blame patients for their disease – <http://ow.ly/paR4i>

(2) Oct 3 Tweet-a-Day for Breast Cancer. Vitamin D good for bones – what about cancer? Find data at: <http://ow.ly/pudgz>

(3) Noticed today I've got quite a bit more gray hair. Ah, well: I've considered it a race between graying & accelerating baldness

Tweets constituting replies are addressed at other MDs, institutions, patients and 'ordinary' users as well. The messages comprise social comments, acts of politeness, such as thanks, wishes, compliments, which can serve the purpose of community enhancement and integration. The second major function of replies involves exchanging information and opinions, clarification of information and exchanging experiences concerning medical practices:

(4) @user @user @user @user Thanks for the mention! Inspired by your work too--please keep in touch!

(5) @user Heard you did a great job in SWOG social media meeting. Thanks! Had conflict with breast working group

(6) @user no, common serum tumor markers are CEA, CA-125, CA19–9

Retweets comprise messages published by health-institutions, organizations, societies, as well as other MDs. The major purpose of retweets in this case involves disseminating news and information. Retweeting may also be used in order to recognize the expertise of other MDs. Retweeted messages are often accompanied by comments evaluating the forwarded message. For instance:

(7) RT @user: ALK-positive NSCLC–patient's story opens eyes, 9/13:58 | CAP TODAY <http://www.captodayonline.com/alk-positive-nsclc-patients-story-opens-eyes-91358/>

(8) Helpful. RT @user: User, MD, discusses mgmt of adverse events (AEs) from treatment w/immunotherapies <http://flip.it/hV8sk>

Tweets comprise messages posted from Twitter chats (6%) and conference venues (4%) as well. A relatively high frequency of tweets from Twitter chats confirms previous observations that the medium has become a popular channel for online discussions concerning health care issues (cf. Sugawara *et al.* 2012). Such chats constitute an important tool of health care communication as they offer a floor for discussion for different audiences, uniting both professionals, as well as non-professionals, such as patients and care givers. Among the analysed posts there occurred messages from chats concerning health care and social media, breast cancer and lung cancer, among others (marked by the following hashtags: #hcsm, #bcsm, #lcsm, #gyncsm):

(9) Of my new #ovariancancer patients this week, 100% had a delay in diagnosis. Raising awareness is such a priority. #gyncsm

(10) How much of a problem is concept of randomization? Some pts don't want to be subjected to randomization, even if both arms are OK. #lcsm

Conference tweets comprise tweets disseminating news on conference presentations or updates on the research discussed at the conferences. The messages also involve comments evaluating the presentations, which may be aimed at initiating a discussion, as well as questions directed at speakers and participants. A small number of conference tweets involve self-promotional tweets, in which MDs inform the audience on their participation in a conference and the presented research:

(11) #epatient User: with pancreatic cancer, the outcome is known. Speaks to importance of healing when curing isn't possible #MedX

(12) Tweeting from WE CAN breast/cervical cancer advocacy conf in Uganda. #bcsm followers, share support of our African sisters on #WECANAfrica

(13) User postulate that the ER+ metastatic breast cancer become dependent on androgen pathway when estrogen becomes low #AACRBC13

These results are in line with the previous research (Desai *et al.* 2012, McKendrick *et al.* 2012), which proved an increase in the use of Twitter during medical conferences. Twitter backchannels are seen as an important information and knowledge dissemination tool, spreading news to both participants and non-participants of the meetings, and increasing the audience's awareness of the medical problems discussed. Backchannels also perform a social function, integrating the participants of the conferences, as well as an important promotional function, disseminating news on the conferences to a wide audience.

In general, tweets published by MDs can be seen to perform three major functions: dissemination of information and knowledge, interaction, discussion and community enhancement, as well as self-promotion. Twitter serves MDs as a channel used for constructing and mediating news and knowledge concerning health care (both scientific and popular-science information), results of medical trials, as well as up-to-date news on medical research. Posting news from mass media or medical websites may also be seen as a form of promoting a healthy life-style and raising others' awareness of health issues. Tweets, in particular addressed messages and chats, serve the purposes of interaction, communicative connection (Page 2012: 426) and discussion. They create a possibility of interaction concerning medical research, discussion of treatment and patient care, which helps to mediate and construct knowledge. Moreover, tweets may be seen to help to create and maintain a community of users – posting public messages directed at other MDs with thanks for recognition, congratulations, wishes, invitations to events helps to establish and improve community relations and bonds. Posts also comprise instances of interaction with patients, giving others an insight into patients' experiences, and reflecting the practitioner's relationship and involvement in treatment practices.

Tweets also serve as a means of fulfilling self-promotional objectives, in that they are tools of self-presentation, increasing self-publicity and presenting one's achievements and medical practice. Tweets, namely, comprise updates on one's professional activity, publications or participation in conferences and meetings. For instance:

(14) New patient flying in to see me for consultation next week. Always nice to know they really value my perspective that much

(15) My breast clinic is starting now. Wish the best for me any my patients

(16) Speaking to the county medical society tonight about social media. Hoping for an interesting discussion

5. Linking patterns

Hyperlinking has been observed to perform important functions in blogging and microblogging (Kim 2000, Thelwall 2003, Ali-Hasan/Adamic 2007, Luzon 2009, Myers 2010). Disseminating and exchanging links represents the essence of communication in Twitter and constitutes one of its social functions (Page 2012, Zappavigna 2012). Links constitute a significant component of the analysed tweets as well, as nearly 29% of the updates contained hyperlinks. The analysis of the content of links has revealed a considerable diversity of the sources to which MDs refer the addressees. The table below presents the most frequent types and content of links, and their rhetorical function, investigated with reference to Luzon's (2009: 86) analysis of links in academic weblogs.

Linked source	*%*	*Rhetorical function*
Medical society/ organizations' websites and blogs (e.g. ASCO)	24%	Disseminating information Dissemination of medical knowledge Community formation and integration Promotion
Medical journals (NEJM, JAMA)	22%	Dissemination of information and knowledge Crediting medical discoveries Referencing and citing
Mass media (Reuters, New York Times, Washington Post, etc.)	15%	Disseminating information Popularization of medical knowledge Promotion of healthy life-style Increasing public awareness of health matters
Medicine-oriented websites (e.g. Oncology Tube, Health Day)	14%	Dissemination of information Popularization of medical knowledge Promotion of healthy life-style
Other MDs' personal homepages, blogs	11%	Community formation and integration Crediting information
Organizations/institutions MDs are affiliated with (MD Anderson Centre)	7%	Promotion Enhancing credibility Identity management
MDs' homepages, blogs	5%	Self-publicity Enhancing credibility Identity management
Other	2%	Disseminating news Humour

Table 1. Content and function of links.

Links reflect the filtering function of tweets. Their primary function is to provide extra information and refer the reader to further external materials. Similar to their function in academic and scientific blogs, in microblogs links may serve as tools of knowledge and information dissemination (Luzon 2009: 85). The links contain content aimed at various audiences, both healthcare professionals and non-professionals. By spreading hyperlinks MDs share medical knowledge, credit medical discoveries and trigger discussions concerning health care and medical practice. External links to news media articles may serve the purpose of popularizing medical knowledge or recent findings concerning health and medicine, and promoting a healthy life style. Doctors also link to nonprofit healthcare organizations and societies, with the purpose of disseminating information for both practitioners and patients concerning testing, treatment, and funding of medical care. Links may be seen to perform the function of community integration as well. References to the content created by other MDs (e.g. articles, blogs) contribute to community building and strengthening bonds with others (cf. Luzon 2009: 81). Links also include references to the author's blog, homepage or publications, performing a self-promotional function, which helps to enhance the authors' reliability as medical doctors. Linking, thus, may be compared to referencing and quoting practices in other professional genres, and as such can be interpreted as a means of establishing and confirming one's professional identity and credibility (Luzon 2009). Links may inform on the tweeter's interests, expertise, authority, affiliations, and quite importantly, opinion and attitude towards the issues tweeted about (Page 2012: 109).

The form of the captions annotating the links is worth noting. In the analysed corpus, the captions perform two main functions, namely, abstracting the content of the linked text and/or providing the tweeter's evaluation of this content (cf. Page 2012: 110–111). The captions created by MDs most often differ from the original headlines of the referenced content in their discursive and pragmatic shape, with a visibly higher impressive and informative potential. It can be seen that in contrast to the original headlines the captions created by the authors exhibited a higher degree of expressiveness and dialogicality. The persuasive value of the headlines is enhanced by the use of direct references to the audience (pronoun *you*), questions directed at addressees, exclamations, imperative forms, evaluative vocabulary, as well as statistical data:

(17) Is your physician's electronic medical record system selling your info to drug & device companies? <http://bit.ly/1dyXR43h/t@user> [Original headline: The hidden cost of free EMR systems]

(18) Using a tiny robot to treat brain tumors? Great idea, but would ditch the maggot reference if u want buy in! @user <http://n.pr/1h8K5oW> [Original headline: Why Brain Surgeons Want Help From A Maggot-Like Robot]

(19) Half of med students still receiving drug company gifts in last year--are you kidding me? @user <http://well.blogs.nytimes.com/2013/10/03/for-med-students-love-from-the-drug-rep/?ref=health&_r=0> ... [Original headline: For Med Students, Love From the Drug Rep]

In addition to the persuasive function, the captions perform an abstracting role as well, as identified by Page (2012). In these cases MDs focus on the informative value of the captions by providing abstracts of the materials behind the links, including the gist of the content behind the link in the caption:

(20) Veterans Health Admin proposes new rule whereby nurses will care for sickest patients without MD supervision/input. <http://bit.ly/177jA1r> [Original title: The latest salvo in the federal government's war on physicians]

(21) Anti-PARP inhibitor BMN 673 study shows high response rates in BRCA+ breast and ovarian cancer patients. <http://www.medpagetoday.com/MeetingCoverage/ECC/42081> [Original title: Anti-PARP Study Called 'Flat-Out Successful']

Focusing on the persuasive and informative value of the captions may be interpreted as a means to attract readers to follow the links and become familiar with the content. It is clear that MDs use the medium to disseminate and promote medical research, advances in medicine, and methods of treatment.

6. Multimedia – frequency and functions

Since Twitter is becoming increasingly multimodal, audiovisual elements have started to play an important role in the interaction on this platform and may significantly influence the meaning potential of the posts. The investigation of multimedia has shown, however, that doctors only rarely resort to the use of audiovisual elements. Among the analysed tweets, only 120 posts include an audiovisual element. Among the multimedia present in the corpus, the following are the most frequent:

Audiovisual content	*%*	*Rhetorical function*
Photographs of posters and conference slides	22%	Information dissemination Popularization of medical knowledge and research
Photographs picturing other MDs at conferences	7%	Community formation and integration Crediting medical discoveries
Photographs picturing the self at conferences	5%	Self-publicity Enhancing credibility Identity management
Medicine-oriented videos, graphics, cartoons, photographs of medical equipment, medicines	48%	Disseminating information Popularization of medical knowledge Promotion
Personal-life photographs	8%	Identity management
Other (news, humorous memes)	14%	Disseminating news Humour

Table 2. Content and function of multimedia.

Audiovisuals can be seen to serve a number of purposes. Audiovisual content uploaded from conference venues serves as a means of knowledge and information dissemination, promotion of medical research and medical findings, and thus helps to construct medical knowledge. Photographs picturing other MDs at conferences and group pictures help to enhance community relations and improve interpersonal bonds, but also give credit to others' research. Photographs picturing the self at conferences, though rare, perform an important function of enhancing the microblogger's professional identity, help to picture him/her as a researcher and an active member of the medical community. Audio-visual content comprises as well infographics, audiovisuals concerning public health, photographs of medicines and medical equipment. The purpose of such audiovisual content is to promote products and raise public awareness concerning health care. Within the group of such audiovisuals also medicine-oriented cartoons can be found, which add a tinge of humour and jocularity to the discussions concerning medicine and health care. A small percentage of audiovisual content concerns the tweeter's personal life and comprises photographs of family members and everyday life events. Such content enhances the personal nature of the profile, establishes a warmer and more friendly image of the author. Disclosing personal details may help reveal the tweeter's 'ordinary' face and make the profile more attractive to other users and readers.

7. Discourse patterns

As shown above, the uses to which Twitter is put encompass filtering and distributing information, updating on one's activities, maintaining ties and relationships, i.e. the primary functions of social media in general. This multifunctional nature of tweets is reflected in their heterogeneous nature as regards discourse – as the examples provided above show, a merger of informal interaction with professional and information-oriented communication can be seen on the profiles. As tweets are directed at peers, professionals, patients and the general public, a blending of personal, professional and popularization discourses can be observed. This observation is in line with the conclusions reached by Myers (2014) in his recent analysis of medical tweets. Myers (2014) considers tweets by medical practitioners as hybrid forms in which instances of professional, public, institutional and private discourses can be identified.

Since a comprehensive analysis of all discourse features of tweets is beyond the scope of this chapter, I wish to focus on a single aspect, that is the strategies of expressing stance employed by MDs. Stance-taking is a crucial component of institutional and professional discourse, where it helps to establish and communicate professional expertise, but also of private and popularizing discourses, where it can function as an important strategy directed at stamping one's authority, as well as at engaging and attracting addressees (Luzon 2013). An initial observation proves that medical doctors apply various stance-taking strategies and that Twitter functions as an important channel for communicating opinions and attitudes. That stance-taking plays a crucial role in medical discourse in Twitter was also confirmed by Myers (2014). In Myers' (2014) corpus, namely, strategies expressing stance and attitude (i.e. negativity and deontic modality) constituted the key semantic categories.

7.1 Stance-taking strategies

A variety of strategies expressing stance can be seen in the discourse of tweets. Tweets reveal authors' stance concerning events, publications, contents of the linked texts, or attitude to other tweeters. Practices of expressing opinions bear a close resemblance to the practices present in blogging and microblogging (Myers 2010). Evaluation is often expressed in the context of sharing hyperlinks and retweeted material. Retweeting can be considered a form of quotation and analogically to the role of quotation and referencing in professional and academic discourse it may function as a stance-taking strategy. It can be assumed, following Zappavigna's (2012: 59) view, that evaluation may in this case be expressed both in an implicit and explicit way. In the case of the former, the sheer act of retweeting and sharing a link may indicate the user's positive evaluation of the content and a wish to share it. Evaluation is here implicit as the link or retweet is not accompanied by the user's comment. The act of retweeting may indicate the author's agreement with, support of the claim presented in the retweeted message, or may serve as a means of triggering a conversation by forwarding topics for a debate:

(22) RT @user: We are trying new idea of screening/testing patients remotely for RET/FGFR abnormalities so that patients only travel if need

(23) RT @user: Smaller, flexible trials mean more options for patients & faster scientific answers: <http://mobile.reuters.com/article/idUSBRE98P05N201309>

(24) RT @user T1 Do not think sequencing will solve all. So many heterogeneity in cells. One in a million cells could be the bad one #mmsm

Evaluation, however, is more often expressed explicitly and involves expressions of both attitudinal and epistemic stance. An expression of attitude in the tweets comprises evaluation of the content as regards its value, importance and accuracy. Tweeters evaluate others' research, publications, online materials, news, as well as tweets and statements posted by other MDs, patients and tweeters in general. Positive stance, prevailing over negative evaluation, is expressed in various ways, differing in syntactic and lexical complexity. In most cases, authors express attitude by means of adjectives and noun phrases with adjectives premodifying nouns indicating the type of content being evaluated, as well as attitude verbs (e.g. *agree*). The adjectives differ in the emotive load and expressive value, as well as in the degree of formality, involving neutral, and highly expressive and emotional, as well as colloquial evaluations:

(25) Excellent review by @user: How can social media improve oncology care? <http://ow.ly/oDARZ>

(26) Cool video from Iceland. MT @user: Really creative <http://huff.to/GJIF92> "This Road Leads to Breast Cancer Awareness"

(27) Awesome spoof <http://clinicaltrials.gov> listing for James Lind's original clinical trial in 1757. Created by @user <http://ictd2014.lillycoi.com/>

In the case of verbs, instances of subject ellipsis are frequent, which may result from space restrictions. Such ellipsis, however, may actually strengthen the force of the user's stance and the value of the statement with which the tweeter agrees. In selected cases, expression of stance by means of a verb with subject ellipsis was followed by a justification of the author's opinion:

(28) Agree! MT @user: Just want to take a step back: it's great that twtcht is a rare place for docs/pts/cgivers to all come together #lcsm

(29) Agree. RT @user always remember about it. Inflammatory breast cancer doesn't show in mammograms. It's a … <http://tl.gd/mp59s3>

(30) @user Agree. I do not deny medicine is a business but how we operate and what we need to achieve require the highest ethical standard

Alignment with or objection to an idea, approval or criticism also takes the form of a single *yes* or an interjection. In these cases, stance is expressed in an informal, highly expressive and conversational tone (cf. Myers 2010: 111–112):

(31) Yes! RT@user: @user It is reasonable that #empowered pts can do research on their own & introduce it to their docs? #lcsm

(32) Ugh MT @user: Pts discouraged about cancer clinical trials: ~60% by oncologist & ~50% by family physician <http://ow.ly/psYbB>

As the examples presented above show, attitudinal markers comprise highly subjective and strongly evaluative expressions. Though justification of opinions can be found, it is infrequent, which may be explained by the technological determinants of the medium and constraints on the length of the messages. However, this strategy plays an important pragmatic function. Such wording helps to convey the message in a concise but clear way. Evaluation of the content, expressed succinctly, in the front part of the tweet, makes the evaluation more explicit and conspicuous and immediately positions the reader as to the information and content of the message. A higher frequency of positive evaluation may be conditioned by the medium, with its main role encompassing the establishment and maintenance of bonds and solidarity. Such comments play a crucial relational work (Page 2012: 114) and social function, associated with building solidarity with other tweeters (Mauranen 2002).

Projection of epistemic stance proves particularly frequent in Twitter chats, which is understandable since it is in chats that the interlocutors discuss different issues concerning healthcare and it is here that the need to stamp one's authority and express the viewpoint clearly is significant. Doctors explicitly signal their opinion using first person pronouns and verbs indicating stance. The most common way of expressing stance was the use of verb and complementation, which is a typical means of expressing opinions in blogging discourse (Myers 2010).

In this way bloggers, as Myers (2010: 101) observes, mark an individual character of the opinion in case other users did not share this view. For instance:

(33) @user I think pt pref is always part of equation, but not necessarily overriding all evidence or anticipated value. #lcsm

(34) I predict that there will be no major impact to TNBC outcome unless patients are willing to participate in clinical trials.

(35) @user I do think that can be a barrier-should we give up some purity of data for more opportunity for participation? #lcsm

As the examples above show, verbs expressing stance tend to be modified (e.g. "I do think", "I actually think"), which makes the opinions stronger and more salient. Worth noting are markers of stance expressed in the first person plural. The inclusive *we* stands for the group encompassing all medical practitioners. Such expressions show that MDs express the views speaking on behalf of the community of professionals. Stance in these cases is often expressed by means of modal and semi-modal verbs, expressing deontic modality, obligations and duties lying on the group, and norms shared by the community (cf. Myers 2014). For example:

(36) We need to improve the speed of trial enrollment process. Or come up with a totally new enrollment process

(37) Palliative care is prob best as a specialty for difficult sx mgment/end of life, as med oncs we should be practicing palliative care #lcsm

(38) RT @user T2 Sometimes research and findings come out of the blue. We have to stay curious an awake. Just like with penicillin! #mmsm

Moreover, authors' stance is visible in statements they make concerning the current and desired state of affairs in health care. In the examples below, by using modal verbs expressing deontic modality, they voice the importance of pursuing a particular course of action in order to improve standards of medical care and patient treatment:

(39) Goals of care and expectations should be spelled out from the get go in advanced disease and importantly pt values and preferences #lcsm

(40) Medical care needs to begin with reforming pt-doctor communication @user #MedX

Expressions of negative evaluation in which MDs disalign themselves from the statements have also been identified. They help doctors mark status, enhance their professional authority and credibility:

(41) MT @user disagree. Life is incurable condition too. Everything we do is "controlling" human condition. Trick is nontoxic tx #mmsm

(42) MD says apps with skin pictures can mitigate shortage of dermatologists. <http://bit.ly/16C3mJx> Dubious. In derm, context is key to dx…

(43) MT @user T2 – lvl of response, from pt perspective, best QoL w/ least invasive/ toxic/ side-effects…medical system might c it diff #mmsm

MDs reject the validity of others' views with a different force, both directly and indirectly. The use of adjectives and modal verbs reduces the strength of criticism, which might be seen as a strategy to avoid antagonizing others. Frequent occurrence of the adversative conjunction *but* is worth noting at this point. As Myers (2010: 110–11) claims, the use of *but* is a common stance-taking strategy in the discourse of blogs. It helps to reduce the force of the opinion in that it indicates that the speaker considered one interpretation of the problem, but wishes to present his/her individual viewpoint and interpretation as well:

(44) To clarify, I'm a big fan of involved pts, but I see some who exemplify why it's great, & some who highlight why many docs resist. #s4pm

(45) @user @user has great promise but will lead to huge costs for speculative Rx along w/testing: we need some OUTCOMES DATA.

(46) @user I'm not a dermatologist. But I know that skin photos can be very misleading without full context and controlled lighting, etc.

Moreover, frequent instances of negation can be seen, which was identified by Myers (2014) as another strategy of projecting stance. According to the scholar, the use of the negative in this case may indicate that the author follows the opposing view. For instance:

(47) @user @user But we don't have society where pt decides how to allocate limited resources to themselves. No reason to self-limit #s4pm

(48) Don't kid yrself. Docs not aware either. MT @user: I think better hosps test for ALK & EGFR, though most pts NOT aware of ROS1 #lcsm

(49) @user It's not easy--needs partnership between doctor and pt, and pt also has to do part to tell good story #MedX

The analysed tweets also comprise messages containing expressions of feelings and emotional reactions. Authors express both positive and negative emotions, which can be interpreted as a wish to establish solidarity and create or maintain bonds with others, as can be seen in the examples below:

(50) I'm impressed by ALK & ROS pts online. RT @user: T2: sharing trial options in social media seems 2 be effective for some pts #lcsm

(51) Sad/frustating. MT @user: For me, it's more about fighting insurance to cover trials vs. finding them hasn't been issue. #lcsm

(52) Excited to join the faculty of George Washington University and looking forward to working with @user!

It is in the expressions of stance that the inherently dialogical character of tweets is particularly clear (cf. Zappavigna: 2012: 63). In the case of retweets and linking, the dialogue takes place in a single tweet, as the original tweet is combined with the retweeter's message (Page 2012: 113). In these cases, within the confines of a single tweet MDs enter into a dialogue with the original retweeted statement and supplement it with their own view. Instances of both aligning and disaligning oneself from the statements can be observed. MDs explicitly agree, disagree, deny the validity of the statements or distance themselves from the opinions.

The patterns of evaluation and stance and the frequency of their respective types reveal an interweaving of a few factors – the influence of the medium, the audience and the author's motivations. Infrequent justification of opinions, hedges, concise expression of evaluation may result from the technological constraints put on the length of the message. Such wording of stance, however, makes it more direct and enhances its persuasive potential. Comments expressing stance are not only aimed at disseminating tweeters' opinions, but also at showing their expertise and critical evaluation of the content and phenomena tweeted about. The tweeters express their support or disalignment from the content they evaluate. Though justification is rare, in selected cases MDs substantiate their opinions with personal experiences and additional comments. The evaluative remarks also help to initiate a discussion concerning the content of tweets and in this way constitute a conversational strategy.

8. Conclusions

The content of tweets shows that MDs' profiles are aimed at a diversified audience, involving both the medical community, patients, as well as the general public (cf. Myers 2014). Among the main purposes of tweeting dissemination and negotiation of medical knowledge, knowledge translation between experts and the public, interaction and discussion of health issues, and promotion of the self can be identified. Doctors tweet to gain, explore and contribute new information to the community, to discuss health care news, reports and findings, to share experiences and advice, evaluate health care services and treatment practices, and promote a healthy life style. A frequent use of Twitter as a conference backchannel has also been observed, in which case it serves as a tool of contributing new information to the community. A growing use of Twitter chats was confirmed as well – chats gathering both medical doctors, patients and representatives of health care institutions. Finally, Twitter serves as a tool of self-promotion, enhancement of identity as a medical doctor/researcher.

References

Ali-Hasan, Noor / Adamic, Lada 2007. Expressing social relationships on the blog through links and comments. *Paper presented at the International Conference on Weblogs and Social Media, Boulder, CO.* <http://www.personal.umich.edu/ladamic/papers/on/onlinecommunities.pdf>.

Chaudhry, Aafia / Glode, Michael / Gillman, Matt / Miller, Robert 2012. Trends in Twitter Use by Physicians at the American Society of Clinical Oncology Annual Meeting, 2010 and 2011. *Journal of Oncology Practice* 8/3. <http://jop.ascopubs.org/content/early/2012/04/17/JOP.2011.000483.short>.

Desai, Tejas / Shariff, Afreen / Shariff, Aabid / Kats, Mark / Fang, Xiangming / Christiano, Cynthia / Ferris, Maria 2012. Tweeting the Meeting: An In-Depth Analysis of Twitter Activity at Kidney Week 2011. *PLoS ONE* 7/7. <http://www.plosone.org/article/info%3Adoi%2F10.1371%2Fjournal.pone.0040253>.

Lovejoy, Kristen / Saxton, Gregory 2012. Information, Community and Action: How Nonprofit Organizations Use Social Media. *Journal of Computer-Mediated Communication* 17, 337–353. <http://onlinelibrary.wiley.com/doi/10.1111/j.1083-6101.2012.1576.x/full>.

Kim, Hak Joon 2000. Motivations for Hyperlinking in Scholarly Electronic Articles: A Qualitative Study. *Journal of the American Society for Information Science* 51, 887–899.

Luzon, Maria Jose 2009. Scholarly Hyperwriting: The Function of Links in Academic Weblogs. *Journal of the American Society for Information Science and Technology* 60/1, 75–89.

Luzon, Maria Jose 2013. Public Communication of Science in Blogs: Recontextualizing Scientific Discourse for a Diversified Audience. *Written Communication* 30/4, 428–457.

Machin, David 2007. *Introduction to Multimodal Analysis*. London: Bloomsbury.

Mauranen, Anna 2002. 'A Good Question'. Expressing Evaluation in Academic Speech. In Cortese, Giuseppina / Riley, Philip (eds)

Domain-specific English. Textual Practices across Communities and Classrooms. Bern: Peter Lang, 115–140.

McGowan, Brian / Wasko, Molly / Vartabedian, Bryan / Miller, Robert / Freiherr, Desirae / Maziar Abdolrasulnia 2012. Understanding the Factors That Influence the Adoption and Meaningful Use of Social Media by Physicians to Share Medical Information. *Journal of Medical Internet Research* 14/5. <http://www.jmir.org/2012/5/e117/>.

McKendrick, Douglas / Cumming, Grant / Lee, Amanda 2012. Increased Use of Twitter at a Medical Conference: A Report and a Review of the Educational Opportunities. *Journal of Medical Internet Research* 14/6. <http://www.jmir.org/2012/6/e176/>.

Moorhead, Anne / Hazlett, Diane / Harrison, Laura / Carroll, Jennifer / Irwin, Anthea / Ciska Hoving 2013. A New Dimension of Health Care: Systematic Review of the Uses, Benefits, and Limitations of Social Media for Health Communication. *Journal of Medical Internet Research* 15/4. <http://www.jmir.org/2013/4/e85/>.

Murthy, Dhiraj 2013. *Twitter*. Cambridge: Polity Press.

Myers, Greg 2010. *The Discourse of Blogs and Wikis*. London: Continuum.

Myers, Greg 2014. Social Media, Scientific Research and Professional Practice. *Paper presented at the Cerlis 2014 Conference The Language of Medicine: Science, Practice and Academia*, Bergamo 19–21 June 2014.

Neiger, Brad / Thackeray, Rosemary / Burton, Scott / Thackeray, Callie / Jennifer Reese 2013. Use of Twitter Among Local Health Departments: An Analysis of Information Sharing, Engagement, and Action. *Journal of Medical Internet Research* 15/8. <http://www.jmir.org/2013/8/e177/>.

Page, Ruth 2012. *Stories and Social Media. Identities and Interaction*. London: Routledge.

Scanfeld, Daniel / Scanfeld, Vanessa / Larson, Elaine 2010. Dissemination of Health Information Through Social Networks: Twitter and Antibiotics. *American Journal of Infection Control* 38/3, 182–188. <http://www.ncbi.nlm.nih.gov/pubmed/20347636>.

Sugawara, Yuya / Narimatsu, Hiroto / Hozawa, Atsushi / Shao, Li / Otani, Katsumi / Akira Fukako 2012. Cancer Patients on Twitter: A Novel Patient Community on Social Media. *BMC Research Notes* 5:699. <http://www.biomedcentral.com/1756-0500/5/699>.

Thackeray, Rosemary / Neiger, Brad / Smith, Amanda / Sarah Van Wagenen 2012. Adoption and Use of Social Media among Public Health Departments. *BMC Public Health* 12/242. <http://www.biomedcentral.com/1471-2458/12/242>.

Thelwall, Mike 2003. What is this link doing here? Beginning a Fine-grained Process of Identifying Reasons for Academic Hyperlink Creation. *Information Research* 8/3. <http://www.informationr.net/ir/8-3/paper151.html>.

Van Eperen, Laura / Marincola, Francesco 2011. How Scientists Use Social Media to Communicate their Research. *Journal of Translational Medicine* 9/199. <http://www.translational-medicine.com/content/9/1/199>.

Zappavigna, Michelle 2012. *Discourse of Twitter and Social Media*. London: Continuum.

Carol Berkenkotter/ Cristina Hanganu-Bresch /
Kira Dreher

'Descriptive Psychopathology' in Asylum Case Histories: The Case of John Horatio Baldwin

1. Introduction

Psychiatry in Great Britain at the turn of the 20th century underwent a nosological paradigm shift strongly influenced by the systematic efforts of German psychiatrist Emil Kraepelin (1856–1926) to 'carve nature at the joints' by separating mental illnesses into two major categories: those of thought and those of mood disorders. In the English-speaking world, Kraepelin's categories were first debated academically, but they eventually permeated psychiatric vocabulary and practice and took on legal and forensic implications as they became ensconced in regulatory literature. Asylums were still at the forefront of psychiatric practice in the early 20th century; thus, documenting the practices of asylum doctors can offer a window into the early process of adopting the new nosology. In this chapter we focus on one of the key terms of the Kraeplinian nosology – Manic Depressive Insanity (MDI). We analyze its adoption in the clinical practice of one English asylum (Ticehurst) by looking in detail at the documented case history of the first patient formally diagnosed as 'manic-depressive' at that institution. Our goal was to chart the case notes documenting that patient's symptoms longitudinally to see whether we could discern a pattern exhibiting the main characteristic of MDI, the cycling between mania, depression, and, occasionally 'lucid intervals', a pattern that could be visible in a retrospective historical analysis, but which attending doctors failed to perceive until the MDI diagnosis was adopted by the psychiatric community in Great Britain. We set that analysis against the backdrop of the larger debate surrounding the new diagnosis category by using the notion of 'enregisterment' described by Wilce as "the process by which a linguistic register emerges and solidifies as a recognized, ideologically construed set of forms" (2009: 205). Thus, we are contrasting two parallel processes pertaining to Kraeplinian enregisterment in academia and practice using MDI as an illustrative category. In what follows, we first provide background and context by explaining the notion of enregisterment as it applies to the shift in psychiatric vocabulary and practice in the early 20th century. After briefly describing the Ticehurst Asylum corpus and its value for medical history and anthropology, we then present the case of John Horatio Baldwin, as documented at Ticehurst, and our discourse analysis of his case notes, focusing on documented instances of mania and depression that provide depth to his case and justify his (late) diagnosis. Finally, we discuss the results of our analysis by interpreting them as an illustration of the uptake process that solidified the category of 'manic depression' in the psychiatric vocabulary for the better part of the 20th century. By 'uptake' we mean the process by which a text 'invites' interpretation from successive texts that follow it. The question we raise is why is it that the diagnosis of 'maniacal depression' is employed by Ticehurst physicians so late – 1918 – when it had been a term of art in the psychiatric literature nearly two decades earlier?

To answer this question we are enlisting – at the theoretical level – the concept of 'enregisterment' popularized by Agha (2003), who used it to describe the evolution of Standard British English or Received Pronunciation (RP). Agha defines enregisterment as "processes through which a linguistic repertoire [i.e. register – our note] becomes differentiable within a language as a socially recognized register of forms" (2003: 231). Such processes have discernible socio-historical roots that can help explain the ever-shifting 'cultural value' (2003: 232) assigned to a certain discursive practice. Drawing upon Agha, Wilce (2008, 2009) points out that analogously the 'medical register' plays a role in the professionalization and credibility of a group of people or practitioners, such as, for example, psychiatrists or expert witnesses. At the center of the enregisterment process for specialized discourses such as that of psychiatry lies the primacy of classification: "the self-conscious development of a set of labels, knit together in hierarchies, uniquely characterizes the self-invention of the natural sciences in early modernity" (Wilce 2008: 92). Wilce points out psychiatry's fascination with natural kinds, stemming from what he calls its 'science envy' (2008: 93). In other words, while Agha's enregisterment analysis of 'received pronunciation' (RP) focuses on a speaker's class affiliation in Britain, Wilce believes a similar analysis of psychiatric discursive reform should focus on the 'will to professionalize' borne out of the envy/frustration experienced in the context of the apparent success of other natural sciences at the end of the 19th century. The many texts driving psychiatry's nosology-bound enregisterment processes include, according to Wilce, medical journal articles, hospital records, and psychiatric textbooks. Although efforts to describe and conceptualize mental illness in a systematic fashion abounded, they did not succeed until the years after Kraepelin made a rigorous effort to establish 'biological taxonomies' in his 1899 edition of his textbook on clinical psychiatry. Thus, Wilce concludes,

> [T]he Kraepelinian revolution spawned new *scientizing* [emphasis ours] uses of language that came to define the psychiatric register. Registral consequences are still being felt through successive iterations of the Diagnostic and Statistical Manual of Mental Disorders (DSM), in use to a greater or lesser extent around the world. (2008: 93–94)

While Agha and Wilce focus on 'speech chains' as the main processes enabling enregisterment,[1] we prefer the term 'uptake' from speech-act theory due to its vectorial quality that captures the dynamic and transformational nature of the process. Following Austin (1962) and Freadman (2004) we call 'uptake' in this context the process through which an initial document or series of documents becomes transformed into practice – in other words, the path through which a discursive construct, through a series of 'interpretant texts' (Freadman 2004), affects psychiatric practice, by which we mean patients' confinement, treatment, and release, doctor's duties, and institutional habits. In this case, the uptake that leads to the concept of manic-depressive insanity becoming

---

1 A speech chain, which is the main mechanism of social transmission of RP, according to Agha (2003), is defined as "a historical series of speech events linked together by the permutation of individuals across speech-act roles in the following way: the receiver of the message in the (n)th speech event is the sender of the message in the (n+1)th speech event" (2003: 247). Wilce (2008, 2009) uses the same term to explain enregisterment of psychiatric vocabulary.

ensconced into psychiatric practice in the first half of the 20th century in Britain would involve the following:

Genre	*Authors*	*Audience*	*Time frame*
Textbook, lectures	Emil Kraepelin	German-speaking psychiatrists	1899
English translations	Defendorf, Johnstone	English-speaking psychiatrists	1902, 1904
Psychiatry textbooks Academic articles	Psychiatrists, researchers	English-speaking psychiatrists	Early 1900s
Clinical practice genres: medical certificates, statements, case notes, etc.	Practitioners/ clinicians	Asylum/practice supervisors, commissioners in lunacy, other psychiatrists	Early 1900s
Official nomenclatures	Professional organizations (e.g. Royal College of Physicians)	Psychiatrists, regulators, legislators	1918

Table 1. Uptake of 'maniacal-depressive insanity' diagnosis in British psychiatric literature and practice.

Although most psychiatrists gradually adopted the Kraeplinean nomenclature, a practice which provided them with a more systematic approach to depicting what often seemed like disparate symptoms in search of a concept, many continued to record those symptoms in detail in an effort that, as William Sargant (1967) argued, perhaps reflected a sense of clinical impotence meaning that where cure was still elusive, the act of recording patient symptoms in minute detail offered a sense of purpose and supplanted a form of action (writing) for healing.

We wanted to see how, in everyday practice, psychiatrists recorded and made sense of the symptoms for a condition – manic-depressive insanity – what we have elsewhere called 'symptoms in search of a concept' (Berkenkotter/Hanganu-Bresch 2011b). The corpus of documents from Ticehurst Asylum in Sussex, England (1845–1917), which we have described in detail elsewhere (Berkenkotter/Hanganu-Bresch 2011a), offered an excellent opportunity to document this process. The considerable material resources and the wealthy clientele of the asylum allowed

> the superintendent and staff physicians to maintain contact with the individual patients, and to write up these contacts in detail, making it possible to determine – as time went by – the trajectories of the patients' illnesses over several months or years. (2011a: 226)

The case we are about to describe occurs over the time frame in which the term *manic depressive insanity* as a distinct diagnosis is gradually accepted and adopted by the psychiatric community (previous attempts at labeling it notwithstanding – see Baillarger 1854; Falret 1854). Kraepelin points out two major criteria for distinguishing between MDI and other kinds of mood disorders (involuntary melancholia): cycles and lucid intervals. Berrios (1996) adds that a longitudinal perspective is important too:

> Up to the eighteenth century, insanity (lunacy, madness, vesania) was an opaque concept which predicated of the insane a state of existence, rather than of mind. The obvious problem with this view was to explain clinical remissions. For this, the notion of' 'lucid interval' was created which accounted for 'normal' behavior without abandoning the view that the person remained mad at a deep level [...]. Madness itself was only given a temporal context during the nineteenth century, when 'time' became for the first time, a dimension of mental disorder. Adding a time dimension rendered madness into a longitudinal process. (1996: 301)

Thus, it is important to discuss the patient's history in order to understand how coding it thematically and arranging those themes chronologically might yield fruitful results.

2. A narrative history of John Horatio Baldwin's multiple confinements at Ticehurst, 1911–1925

The Baldwin case history corpus consists of nearly 70 handwritten pages, an institutional narrative spanning his multiple confinements at Ticehurst between June 1911 and his discharge into private care in November 1925. Baldwin, a 52-year-old former wine merchant and widower, was the first patient at Ticehurst Asylum in England to be diagnosed as suffering from 'maniacal depression' in 1918, although Herbert Hayes Newington, Baldwin's chief physician, had presciently identified Baldwin as being most likely a manic depressive patient in April 1913. Baldwin was admitted to Ticehurst six times over the course of fourteen years, with only very brief intermissions between each admission (see the Appendix for a list of all of Baldwin's confinements).

We devote the next several pages to presenting an overview of Baldwin's mood swings beginning with brief descriptions of his first and second confinement at Ticehurst from June 1911 to November 1912, and from February 1913 to April 1913 respectively. It is during this period that the case notes describe some of the more flamboyant maniacal elements of Baldwin's behavior and speech.

Necessary for Baldwin's confinement are two legal testimonies, or Medical Certificates, written by physicians/experts who attest to the extremely erratic behaviors and speech having occurred before at other institutions. These medical certificates describe Baldwin as "having an 'intense' manner, lying frequently, being prone to extravagant spending, and displaying poor impulse control" (George W. Potter MD, Cheapside, London). They also describe his previous 'attack of melancholia' lasting about two years (DR. Geo. H. Savage, MD, 26 Devonshire Place W.).

Other legal documents written by Ticehurst physicians shortly after the patient is confined include the Medical Statement written by Ticehurst's Medical Superintendent H.H. Newington. This document has also medico/legal status as it corroborates what the writers of the medical certificates had testified:

> Medical Statement: "He [Baldwin] is excitable, garrulous, and finds it difficult to keep to the thread of conversation. [...] He refers everything to himself and his own feelings. He says that the 'Medical Syndicate, Savage [the second Medical Certificate writer] and Co. have conspired with his son and daughter to shut him up for life. He even hopes that his son will fail in his forthcoming examination as a punishment. He is not of sound mind and judgment: with respect to Bodily Health and Condition they are both good." Dated the 30th Day of June 1911, Signed H.H. Newington.

Together these three documents argue that Baldwin is displaying the behavior and speech of someone who suffers exultation, excitement, and grandiosity characteristic of mania. All of these behaviors constitute a well-detailed description of someone who suffers from mania, but who also possesses personal idiosyncrasies that play into this disorder, such as Baldwin's obsession with the female sex.

Over the course of several months, the case notes by the Ticehurst physician, Herbert Hayes Newington, chart Baldwin's behavior and general mental and physical state, concluding in periodic 'medical statements' that "[H]e is not of sound mind & judgment" – a speech act in the medico-legal jargon, used arguably in the absence of a specific diagnosis. This phrase also demonstrates that at the time, psychiatric terminology was at the cusp between being aligned with law and being aligned with medical science.

In the case notes Baldwin's mood changes are documented in detail, as can be seen in the following entry:

> 30 April, 1912: He complains of sleeping badly on account of thinking about Miss Stevenson who he asserts he loves more than anybody in the world. He asked me why he could not be discharged and I told him it was because he was not yet the normal Baldwin, as shown by his proposed ridiculous speculations, the instability of his kaleidoscopic ideas, and the impression he gave others that he was at times 'inebriated with his own verbosity'. He denied nothing but said that he was now fit for discharge and he ought to be allowed to do as he liked just as a thief who had served his time could return to his thieving ways until caught again.

A second example of Baldwin's manic behaviors can be seen in the case note dated 30 May 1912:

> In spite of having an allowance & promising not to exceed, he runs up little bills while on parole & has pawned his watch. Though he had written his daughter to tell her that he had pawned his watch to help an exhausted female home in a carriage, and though his attendant had seen a few days ago the actual pawn ticket, he solemnly assured me this morning when I told him that I know that he had pawned it, that he had sold it to an attendant here who had left a long time ago, and that it was in America now. Such evasions show a remarkable weakening of intellect and common sense. Signed, H.H.N. [Herbert Hayes Newington]

Not only do the case notes depict specific examples of manic behaviors, but the reader also finds Baldwin's own correspondence with family members attesting to his unstable state of mind. One such example appears in the case notes in a "copy of card addressed to Miss Baldwin, May 12 1912." This card is an example of 'reported speech' or the direct representation of the patient's own words.

> Am writing Dr. Alexander Mitchell to tell him the result of my proposal to you. Dr. S. Newington [Samuel Newington] would have been quite agreeable. After all, I am asking for rights (and not favours) and your brother solely that he can pass his examination in June is depriving me of them. You speak not truly when you say you can't help me. You mean you won't, & I swear to the Almighty I – you & Disown you although my bounty – keep you from the streets and becoming a harlot [...] If I marry again the inhuman conduct of yourself & brother towards me will be the sole cause.

Placed as it is among the case notes, such examples of reported speech reinforce the examples in the case notes of Baldwin's disturbed ideation during a manic phase. Elsewhere the reader finds documentation of Baldwin's depressive episodes. For example,

> 8 March, 1913: He has had no narcotic for several nights: he continues to be depressed & anticipates all sorts of calamities, e.g., that his son will break down and be certified & sent to Virginia Water [Asylum].

As Baldwin moved in and out of the asylum, the circular nature of his symptoms did not escape the trained eyes of the senior psychiatrist, Dr. Hayes Newington, who, in April 1913, wrote a lengthy note regarding the diagnosis of this case, which he deemed as being 'particularly interesting'. Newington described in detail Baldwin's melancholic moods followed by 'well' stages and then 'maniacal' behaviors (of particular concern to him and Baldwin's son, actually, were Baldwin Senior's tendency to self harm, such as eating glass, as well as his preoccupation with the fair sex and his masturbatory habits).

Thus, the doctor wonders,

> As these symptoms became more marked the question of diagnosis came to be premier – was it melancholia or simply depression as a forerunner of excitement in manic-depressive insanity?

While Baldwin's son, citing his father's 'disturbing' behaviors, wants him again 'certified', Hayes Newington seems resistant to the idea, writing:

> I have regarded and now still regard certification in this case as a great evil. It would destroy the patient's hope of better things, and the change from his easy and liberal treatment to that which he knows would be entailed of certification would probably result in an acute break-down. This would be in any case a disaster, but still more disastrous if it thereby defeated the hope, which I have, that rest and careful medical treatment will tend to break up the tendency, that undoubtedly exists, to confirmed manic-depressive insanity. (154–175)

Newington is hesitant to apply the new and 'interesting' medical diagnosis, possibly because of its long-term implications: MDI is a longitudinal disease with a bleak outcome, and he is still hoping they were just witnessing curable episodes rather than a lifetime illness. Still, it is the first time that a Kraeplinian register is encroaching on the old, vague, all-encompassing label 'of unsound mind'. This first attempt to organize symptoms into a diagnosis is not, however, formalized in either the medical statements or in the medical certificates until five years later. This may be due to a possible resistance by Newington to Kraeplinian nomenclature. In 1909, he had in fact participated in a Medico-Psychological Association meeting during which he argued against adopting another Kraeplinian category, 'dementia praecox'. While we cannot extend Hays Newington's perspective on dementia praecox to manic-depressive insanity, we can speculate that a resistance to Kraepelin's wide-ranging disease groups could explain his delay in identifying Baldwin's condition as manic-depressive insanity for two years after his entry to Ticehurst, as well as his hesitation to ascribe the new diagnosis formally.

Meanwhile Baldwin is hospitalized again from 1916 through 1918, escapes on July 12, 1918, then is readmitted a few days later on July 18th the same year. This is when, in the wake of Newington's death in 1917, Newington's successor, Colin McDowall, rather matter-of-factly states in the 'Medical Statement' that "He is suffering from maniacal depressive insanity." While at the moment of his admission Baldwin is described as being manic (making rash decision, such as marrying a housemaid in the month during which he was out of the asylum), he is soon described as 'depressed'. In fact, McDowall convincingly notes now that "The depressed phase has begun" (July 25th). The same diagnosis is repeated in the August 19th Medical Statement:

> He is suffering from maniacal depressive insanity. At one time he is noisy, excitable and inclined to be abusive. After this period has passed he becomes depressed, morose and despondent. At present Mr. Baldwin is despondent and looks upon the dark side of everything. He is agitated at times and worried regarding his future.

A similar statement is made nearly one year later, in June 1919:

> June 26 Special Report. He is suffering from maniacal depressive insanity. He is quite unreliable. Says one thing today, tomorrow another. He has periods of depression and periods of escalation. He is just recovering from the depressive stage of his malady.

These two descriptions of Baldwin's illness now follow an easily recognizable pattern that neatly captures the cyclical nature of mania/ depression, a pattern that had been difficult to discern seven years prior, with his first hospitalization. These descriptions are strikingly different from Hayes Newington's first Medical Certificate (reproduced above), which carefully avoided any diagnosis other than the standardized and vague medico-legal jargon 'not of sound mind and judgment', a catchall diagnosis justified by the accumulation of specific behavioral descriptions that obscure rather than reveal a pattern; that Certificate was essentially an accretion of observational details meant to buttress the hollow nature of the diagnosis. By contrast, McDowall's clinical descriptions are entirely devoted to revealing the pattern of the disease, which seems to satisfyingly mirror its textbook description. In fact, we know that McDowall was intimately familiar with the clinical description of the disease from his review of a French monograph devoted to this topic, which he had published in the *British Journal of Psychiatry* in 1908 (McDowall 1908). Thus we would argue that by 1918 the term 'manic-depressive' insanity had become a term of art ensconced – or rather, *enregistered* in the vocabulary of practicing psychiatrists, and as such, the patterns that used to be obscured by a thick layer of pathological description emerge once the stencil of the Kraeplinian categories is applied.

Similar descriptions appear sporadically throughout Baldwin's final seven-year hospitalization at Ticehurst. Baldwin is eventually discharged to the care of a Mrs. Wells of Heathfield Hotel in November 1925 and leaves Ticehurst for the last time.

3. Discourse analysis of Baldwin's case notes

We transcribed the entirety of Baldwin's Ticehurst case notes and decided to code them based on inductively built categories; in particular, we discussed code categories and conducted extensive norming sessions in order to smooth disagreements. In the end we created a coding scheme for several categories, out of which we have decided to focus on the most important for our purposes of tracking Manic-Depressive Insanity. These categories include symptoms of mania, depression, and lucidity. All categories were coded by T-Unit – a complete independent clause with all of the dependent clauses or phrases attached.

3.1 Symptoms of mania

This category identifies any T-unit describing a symptom of mania. No distinction was made between general descriptions of mania symptoms (e.g. "he is very talkative") and more specific behavior descriptions indicating mania (e.g. "he abusively spoke to his attendant this morning"). Note that grandiosity is a common symptom of mania in this patient. This category includes mischief and inappropriate behavior, such as Baldwin's extravagant dress and amorous tendencies.

(1) He is undergoing an attack of active recurrent mania. He is excited, very coarse and abusive. He never ceases talking. (Medical Statement, February 21st, 1916)

3.2 Symptoms of depression

This coding category includes neurotic worry, such as Baldwin's back-and-forth fears regarding leaving Ticehurst as well as his anticipating legal and financial trouble.

(2) Was in a very depressed condition, said he felt to be so but could give no reason for it. (Medical certificate #1, 30 May, 1913)

This category also includes suicidal thought and/or reported speech/behavior.

(3) He states that two days ago he swallowed a large quantity of broken glass. He says he felt impelled to swallow it and could not help himself. (Medical certificate #2, 30 May, 1913)

3.3 Improvement, or possible lucid interval

This category applies to case notes that describe improved or lucid behavior. No distinction was made between direct statements of improvement ("He is improved") and descriptions of behaviors that provided evidence of improvement ("This patient is quieting down").

4. Results

The results of our coding (Tables 2 and 3, below) reflect the alternating pattern of symptom reporting in the case notes – for example, where few depression symptoms are reported, or manic symptoms are frequently reported, and vice-versa. There is also a tendency to over-report manic symptoms by comparison with depression or improvement symptoms – an understandable tendency if we consider that each hospitalization is usually the result of a manic episode during which the patient is in crisis and psychiatric staff must manage varied manifestations of mania. We are showing these data in both 1- and 2-year increments: the 1-year breakdown of data provides a 'natural' division while the 2-year breakdown of data reveals a more pronounced clustering of symptoms on either side of depression or mania.

	Depression	*Mania*	*Improvement*
1911	0	42	11
1912	0	32	10
1913	24	0	32
1914	10	0	12
1915	3	0	7
1916	0	50	14
1917	0	10	2
1918	23	1	1
1919	23	0	0
1920	17	0	6
1921	4	0	5
1922	1	23	7
1923	1	2	2
1924	3	46	6
1925	0	22	1
Totals	109	228	116

Table 2. Frequency of depression, mania, and improvement symptoms as recorded in Baldwin's case notes in 1-year increments, 1911–1925.

	Depression	*Mania*	*Improvement*
1911–1912	0	74	21
1913–1914	34	0	44
1915–1916	3	50	21
1917–1918	23	11	3
1919–1920	40	0	6
1921–1922	5	23	12
1923–1924	4	48	8
1925	0	22	1
Totals	109	228	116

Table 3. Frequency of depression, mania, and improvement symptoms as recorded in Baldwin's case notes in 2-year increments, 1911–1925.

To get a better sense of the symptom reporting patterns, we have created charts for each of Baldwin's hospitalizations, which we compiled into a single chart to better show the longitudinal aspect of his disease. Below are graphs documenting the frequency of our three main categories in Baldwin's coded case notes across 1- and 2-year increments.

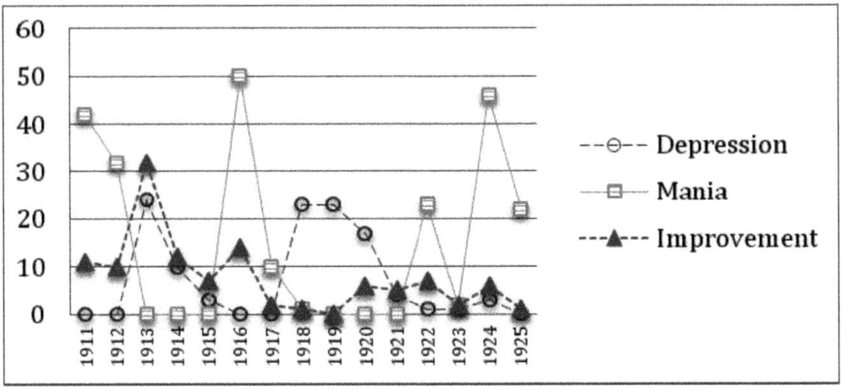

Figure 1. Coded Symptom Frequency (1-year Increments).

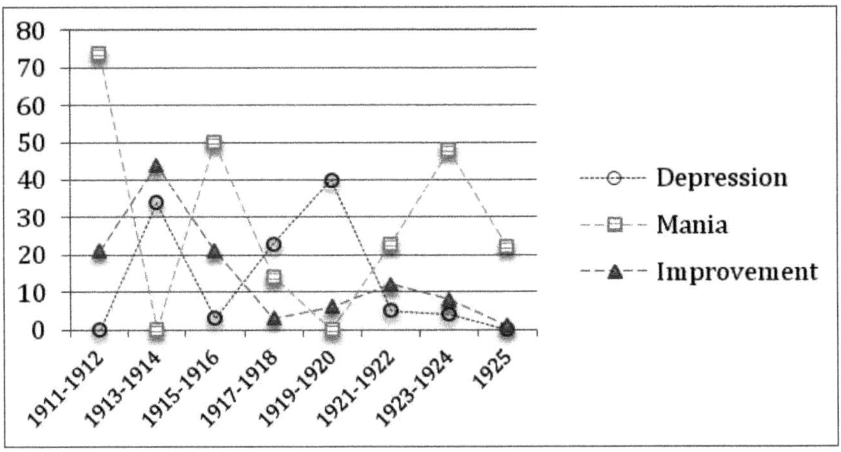

Figure 2. Coded Symptom Frequency (2-year Increments).

Note that these two graphs represent the frequency of case notes documenting the manic, depressive, and lucid interval symptoms rather than the intensity of the symptoms of the day-to-day order or number of symptoms. This distinction is important because the two graphs confirm that to the physician-writers at Ticehurst the ebb and flow of mania and depression can be visually organized in a predictable, recognizable manner for someone who understands and accepts the concept of manic depression.

5. Discussion

The charts in Figures 1 and 2 validate the eventual diagnosis and echo earlier visual representations of the disease that are attempted in the psychiatric literature (e.g. Paton 1905). Nevertheless, two patterns can be seen to be salient in this visual representation:

1. The apparent disproportionate reporting of manic episodes versus depressive or lucid intervals, especially during the first hospitalization. This asymmetry can possibly be explained by the certificating physician's need to foreground the more sensational, visible aspects of manic behavior necessary for certification. As the case progresses and the diagnosis becomes more clear, the manic and depressive symptoms seem to be more balanced – or at least more routine except toward the end of Baldwin's final hospitalization (which most likely occurred at the end of a manic cycle). We may also speculate that what we have been calling the enregisterment of 'manic depression' in psychiatric vocabulary has a 'normalizing' effect on the way psychiatric symptoms are reported in the case notes, by which we mean that they offer a lens (a 'terministic screen' in Burkean rhetorical parlance) that speeds the process of pattern recognition in interpreting widely divergent behaviors. Thus what was once a 'highly interesting case' for Newington in 1913 becomes relatively routine for MacDowell in the 1920s. Consequently, the volume of the observational notes decreases sharply during the last seven-year hospitalization, in contrast with the rich details accumulated during the first few hospitalizations.

2. The case notes reporting improvement or 'lucid intervals' decrease considerably after 1918, the year Colin MacDowell first officially diagnoses Baldwin. In fact, they are highest in 1913, the year Hayes Newington, the older physician who dies in 1917, has the prescient insight into Baldwin's condition. Hayes Newington had also been opposed to 'certifying' Baldwin as 'unsound' at the time, despite his considering him a good candidate for the diagnosis of manic-depressive insanity, arguing that this certification would hinder the patient's recovery. We may in fact look at this as a stage in the uptake process where the gravity of manic-depressive insanity may be a concept still in flux, and recovery is still thought possible. The other possibility, of course, is that as patients became chronic, the number of lucid intervals diminished. Conversely, McDowall, operating under a new nomenclature that officially includes MDI as a diagnosis of insanity, may be less inclined to report on 'lucid intervals', except on rare occasions. In fact, the sporadic nature of entries in Baldwin's case history between 1918 and 1925 (by comparison with his previous five hospitalizations) suggests that Baldwin has become a chronic long-term – incurable – patient, like those Trevor Turner (1989) calls 'hardy perennials'.

6. Conclusion

We could tentatively interpret these results as a visual representation of the 'subjectivity' of the medical/psychiatric gaze that can only see what the available linguistic and conceptual framework allows it to see. To the doctors attending to Baldwin's case, the circularity or the longitudinal evolution of the disease becomes visible when a relevant category comes along to help them interpret it. The concept of 'maniacal-depressive insanity' is thus used to definitively tame a tangled array of symptoms encompassing over time the totality of the patient's experience.

The narrative and extensive nature of the case notes allows for the flashes of insight into Baldwin's case, such as Newington's realizations; this is possible because the concept of MDI is in the zeitgeist, so to speak, and it is ready for its uptake from hypothetical nosology to practical experience. The analysis of this case is, we believe, the first time researchers using archival data (case notes/histories) have been able to track the detailed documentation of a patient's manic-depressive symptoms over time, thus providing a snapshot of the enregisterment process that resettled psychiatry's foundations in the early 20th century. Indeed, Baldwin's case reflects the transition from a medico-legal register to a Kraeplinian register.

References

Agha, Asif 2003. The Social Life of Cultural Value. *Language & Communication* 23, 231–273.

Austin, John L. 1962. *How to Do Things with Words*. Cambridge, MA: Harvard University Press.

Baillarger, Jules 1854. Notes Sour un Genre de Folie Dont les Accés Sont Caractérisé par Deux Periods Régulaires, l'Une de Depréssion, l'Autre d'Excitation. *Bulletin de l'Académie de Médicine* 19, 340–352.

Berkenkotter, Carol / Hanganu-Bresch, Cristina 2011a. Occult Genres and the Certification of Madness in a Nineteenth Century Lunatic Asylum. *Written Communication* 28/2, 220–250.

Berkenkotter, Carol / Hanganu-Bresch, Cristina 2011b. Symptoms in Search of a Concept. Paper presented at Madness and Identity Conference, Oxford, September 2011.

Berrios, German E. 1996. *The History of Mental Symptoms: Descriptive Psychopathology since the Nineteenth Century.* Cambridge: Cambridge University Press.

Falret, Jean-Pierre 1854. Mémoire sur la Folie Circulaire. *Bulletin de Académie de Médicine* 19, 382–415.

Freadman, Anne 2002. Uptake. In Richard Coe / Lorelei Lingard / Tatiana Teslenko (eds) *The Rhetoric and Ideology of Genre: Strategies for Stability and Change*, Creskill, NJ: Hampton Press, 39–53.

McDowall, Colin 1908. *The Intermittent Psychoses [Les Folies Intermittentes], Maniacal Depressive Insanity. (La Psychose Maniaque Depressive)*. By Drs. Denny, Physician to the Hospital of Salpetriere, and P. Camus, House-Physician of the hospitals of Paris. *British Journal of Psychiatry* 54, 585–586.
Paton, Stewart 1905. *Psychiatry: A Text-Book for Students and Physicians*. Philadelphia: J. B. Lippincot Company.
Sargant William W. 1967. *The Unquiet Mind: The Autobiography of a Physician in Psychological Medicine*. London: Heinemann.
Turner, Trevor 1989. Rich and Mad in Victorian England. *Psychological Medicine* 19, 29–44.
Wilce, James M. 2008. Scientizing Bangladeshi Psychiatry: Parallelism, Enregisterment, and the Cure for a Magic Complex. *Language in Society* 37, 91–114.
Wilce, James M. 2009. Medical Discourse. *Annual Review of Anthropology* 38, 199–215.

Appendix

List of Baldwin's hospitalizations at Ticehurst

Hospitalization 1: June 24, 1911 – Nov. 20, 1912
Hospitalization 2: Feb. 15, 1913 – Apr. 10, 1913
Hospitalization 3: Apr. 14, 1913 – June 1, 1913 (as voluntary boarder)
Hospitalization 4: Jun. 1, 1913 – Jan. 21, 1916 (change in status to 'certified patient')
Hospitalization 5: Feb. 16, 1916 – Jul. 12, 1918
Hospitalization 6: Jul. 18, 1918 – Nov. 9, 1925

Syelle Graves / Rebecca Burson / Victor Torres-Collazo

Dialectal Variation and Miscommunication in Medical Discourse: A Case Study

1. Introduction

This study explores the case of a minority English-speaking patient who was misdiagnosed with mental illness, leaving her actual neurological illness, Stiff Person Syndrome (SPS), unobserved for over ten years. We hypothesize: 1) that this patient's minority-affiliated speech variant, African American Vernacular English (AAVE), contributed to her being misdiagnosed – by multiple doctors – for a decade, 2) that dialect discord in general can both influence how a physician conceptualizes the symptoms of a patient, and exacerbate the ambiguity that can occur when describing symptoms, and 3) that medical school training may emphasize limited lexical cues that often vary from actual patient descriptions. We explore an interface of linguistic variation and unconscious bias against unfairly stigmatized language variants, as a cause of misdiagnosis, such that, for example, written records of patient descriptions, which are not phonetic, may even reduce some of the communication barrier. Extant research on doctor-patient communication primarily focuses on successfully conveying information to the patient, making this chapter a step toward filling a gap in the literature on doctors misunderstanding patient descriptions of symptoms, and, on doctor-patient dialect discord.

This study includes: a working definition of language variation and sociolects in §2; a review of the literature on dialect discord and stigmatization in §3; the medical details of the case study, a discussion of some medical training words associated with SPS, and a retrospective medical chart review with doctor reports of the patient's descriptions throughout the period of misdiagnosis, in §4; and finally, an analysis of the patient's linguistic patterns and AAVE features (phonological, morpho-syntactic, lexical, and stylistic) in §5. This speech analysis was done on a transcription of a video interview of the patient, conducted after she was diagnosed correctly; the transcription can be read in full in the Appendix.

2. 'Nonstandard' English varieties and related misconceptions

First, in order to better understand the patient case, it is important to describe the inaccurate understanding, by non-linguists, that 'nonstandard dialects' (language varieties) are 'inferior'. All natural human languages, if spoken by an observable population, are by definition systems of mutually intelligible communication, subdivided into variants that differ stylistically, syntactically, lexically, and – in particular – phonologically. However, historically, non-linguists have overwhelmingly believed many of these varieties to be inferior, simplified, or degraded, even though linguistic analysis in fact indicates that all native speakers of all languages speak rule-governed dialects, and that any negative or positive judgments of said dialects are in fact attributed unknowingly to the groups of people who speak them, and not based on linguistic or scientific factors. While some dialects are regional, others (so-called 'sociolects') are distinguished by the socio-economic status and/or racial/ethnic identity of their speakers.

Of the unfairly stigmatized language varieties of American English, one of the most widely known and studied is one spoken primarily by a large and diverse group of African Americans, usually referred to as 'African American Vernacular English' (AAVE). AAVE is identified by a number of rule-governed features that vary systematically when contrasted with the idealization 'Standard American English' (SAE) or with other varieties of English. These include phonological features such as deletion of final velar stops in gerunds and progressive verbs (e.g., *walkin'*) and metathesis of syllable-final consonant clusters (e.g., *aks* vs. SAE *ask*); morpho-syntactic patterns such as generalization of the third-person singular verb forms to other subject forms (e.g., *They is crazy*) and reduplication of the past tense suffix (e.g., *likeded*) (Rickford 1999).

According to Rickford (1999) and Sclafani (2008), perceptions of stigmatized dialects have changed very little despite extensive representation in linguistic research and literature. They both observe that these perceptions have historically included adjectives such as 'lazy', 'slang', and even 'corrupt'. An additional important point is the common misperception that speakers of nonstandard varieties have a decreased ability to express (or indeed, even to have) abstract thought. Lanehart (1998: 126–127), in her discussion of AAVE's lack of prestige, and its perception as a "bastardized form of English that is spoken because the speakers do not know any better", cites (and rejects) Orr's (1987) report that AAVE is less capable of abstract thought, and that its speakers have a built-in barrier to learning math and science.[1] Cross, DeVaney and Jones (2001) cite Baugh (1999) as observing that "while linguistic prejudice represents an unfortunate form of sociolinguistic pathology, it takes on a particularly destructive form among [...] educators who conclude that students who do not speak mainstream American English have cognitive deficiencies or that they lack the capacity for abstract thought" (2001: 214–215). It is critical to understand that any native speaker of any human language can express any abstract thought, but may do so in a manner unfamiliar to a standard-dialect-speaking interlocutor. The potential for unconscious bias against minority English speakers, and the necessity of understanding the abstract descriptions of emotional and mental symptoms which cannot be tested in a laboratory, may be useful in understanding the reasons behind the misdiagnosis of the patient in this case study in particular.

There is extensive work exploring and justifying the claim that natural human language cannot be inherently illogical (see Labov 1969;

---

1 This is not to say that bidialectalism should not be encouraged in schools; everyone must learn a formal language version in order to read and write successfully in school. Because formal writing does not resemble any speech variety perfectly, even the most 'standardized' speakers cannot write in the informal way that they speak. However, negative judgments regarding the critical-thinking skills of nonstandard dialect-speaking individuals are unfounded, and indeed unsupported by research.

Pinker 1994), in response to people who consciously and overtly criticize certain dialects, or erroneously believe that some language variations are inferior. The case study in this analysis, however, considers the possibility of unconscious/unobserved miscommunication, and possible lack of full mutual intelligibility across dialects that are generally considered to be mutually intelligible. However, it also considers the possibility that some practitioners may unconsciously assume an inability to express abstract thought when they encounter speakers of non-standard varieties. This is something that may stem both from lack of knowledge of linguistics, and from the unconscious bias against speakers of dialects lacking in prestige. In addition, the fact that all speech varieties are just as capable of expressing abstract thought is crucial to an analysis of patients describing abstract and unobservable ('reported') symptoms.

3. Dialects and communication in medical discourse

Most research on the general concept of miscommunication due to dialectal variety and stigmatization focuses largely on the classroom, and on educational implications. For instance, Meier (1999) observes that "teachers' lack of knowledge about [AAVE] features can result in misunderstandings that interfere with effective literacy instruction that cause a child's abilities to be underestimated or assessed properly" (as quoted in Cross/DeVaney/Jones 2001: 214).

Research on the general concept of doctor-patient communication, another closely related area, reveals a plethora of work on doctors effectively communicating *to* their patients. For example, Hasty *et al.* (2012: 44) discuss doctor use of double-modals – which "is a regional feature […] not generally considered to belong to the standard variety of U.S. English" – to soften their medical instructions. In addition, Ferguson and Candib suggest that non-minority doctors "need to be more effective in […] their communication […] with minority patients" (2002: 353). (See also Maynard/Heritage 2005 on patient perception of doctor instructions, and Castro *et al.* 2007 on doctor use of medical jargon when addressing patients).

Though fewer, there are some studies indicating that bias can adversely affect both the diagnosis of and the communication with minority patients. Bell and Mehta (1980), for example, report that black Americans were diagnosed with schizophrenia at a significantly higher rate than white Americans, despite no epidemiologic or genetic evidence that they show a greater predisposition for any type of mental illness. More relevant here, while the authors consider the primary reason for this to be unconscious bias due to race, they also acknowledge the role that linguistic factors may play:

> The language barrier between the patient and physician (many of whom are foreign medical graduates and are unfamiliar with cultural aspects of black patients' language and behavior) makes for further difficulties leading to misinterpretation, and thus misdiagnosis. (Bell/Mehta 1980: 144)

This observation is two-fold: While non-native English speaking doctors understandably may have communication barriers with native-English-speaking patients, there is an added layer of difficulty when such doctors have not been exposed to, and therefore lack familiarity with, the 'nonstandard' English of so many minority patients.

In addition, Schouten and Meeuwesen (2006: 31) come close when they observe findings in a literature review that English-speaking Hispanic patients report being less satisfied with care received from white doctors than white patients do. However, no analysis of the variety of English spoken was conducted (many Hispanic Americans speak a different and also stigmatized English variety), leaving this concept of dialect discord in medical discourse unexplored.

Our finding that the narrow topic of dialect discord in medical discourse is something of a gap in the literature is substantiated by Bennink (2014), who has researched lexical variants in Spanish dialects in medical diagnostics in the United States, and resulting misunderstandings. She reports a variety of communicative difficulties and medical mishaps, and also concurs that although "several studies have been undertaken to comprehend the effect of the language barrier on access to and quality of care […] *this research generally excludes analyzing the effect of* [...] *dialect variants on doctor-patient communication*" (emphasis added). Miscommunication when treating a patient through an interpreter is an expected risk, while miscommunication when faced with dialect discord within the same language is traditionally overlooked.

Yet, while such literature is scant, there is some, in addition to Bennink's (2014) findings. For example, early work by Shuy (1984) reports communication barriers in cross-cultural medical interviews, particularly between black, inner-city, AAVE-speaking patients and their doctors. He observed doctors not making an effort to learn and understand the vocabulary and general linguistic perspective of the 'Vernacular English' speakers, instead relying on the patients to adapt to the doctors' linguistic style. More recent work on dialect discord in medicine includes Balsa and McGuire (2003: 97), who observe that "overt and subtle forms of miscommunication and misunderstanding can lead to misdiagnosis. [...] In mental health care, for example, many studies show that symptom presentation varies across racial and ethnic groups *and can differ from what most clinicians are trained to expect*" (emphasis added). This concept will be addressed in more detail in Table 1 in §4, a discussion of medical school doctor-training 'buzz words', or specific lexical items and phrases, and how these can differ from real patient symptom descriptions.

A final case of research that names dialect discord as a cause of miscommunication in medical discourse is Ashton *et al.* (2003), as follows:

> The race and ethnicity of doctor and patient can affect their ability to communicate and negotiate to a shared model in several ways. *The most obvious is language or dialect discordance.* Even when the interactants speak the same language, they may use and interpret terms, idioms, and metaphors differently. (Ashton *et al.* 2003: 148, emphasis added)

These authors also report a disparity in usage of health services by minority Americans, even when access is not restricted. The authors consider racial bias as one possible cause, along with 'poor communication', which, like we do, they find to be largely unexplored in the literature. Ashton *et al.* acknowledge that there is difficulty in 'proving' bias as a factor, because most doctors intend to treat patients without any (see Teal *et al.* 2012 for more on the unconscious nature of human bias, particularly in medical care). They do also report findings that perceived socio-economic status affected doctors' response to patients and their self-described symptoms. Since these bias-based discrepancies, however, were slight, they conclude that a "communication hypothesis," with some level of unconscious bias, better accounts for the disparity in minority care than bias alone (2003: 146). It seems logical to conclude that the communication barrier partly triggers the bias, in that differences in regional and social language styles (communication) contribute to perceptions of the patient on the part of the doctor (bias).

Ashton *et al.*'s paper illustrates another key point: When the authors, all of whom are doctors and not linguists, refer to 'communicative predispositions' as being linked to commonly known demographic variants such as age and socio-economic status, they include something they call 'linguistic skill' on this list of predispositions. This term calls attention to the tendency in the non-linguist professional community to conflate a lack of education and resources (and therefore, perhaps, a lack of advanced vocabulary) with something akin to 'under-developed language'. As outlined in §2, dialects of a single language pattern themselves differently from each other, leading to some reduction in intelligibility when faced with a speaker of another dialect, but show no scientific evidence of 'underdevelopment' as a linguistic system, nor of lacking in any universal language features. Therefore, barring conditions such as SLI (Specific Language Impairment) or other cognitive deficits, there is no valid reason to hypothesize that minority members speak with any lack of 'skill' or clarity when communicating with other native speakers of that same dialect. Children absorb the language they are exposed to with perfect efficiency, regardless of socio-economic factors, race, and even intelligence, within a normal range.[2] There is, however – clearly – potential for professionals to perceive dialectal differences as reflecting an overall 'lack of linguistic skill' rather than simply a systematically different form of expression.

2 See Pinker (1994) for a detailed description of how SLI is independent of intelligence. Also see cases of the opposite condition/situation: linguistic 'savants' with non-functioning IQs, such as Christopher, as documented by Smith/Tsimpli (1995).

Finally, related to this is the importance of disentangling language from education. It has been established that non-linguists are usually unaware of the fact that, although literacy level does impact spoken language, it does not do so significantly, or at least not in the ways many imagine. So, since minority members are associated with a lower level of socio-economic status – especially when they speak a language variety associated as such – doctors (who often come from a higher socio-economic background with a more standardized language variety) may be inclined to assume a deficit in something similar to what Ashton *et al.* (2003) describe as 'linguistic skill'. There is technically no logical problem with suggesting that people with a college education have more developed analytical skills, a somewhat larger vocabulary, and other professional advantages, when compared to people who do not finish high school. However, written and spoken language are independent of each other, so even an elementary school-educated patient can describe abstract symptoms, and is not lacking in any 'linguistic skill' – only in literacy skills. In addition, successful patient expression of symptoms need not require vocabulary learned only by high levels of education, so while the educational level of the patient may play a small role, it seems that dialectal variation likely plays a larger one.

4. Discussion of a case study

4.1 Medical background

The case-study patient is an African American woman in her mid-forties from Miami, Florida, and an accomplished military professional. For over a decade, she remained misdiagnosed with anxiety when she was in fact suffering from Stiff Person Syndrome (SPS), a rare and progressive neurological disorder of the central nervous system. Although Rose was seen by many physicians (including neurologists), given a complete neurological exam and an MRI, her symptom descriptions did not lead any doctor to give her serologic (blood) testing during the period of misdiagnosis, which would have shown (and later did show) high antibody titers to glutamic acid decarboxylase: evidence of SPS. She was finally diagnosed by author Dr. Burson, who subsequently, along with author Dr. Torres-Collazo, took an interest in her case to try to understand how Rose went misdiagnosed for so long despite engagement with quality medical care. They observed a linguistic nuance in her symptom descriptions, in that although they seemed well-described, they were systematically different enough from doctor expectations that all of her earlier doctors had been unable to identify them. They subsequently videotaped an interview with her, a condensed transcript of which can be found in the Appendix, from which we conducted our linguistic analysis.

Identifying symptoms of SPS include muscle stiffness, rigidity, and spasms – very physical symptoms which differ clearly from psychiatric ones – and it is more common in women than men, but not more common in any race. According to Ciccotto, Blaya and Kelley (2013), the physiologic etiology (reason triggering the symptom set) of SPS is tied to excess glutamate, an amino acid, in the brain, secondary to a deficiency in GABA (gamma-aminobutyric acid), another brain chemical; this imbalance is also shared in many psychiatric disorders, leading to some of the emotional symptoms Rose experienced along with the physical ones. Since she was misdiagnosed with anxiety for so many years, the importance of properly interpreting a patient's description of abstract symptoms like fear and anxiety, which cannot be measured in a laboratory, cannot be overstated.

While establishing a connection between Rose's linguistic patterns and her misdiagnosis may not be completely clear-cut, and we wish to make it clear that we cannot claim definite causality, the possibility that her speech variant contributed to her misdiagnosis warrants consideration, and certainly cannot be ruled out. It is also important to establish the fact that it is not our intention to 'accuse' Rose's initial doctors as negligent or incompetent, or even biased, because attitudes toward language variants are largely both unconscious (as mentioned in §3) and wildly misinformed among members of nearly every profession, and are indeed sometimes observed in speakers of the stigmatized varieties themselves. Interpreting linguistic nuance can be challenging even without dialect discord, and yet it is critical in arriving at a correct diagnosis, especially for illnesses with neuropsychiatric manifestations, like SPS, which can affectively resemble various mental health diagnoses.

Next, it is useful to consider the current diagnostic criteria for SPS in more detail: they include a prodrome (precursor) of episodic stiffness of the axial (trunk) muscles; progression to include stiffness of the proximal (upper limb) muscles; increased lumbar lordosis (lower back curve); response to benzodiazepine; abdominal rigidity; back stiffness; falling episodes; a 'tin solder' walk; painful spasms elicited by triggers (e.g., stress, touch, sudden noise); all with normal sensation, motor function, and intellect.

Some readers familiar with SPS may object that the ten-year timeline for Rose's correct diagnosis is typical of the illness, undermining our premise. While it is true that SPS often takes years to diagnose because it is progressive, meaning that the beginning stages are insidious and often nebulous, we address this as follows: first, it can be acknowledged from Rose's initial presentation of falling that the ten years for which she was misdiagnosed actually started when her symptoms were both fulminant and pathognomonic of SPS. Second, as we have mentioned, Rose was describing SPS in a manner typical of its clinical presentation, leaving the fact that her English belongs to a stigmatized and 'different' variety glaringly relevant as a factor. Finally, we point out that her situation of being in active military duty meant that she had extensive and unlimited access to medical care, including specialists, unlike many members of the undiagnosed population. She had no financial barriers, limits in opportunity to seek treatment, or hesitation to do so, and she also saw multiple neurologists, who by definition should be on alert to catch symptoms typical of a neurological disorder.

4.2 Medical school terminology

In Table 1 below, showing medical terminology and how it compares to quotes from the transcript of Rose's post-diagnosis video interview, we express two key concepts: 1) that Rose does spontaneously describe many of these symptoms of SPS very closely but in her own manner, supporting our hypothesis that her language style played an indirect but definite role in the SPS not being caught, and 2) that one possible contributing factor to this (and other misdiagnoses) is the way medical school trains doctors to limit their diagnostics to a small set of lexical entries and formulaic expressions. We know that lexical choice varies widely from one dialect to another, and even between speech registers or written genres. In medical school materials, students are presented with a limited set of 'buzz-words' with which they are trained to diagnose diseases, even though patients from different linguistic backgrounds may not have those exact terms at their disposal, leading to a delay in recognizing symptom descriptions. This idea with regard to SPS symptoms is outlined in Table 1 below.

	Textbook Diagnostic 'Buzz-Words' for SPS	*Patient's Description*	*Transcript Lines*
1	'Tree trunk' fall (i.e., "Do you fall down like a tree trunk, unable to extend your arms to minimize injury?")	"I'm having problems with [pause] walking. I'm having problems with [pause] falling."	38–39
2	'Tin soldier' posture (i.e., "Do you find yourself standing or walking like a tin soldier?")	"I started walking like a robot. You know, it's like, your left is with your right, but- I was just swingin' my arms- and walkin' like a robot."	12–14
3	'Back stiffness' 'Insidious muscular rigidity'	"…every joint is- stiff."	50
4	"Do the spasms start or get worse when you are doing an activity under pressure such as crossing a busy street?"	"I quit crossing streets, because people watch you when you cross the street."	62–63

Table 1. SPS Symptom 'Buzz Words'.

Rose's use of 'robot' (section 2 in Table 1) to describe her walk is so close to the 'tin soldier' that a doctor may be trained to look for that it is possible that such a similar description was missed by her doctors due to other unconscious factors in the way they perceived her language. In section 4 from Table 1, she mentions crossing the street, just like the 'buzz-words' suggest, but in a different context (avoiding it, instead of reporting that it made the spasms get worse). The fact that her symptom accounts, in an abstract way, are so close to the textbook descriptions heightens the possibility that her original doctors missed the nuances of her descriptions, and the possibility that they were limiting themselves to a finite set of lexical items. The fact that these descriptions were recorded after she had read and learned about the illness is also important, because even having learned about the diagnostic criteria, her narrative style, linguistic patterns, and lexical items are totally different (from the medical terminology) in form, but identical in content.

4.3 Retrospective chart review

Reviewing excerpts from Rose's medical chart, which consists of what her doctors wrote down about what she said to them (provided in Table 2 below) offers several types of supporting information. First, the table includes demographic information about the misdiagnosing physicians, because ethnic and class background are a factor in any sort of bias-related misunderstandings; next, the chart shows that the terminology that Rose used *before* learning about SPS was consistent with the illness, yet still not picked up by all of these physicians; finally, the chart shows how her examining physicians perceived her words, in that they indicated repeated doubt of her experience, and allows us to consider how ambiguity and written language can impact medical diagnosis.

	Date	*Doctor*	*Original Notes on Patient Descriptions*
1	Jun. 5 2006	Hispanic male psychiatrist	• The patient reports significant anxiety regarding being in front of crowds to get an award. She 'freezes' and gets self-conscious
2	Oct. 26 2006	Asian male psychiatrist	• The patient states that when she feels anxious her body stiffens, and then she has a falling episode

	Date	*Doctor*	*Original Notes on Patient Descriptions*
3	Mar. 29 2007	American female of Hawaiian descent neurologist	• Reports significant occupational impairment while on duty in Iraq and currently • Reports using a plastic carton to urinate into to avoid leaving room to go to bathroom, constant falling (reports 30+ falls), needing to hold onto a wall when walking into open spaces, reported inability to cross bridges […] attempted to drive over a bridge, was unable to proceed, and had to be police escorted off bridge (Korea 2001) […] she was told to read a book [about anxiety]; did not feel treatment options adequate for her level of impairment
4	Apr. 2 2007	Female nurse practitioner	• Reports she has experienced one fall since last visit; states she […] became tense and fell. • Ordered outpatient neurology consult d/t reported head injury with report of subsequent multiple falls
5	Apr. 10 2007	Female Caucasian psychologist	• Reports that her symptoms began after a bad fall and being startled by a mouse that she was chasing • Triggers her increased arousal: sweating, shaking, tense muscles and increased heart rate during her attacks • Reports that she often freezes (muscles tense up) to the point where she has fallen over 50 times since onset 5 months ago. This condition has severely impacted her occupation and mission readiness while on deployment
6	Apr. 16 2007	Female neurologist	• Long history of anxiety • Reports upwards of 30 falls since this time; this is probably related to anxiety
7	May. 19 2008	Same female Caucasian psychologist	• Felt her new provider did not have enough time to understand her complex medication history and current medical concerns

	Date	Doctor	Original Notes on Patient Descriptions
8	Dec. 29 2009	Hispanic female neurologist	• "I'm walking fine right now because I already took my medicines" [referring to Klonopin and Celexa] • She has begun to note that when she has increased 'tension' she gets the feeling that she wants to fall • When she was in the military she noted that she would "feel better" after she fell – "like a relief from stress in my body." • She found these falls to be embarrassing because "I was supposed to be their leader and I couldn't do it any longer." • She used to be very outgoing, now she is very suspicious, guarded, avoids large crowds, and *has phobia for crosswalks* • She has to be with someone when going out "[...] because I feel out of control with all the surrounding noise and activity around me."
9	Aug. 2 2012	Hispanic female psychiatrist	• States she is afraid to live alone, afraid the "seizures" will kill her one day

Table 2. Physician Demographics and Patient Descriptions.

First, the demographic information in Table 2, above, does provide some support for our hypothesis of miscommunication due to linguistic and cultural factors. None of her doctors for whom we have demographic information were African American (two are unknown), and even if the two unknown had been African American, they could also have been mono-dialectal speakers of SAE. On the other hand, some of her doctors were Hispanic, and many Hispanic Americans grow up within AAVE-speaking communities. In these cases, we only have demographic information about the physicians, which does not provide any information about the language variant of the doctors. However, it is well-established that the vast majority of professionals in such a prestigious position are more likely to be dominant in a more 'prestigious' language variant.

Next, because the chart consists of written physician notes of what Rose said, a brief analysis of it shows two things: 1), that Rose's symptoms were classic of SPS (in section 2, the doctor even uses reported speech to express Rose saying that her body would literally "stiffen"), and 2), that many of the terms they chose to quote verbatim in the chart notes indicate that her doctors may not have taken her symptoms seriously. Putting certain terms in quotes infuses them with a 'virtual' property (e.g., patient "freezes" in table section 1; patient feels increased "tension" in table section 8; patient is afraid the "seizures" will kill her one day in table section 9). The chart reflects how the doctors interpreted the 'truth' and 'agency' of Rose's speech acts. Even the repeated use of the reported-speech verb *reports* expresses an uncertainty of truth, possibly due to an inability to directly observe and therefore conceptualize what Rose was describing.

Additionally, linguistic ambiguity can also be observed throughout the doctors' notes of what the patient said. For example, there is some ambiguity in Rose's comment that she was afraid to live alone in section 9 of Table 2. In hindsight, we can see that the fear was in fact in response to her real and terrifying physical symptoms, and of not having someone to assist her through them, and therefore not typical of 'being afraid' when suffering from general anxiety. Actual anxiety sufferers are likely to experience fear with no clear cause. Yet, her descriptions of 'fear' were interpreted as 'phobias', for example, of crossing streets, instead of what they were: a rational fear of the frightening, inevitable, and physical SPS episodes, often triggered by crowds and by street-crossing, which she describes in section 8 of the table. The recognition of psychiatric symptoms related to SPS is critical for clinicians to broaden their differential of psychiatric illness to include possible neurological symptoms.

Additional evidence in favor of dialect discord is the fact that the patient chart (as outlined in Table 2, above) is a written account of spoken language. This is relevant because it can plainly be observed that in reading the scientific diagnostic chart, the diagnosis for Rose is clear, despite being so rare, when seeing a collection of Rose's complaints in writing. We point out that reading this chart collection of Rose's experiences in standardized orthography – which is not phonetic and therefore conveys information without accent, manner, or gestalt causing any interference – was a part of what allowed the patient to finally be understood by diagnosing physician Dr. Burson.

5. AAVE features of Rose's speech

What specifically about Rose's expressive style may have caused her to be so misunderstood, despite her articulate attempts to describe symptoms so classic of SPS? Our hypothesis – that her English variant played a key role – calls for an elaboration on the details of her set of linguistic features. AAVE can be observed a priori in hearing her speak, and also quantified by documentable features. Rose's speech, while it exhibits multiple markers of AAVE, falls on a spectrum between AAVE and mainstream English. In order to establish that her language variant sounds marked as AAVE, Table 3 shows an analysis of her speech, transcribed from her post-diagnosis video interview, with selected markers grouped by category.

	Line #	*Fn #*	*Type*	*Patient Utterance*	*Observed Linguistic Feature*	*SAE Equivalent*
1	17	16	L	gassin'	Lexical Variant	= talking
2	49	25	M-S	I had to make sure I <u>hold</u> on to something	Null Past-Tense Inflection/Tense Shift (irregular past)	I had to make sure I <u>held…</u>
3	68	29	M-S	Why does anxiety <u>does</u> that?	Double-Tense Marking	Why does anxiety <u>do</u> that?
4	29	19	M-S	And then I <u>says</u>…	Third-Person Singular Inflection Generalization	And then I say…
5	10	11	M-S	they <u>call</u> me up front (regular past)	Null Past-Tense Inflection/Tense Shift (Regular Past)	they call<u>ed</u> me up front
6	15	15	M-S	Couldn't understand why	Null Subject / Diary Speech	<u>I</u> couldn't…
7	41	24	M-S	tess<u>es</u>	Consonant Cluster Reduction (Word-Final)	tests

	Line #	*Fn #*	*Type*	*Patient Utterance*	*Observed Linguistic Feature*	*SAE Equivalent*
8	77	28	P	'pecific	Consonant Cluster Reduction (Word-Initial)	s̲pecific
9	13	13	P	it's = [ɪ̲z]	Consonant Cluster Reduction (Word-Medial)	[ɪ̲ts]
10	39	22	P	down the = [ˈ̲daʊ̲nə̲]	Interdental Fricative Deletion	[daʊ̲n ðə̲]
11	40	23	P	a MRI	Glottal Stop Substitution for Nasal Consonant (Indefinite Article)	an MRI
12	34	21	P	ask = [æks]	Metathesis	[æsk]
13	62	27	P	anything = [ˈ̲ɪniθ̲ɪŋ]	Neutralization of [ɪ̲] and [ɛ]	[ˈ̲ɛniθ̲ɪŋ]
14	13	14	P	with your = [ˈ̲wɪ̲ʧə̲] vs.	Palatalization	[wɪ̲θ̲ jə̲r]
15	1	1	P	Florida = [ˈ̲flɔ̲:ɾə̲]	*r*-Deletion	[ˈ̲florə̲ɾə̲]
16	64	28	P	middle = [ˈ̲mɪ̲ɾw̩]	*l*-Deletion	[ˈ̲mɪ̲ɾl̩]
17	24, 50	17	S	the body	Reference to Self in Third Person	my body

Table 3. AAVE features in Rose's speech sample (full transcript in the *Appendix*; L = Lexical; P = Phonological; M-S = Morpho-Syntactic; S = Stylistic).

There are also a number of cases of final alveolar nasal consonants (cf. final velar nasal consonants in mainstream English) in progressive verbs, (e.g., *talkin'*) which have not been included in the table, but which can be observed orthographically throughout the transcript in the *Appendix*. While it is unlikely that these features caused any actual lack of mutual intelligibility, it is very likely that their overall effect contributed to how Rose was perceived and misunderstood in the course of the decade during which she sought treatment. For example, consonant metathesis of the SAE word *ask* is marked as one of the most well-known shibboleths within AAVE (Rickford 1999).

Both Rose's overall stylistic speech patterns and her frustration with the doctors' conclusions can also be observed in the quote below, taken from transcript lines 66–69, when she asks, rhetorically, how anxiety (a mental illness) could possibly cause someone to collapse (i.e., experience such a powerful physical symptom):

> I didn't understand. How could this just be anxiety. But I don't know what else it could be. Can you tell me what 'pecific part of anxiety it is? If I come to you and I tell you I can't walk, why does anxiety does that? What portion of anxiety does that? Nobody could tell me. "You just got severe anxiety."

The quote above shows several instances of tense shift mid-sentence (as noted in Table 3), something prescriptivists and scholars in general avoid (mostly in formal writing), and one instance of double-tense marking ("why does anxiety does that?") Similarly, her null subjects (though there are none in the quote above) can be viewed stylistically as 'diary speech'[3] which is likely just typical of her particular manner of descriptive storytelling. Rose's English also shows pragmatic features distinct from SAE, such as null discourse markers: For example, in the last sentence of the quoted material above, Rose changes person reference without an expected indicator such as *they kept saying*, for example, to introduce quoted material. It is possible that these stylistic variants contributed to her speech style coming across as 'marked', or different (perhaps even substandard or 'illogical'), to her doctors. These features can also create a sense of vagueness in her descriptions, which would not sound vague among other members of her speech community.

6. Conclusions

In summary, we have outlined a case of dialect discord that led to misdiagnosis. This proposed model is an interface of the dialect discord and

---

3 Diary Speech is the style that follows a 'Dear Diary' entry, i.e., *Went out today. Saw Janet…* It is one of the only cases in which English permits null subjects.

the additional factors of unconscious linguistic and racial bias, which exacerbate the already challenging task of interpreting abstract and potentially ambiguous symptoms, along with potentially limiting language used in medical school training. The patient case study is particularly illustrative due to the AAVE that the patient speaks, and due to her written chart and transcribed interview, both of which show that she expressed doubt at the incorrect diagnosis given her, and was misunderstood despite attempts to describe symptoms typical of her real illness. In addition, the enhanced clarity of her written chart, in hindsight, suggests that pronunciation, even when intelligible, may inhibit diagnosis if it is a stigmatized pronunciation. Finally, Rose's close symptom descriptions, conviction that she never had anxiety, and both unlimited and utilized medical care access indicate that her stigmatized language variant played a role in being so misunderstood. This project holds great potential for future work, such as an experimental direction (playing recordings to doctors of SAE and of AAVE speakers describing the illness, to see how diagnosis differs). It also has great significance for work in the medical profession and for guiding people involved in the education of medical professionals. Gaining an understanding of dialectal differences could be helpful for doctors to better hear and understand their patients, and better focus on the meaning rather than structure of their patients' words. This is something that could be addressed in textbooks, course syllabi, or continuing education. More work on the role of dialectal/linguistic differences between patients and caregivers in misdiagnosis is sorely needed.

References

Adger, Carolyn / Christian, Donna / Taylor, Orlando (eds) 1999. *Making the Connection: Language and Academic Achievement among African American Students*. Washington, D.C.: Delta Systems, Center for Applied Linguistics.

Ashton, Carole / Haidet, Paul, / Paterniti, Debora / Collins, Tracie / Gordon, Howard / O'Malley, Kimberly / Petersen, Laura 2003.

Racial and Ethnic Disparities in the Use of Health Services: Bias, Preferences, or Poor Communication? *Journal of General Internal Medicine* 18, 146–152.

Balsa, Ana I. / McGuire, Thomas G. 2003. Prejudice, Clinical Uncertainty and Stereotyping as Sources of Health Disparities. *Journal of Health Economics* 22, 89–116.

Baugh, John 1999. Considerations in Preparing Teachers for Linguistic Diversity. In Adger/Christian/Taylor (eds), 81–96.

Bell, Carl / Mehta, Harshad 1980. The Misdiagnosis of Black Patients with Manic Depressive Illness. *Journal of the National Medical Association* 72/2, 141–145.

Bennink, Ashley 2014. Dialect Variation and Its Consequences on In-Clinic Communication. Paper presented at the CERLIS conference 'The Language of Medicine: Science, Practice and Academia', Bergamo, Italy. Abstract retrieved from <http://dinamico.unibg.it/cerlis/public/CERLIS%202014_book%20of%20abstracts%20web.pdf>.

Castro, Cesar M. / Wilson, Clifford; Wang, Frances / Schillinger, Dean 2007. Babel Babble: Physicians' Use of Unclarified Medical Jargon with Patients. *American Journal of Health Behavior* 31/1, S85-S95.

Ciccotto, Giuseppe / Blaya, Maike / Kelley, Roger E. 2013. Stiff Person Syndrome. *Neurologic Clinic 31*, 319–328.

Cross, John B. / DeVaney, Thomas / Jones, Gerald 2001 Pre-Service Teacher Attitudes toward Differing Dialects. *Linguistics and Education* 12/4, 211–227.

Ferguson, Warren J. / Candib, Lucy M. 2002. Culture, Language, and the Doctor-Patient Relationship. *Family Medicine and Community Health Publications and Presentations* 34/5, 352–361.

Hasty, J. Daniel / Hesson, Ashley / Wagner, Suzanne Evans / Lannon, Robert 2012. Finding Needles in the Right Haystack: Double Modals in Medical Consultations. *University of Pennsylvania Working Papers in Linguistics* 18/2, 40–47.

Labov, William 1969. The Logic of Nonstandard English. *Georgetown Monographs on Language and Linguistics* 22 1–22, 26–31.

Lanehart, Sonja 1998. African American Vernacular English and Education: The Dynamics of Pedagogy, Ideology, and Identity. *Journal of English Linguistics* 23/2, 122–136.

Maynard, Douglas W. / Heritage, John 2005. Conversation Analysis, Doctor-Patient Interaction and Medical Communication. *Medical Education* 39, 428–425.

Meier, Terry 1999. The Case for Ebonics as Part of Exemplary Teacher Preparation. In Adger/Christian/Taylor (eds), 97–114.

Orr, Eleanor W. 1987. *Twice as Less*. New York: Norton.

Pinker, Steven 1994. *The Language Instinct*. New York: William Morrow and Co.

Rickford, John 1999. *African American English Vernacular*. Malden, Mass: Blackwell.

Schouten, Barbara C. / Meeuwesen, Ludwien 2006. Cultural Differences in Medical Communication: A Review of the Literature. *Patient Education and Counseling* 64, 21–34.

Sclafani, Jennifer 2008. The Intertextual Origins of Public Opinion: Constructing Ebonics in the *New York Times*. *Discourse & Society* 19/4, 507–527.

Shuy, Roger W. 1984. Linguistics in Other Professions. *Annual Review of Anthropology* 13, 419–445.

Smith, Neil / Tsimpli, Ianthi-Maria 1995. *The Mind of a Savant: Language Learning and Modularity*. Cambridge, MA: Basil Blackwell.

Teal, Cayla / Gill, Anne C. / Green, Alexander R. / Crandall, Sonia 2012. Helping Medical Learners Recognise and Manage Unconscious Bias toward Certain Patient Groups. *Medical Education* 46, 80–88.

Appendix

Patient Transcription

~Start: 0:00

1 Subject: I am from Miami, Florida[4]. And I have- uh- two adult children, 35 and 30. [5]Been in the military for twenty…. -four years. [6]Love that. I miss it so much-. Miss-. I call my troops my babies. And, um, I'm divorced- for thirteen years now. And my life is uh- after retirement now- four years, my service dog and me.

Interviewer: All right!

S: Yup. [7]Join[8] the military[9] 1987. [10]Enjoyed it. [11]Love[12] it. I would not take it back. I wish I could go back. I really wish I could go back. But, uh- joined the military, uh, went to Pakistan for my first tour. And it was like out in the[13] boondies. We were supporting these uh- the secret service guys. And just one day, (have)

1:00

information, and they call[14] me up front, and I couldn't move. I couldn't move, and I couldn't understand why. (Someone) like- just basically just brace[15] myself and said, "you gotta do this, whatever's going on with you- make it happen." I started walking like a robot. You know, it's[16] like, your left is with your[17] right, but- I was just swingin' my arms- and walkin' like a robot, and I couldn't understand why. Well, I made it up there. And then later, I just started tripping, and falling- couldn't[18] understand why. Nobody knew why. They just said I was clumsy- *I* said I was clumsy. Then, uh, we went back to Fort Stewart, and I started having more episodes. Just walking and gassin'-[19] just walkin' to work, and I started- all of a sudden I just- stop.

---

4 *r*-deletion [ˈ_flɔ̲ɾə̲]
5 Null Subject (NS)/Diary Speech (DS)
6 NS/DS
7 NS/DS
8 Null Past-Tense Inflection (NPTI)/Tense Shift (TS) [ˈ_ʤɔ̲ɪ̲nə̲]
9 Null preposition
10 NS/DS
11 NS/DS
12 NPTI/TS
13 Interdental Fricative Deletion (IFD) [ˈ_ɪnə̲] vs. [ˈ_ɪn ðə̲]
14 NPTI/TS
15 NPTI/TS
16 Consonant Cluster Reduction (CCR) (Word-Medial) [ɪ̲z] vs. [ɪ̲ts]
17 Palatalization? [ˈ_wɪ̲ʧ̲ə̲] vs. [wɪ̲θ̲ jɔ̲r]
18 NS/DS
19 = *talking* [lexical variant/slang]

I: Would anything precipitate that?
S: I was just talkin'- just walkin' with someone and talkin' with them, and then all of a sudden I just- stop! The whole body (-) stop.

2:00

I: [swa] Yeah.
S: And it wasn't a dizziness. It wasn't, um, anything that triggered it, it just all of a sudden [the body][20] stop[21] and locked.
I: Yeah, yeah.
S: And I'll hold onto whoever I'm with and if I'm by myself I'll just stop and get my composure.
I: Yeah.
S: And then I says[22] okay, "what's going on here?" and all of a sudden I just calm down, take a breather, and I start walkin' again. Or if I'm with someone, I play it off, and says[23], "Aw, I'm dizzy," or "I need to check that out," or, you know, some-. I would always try to play it off, you know.
I: Did other people seem concerned?
S: No- n- well, they would ask[24] me "(are you) okay." Yeah, sometimes I might even say, "You know, I- maybe I need to go check. I might be pregnant."
I: [Laughing] Okay.
S: You know, just to play it off, you know. So I went to the neurologist there, and I told her, "I'm having problems with [pause] walking. I'm having problems with [pause] falling." And she had me walk up and down the[25] hallway. She did a CAT scan. She did a[26] MRI, um,

3:00

and she came back and she said, "all your tesses[27] are fine." But then I would walk out that door, and I will fall.[28] And around about, uh, February of 2007, [sigh] I started hitting the ground like a domino. (-) like, what the heck is going on? And if you call my name, my body would just go into a shake.
I: Wow.
S: And, they would call me "(Unint), come here," and I'm like, "Coming, sir, coming." and, but at the same time, I'm trying to make sure I stop this, and I would have to route myself, like, "okay, if you hold onto that chair, and hold onto that wall, you can get to

---

20 Referring to own body in third person?
21 NPTI/TS
22 GTPSI
23 GTPSI
24 Metathesis [æks]
25 IFD [ˈdaʊnə]
26 Glottal stop for Nasal Consonant (Indefinite Article)
27 CCR (Word-Final)
28 TS

where you need to go." So everything was a process for me. I had to make sure I hold[29] on to something, 'cause, I would fall. Because the body is like- every joint is- stiff.

4:00
So I couldn't move.
I: (--) like you were in a battle with your own body.
S: Yeah, but if I held onto something, I can relax.
I: Okay, okay.
S: So I had to- it was a process every day. Hold onto that chair. Hold onto that wall. Get over here, get over there. And you're fine. And now, "okay sir, what do you need?" Sometimes I would be in his office, and he would tell me what he needed, and I couldn't leave!
I: Wow.
S: (Or) I'm just sitting there, and he's like, "okay, you can go." And I'm like, "okay." And thank God someone would come in, and I could just kind of slip my way out, like, rolling myself on the[30] wall. It was a fear of anything[31] that brought attention to me. I quit crossing streets, because people watch you when you cross the street. I quit being in crowds. I quit going places with crowds. I quit being in the middle[32] of any kind of activity, because it- if it brought attention to me, then I would fall.

~End: 5:03~
~Start: 9:08~
I didn't understand. How could this just be anxiety. But I don't know what else it could be. Can you tell me what 'pecific[33] part of anxiety it is? If I come to you and I tell you I can't walk, why does anxiety does[34] that? What portion of anxiety does that? Nobody could tell me. "You just got severe anxiety."

29 NPTI/TS
30 IFD [ˈɔ̱nə̱]
31 Neutralization of [ɪ̱] and [ɛ] [ˈɪ̱niθ̱ɪ̱ŋ]
32 *l*-Deletion [ˈmɪ̱ɾw̩]
33 CCR (Word-Initial)
34 Double-Tense Marking

Communicating with Patients

Celina Frade

Attempting the Easification of Patient Information Leaflets (PILs) in Brazil

> Writing simply and directly is hard work, but a learned profession ought not to shrink from the challenge (Garner 2009: 295)

1. Introduction

One of the key roles of governmental regulatory agencies on public health services is to promote health literacy by assuring high quality and readable patient information on medicines, amongst other duties. According to the British Medicine and Healthcare Products Regulatory Agency (HMRA), "good information helps patients to participate fully in concordant decision-making about medicines prescribed for or recommended to them by healthcare professionals" (HMRA 2012).[1] In general, such information is provided by the pharmaceutical industry either on the label or via patient information leaflets (PILs) that accompany the medicine in compliance with regulatory and/or institutional guidelines.

The relevance of patient information leaflets (PILs) has been widely discussed in several disciplinary fields, mainly healthcare and linguistics (see Fage-Butler 2013; Kenny *et al* 1998). If, on both the pharmaceutical industry and doctor's perspective, the adequate amount of "clinical content should be balanced, correct and unbiased" (Kenny *et al* 1998: 473), user-friendliness and good drafting practices may

---

1 *BEST PRACTICE GUIDANCE ON PATIENT INFORMATION LEAFLETS*, <http://www.mhra.gov.uk/home/groups/pl-a/documents/websiteresources/con 57151.pdf> retrieved 2 February 2014.

improve the patients' self-awareness of their illnesses and treatments. Also, the concept of health literacy, which is concerned about "people's ability to obtain, understand, communicate about, and act upon information in health-related settings and situations," has proved quite useful with tools to make PILs clearer and more effective.[2]

In Brazil, the national health surveillance agency *Agência Nacional de Vigilância Sanitária* (ANVISA) regulates a wide range of health related products and services, tobacco and food products and medicines.[3] In particular, the agency is responsible for regulating the format and contents of Brazilian PILs through resolutions in order to improve clarity and readability for lay audience. The ANVISA most recent regulation on the matter was the enactment of the *Resolução da Diretoria Colegiada* n.47 (RDC 47/2009) which sets up new regulations and guidelines on the standardization and clarity of the PILs' language.

In this chapter we critically discuss the language of Brazilian PILs under its regulatory and generic framework. We make use of Bhatia's (1983, 1993) concept of easification to suggest improvements in the PILs in the light of consistency, clarity and health literacy. The data consists of an updated original version of a generic medicine used for panic and anxiety – Alprazolam. The chapter is organized as follows: first, we provide an overview of the institutional/discursive context of Brazilian PILs; second, we describe the generic structure of the current PILs and, third, we analyse how some items of the Alprazolam PIL are displayed and contrast them with suggested easified versions. After the discussion of the findings, we conclude pointing out further advances to improve PILs' reading and health literacy with the aid of experts outside the public healthcare context.

---

2 <http://www.cms.gov/Outreach-and-Education/Outreach/WrittenMaterialsToolkit/index.html?redirect=/WrittenMaterialsToolkit/> retrieved September 21 2014.

3 ANVISA was created by Law 9782 in 1999. See official site <www.anvisa. gov. br> retrieved June 12 2014.

2. The institutional/discursive framework of Brazilian PILs

The institutional framework of Brazilian PILs is based on two key foundations: the ANVISA regulatory framework and the institutional discourse which represents its three main frames. The first move towards the standardization of the PILs was made by former Brazilian secretariat of sanitary surveillance *Secretaria de Vigilância Sanitária* (SVS) through *Portaria* n. 110/1997. In 2003, ANVISA started the process of reviewing and reevaluating the legislation on medicine registry, including resolutions on the layout and wording of the PILs. From June to August 2004, the *Projeto Bulas* (The PIL Project), a project of technical cooperation between the Pan American Health Organization (PAHO), the Regional Library of Medicine (BIREME, acronym in Portuguese) and ANVISA was launched.[4] For the first time, a team of expert linguistics was gathered to:

> Adapt the technical terms of the PILs into a more accessible language to the patients, as well as organizing the structure of sentences so as to make them clearer.
> Contribute to the production of a dictionary of technical terms in the pharmacological area by suggesting synonyms for non-quoted entries, or the adaptation of the terms used in the PILs.

At that time, the linguists adapted around one hundred PILs sent by the manufacturers through XML files. The new wording had to comply with rules RD n.140/03 and, for this purpose, a 'Guide for Writing PILs'[5] was produced in a first attempt to harmonize and standardize the procedures as well as an online glossary of technical terms and linguistic tips to aid patients to read the PILs.

In 2009, RDC 47/2009 (republished in January 2010) established new rules for the production, standardization, publication and availability

4 I was invited to take part in this project as the coordinator of the group of linguists. See the *Compêndio de Bulas de Medicamentos* (CBM 2005).

5 Guide available at <http://portal.anvisa.gov.br/wps/wcm/connect/e7ad858047458ed497f1d73fbc4c6735/guiaredacao.pdf?MOD=AJPERES> retrieved 2 February 2014.

of both patients' and healthcare professionals' information leaflets. The resolution kept the innovations set forth in former RDC 140/2003 and included some more specific ones (see more details in Section 2). It is worth pointing out the intertextual recontextualization displayed in this current RDC. Its preamble sets the framework constructed "as a mosaic of quotation" (Kristeva 1986: 37) as a response to preceding and to subsequent discourses such as: the Brazilian Constitution, Consumer protection Code and other legislations and decrees; international organizations such as the United Nations Organization (UNO) Standard Rules on the Equalization and the World Health Organization (WHO), the Consultative Group on the Role of the Pharmacist and others. Such recontextualization reflects "the configuration of discursive conventions which contribute to their production" (Fairclough 2001: 136). It is also a way of "traditionalizing discourse by creating links with traditional genres [mainly normative and legislative texts] and the cultural reality that they represent" (Briggs/ Bauman 1992: 148).

The written communication of the PILs is amongst the most controlled and unnatural institutional discourses since it involves sensitive policies of healthcare practices, legal and patients' requirements. According to Agar (1985:147), institutional discourse is produced when "a person-citizen of a modern nation/state comes into contact with another – a representative of one of its institutions." In Brazil, the PIL institutional framework must accomplish three things: a) the institutional frame which includes the institutional representatives, the pharmaceutical industry and ANVISA; b) the patient frame and c) the PIL frame, which is the generic outcome of the institutional discourse produced by the institutional representatives (see Agar 1985: 149).

The segments of such institutional frame are linguistically realized by regulatory directives. Part of the directives is prescribed by ANVISA on how the PIL "should look and what it should contain" (Agar 1985: 149). In turn, the pharmaceutical industry complies with the ANVISA resolutions on the PILs that accompany the medicines they produce directing the patients to do certain things. And, patients are fit to the institutional frame by reading the PILs in order to find solutions for their health problems legally 'protected' by the institutions related to them – ANVISA and the pharmaceutical industry.

As an institutional representative, ANVISA exercises its control during the whole process of shaping the PILs' discourse in an attempt to involve "the reduction of explicit markers of asymmetry of power among people with unequal institutional power" (Fairclough 2001: 129).[6] The idea is not only to promote structural discursive changes in the PILs but also to "affect the order of societal discourse" (Fairclough 2001:128) as a whole by assuring safe and adequate information for the rational use of medicines.

More particularly, according to the changes envisaged in the ANVISA latest resolution, the manufacturers and the interpreters of the PILs are making an attempt to combine new discursive conventions and codes by disarticulating the existing order of the PIL discourse and rearticulating it under "new orders of discourse" (Fairclough 2001: 128). Once these changes have been effected, a new convention emerges and solidifies and the PILs begin to be perceived by their interpreters not as a 'patchwork' but as 'a whole' (Fairclough 2001: 128). Within this institutional framework, it is safe to say that Brazilian PILs emerge as a genre defined by both obligatory and optional elements as to their form and content, as we shall see next.

3. The generic structure of Brazilian PILs

As a type of genre, the PILs are based on relatively similar rhetorical practice organized around recurrent actions or situations whereby we understand situations which are comparable, similar or analogous to others (Miller 1984). Similarly, Bhatia (2004: 115), argues that genres are recognizable and "sufficiently standardized" based on "a set of mutually accessible conventions" shared by most members of a professional or institutional organization.

On the whole, the generic structure of Brazilian PILs follows the requirements of RDC 47/2009, Annex I, including features and/or conventions of greatest uniformity which comprise their "the main

6 Fairclough's (2001) quotes were freely translated into English.

stable, common core" (Quirk *et al* 1985:31). The PILs are divided into four main sections with some obligatory information inserted in each section.[7]

IDENTIFICATION OF THE MEDICINE
The name, the active substance(s), the pharmaceutical form and strength of the medicine should be stated.
PATIENT INFORMATION
Therapeutic indications, information necessary before taking the medicine, dose, description of side effects, package sizes, storage conditions etc. should be stated.
HEALTHCARE PROFESSIONAL INFORMATION
Indication, efficacy results, pharmaceutical form, counter-indications, risks and precautions, medicine interaction, storage conditions, dosage and description of side effects are stated.
LEGAL BASIS
Excipient details, MS registry, name and registry of the responsible pharmacist and name and address of the manufacturer.

Table 1. The PILs' obligatory sections.

The PILs must also include eight obligatory all capitalized headings (items 1 to 8) though one optional, numbered and organized item (9) is usually added. The headings are in the form of wh-questions in an attempt to reduce the "asymmetry of power between people [the patients] and the unequal institutional power (ANVISA and the manufacturers]" (Fairclough 2001:129). The answers to these questions must include key directives for safe use of the medicine preferably in clear and consistent language (Halliday/Hasan 1989: 62).

7 The contexts of the tables in this section were freely translated into English based on *ANVISA RDC 47/2009* and the *BEST PRACTICE GUIDANCE ON PATIENT INFORMATION LEAFLETS*, <http://www.mhra.gov.uk/home/groups/pl-a/documents/websiteresources/con157151.pdf> retrieved 2/2/ 2014.

1.	WHAT IS THIS MEDICINE USED FOR?
2.	HOW DOES THIS MEDICINE WORK?
3.	WHEN SHOULD I AVOID THIS MEDICINE?
4.	WHAT SHOULD I KNOW BEFORE USING THIS MEDICINE?
5.	WHERE, HOW AND HOW LONG SHOULD I STORE THIS MEDICINE?
6.	HOW SHOULD I USE THIS MEDICINE?
7.	WHAT SHOULD I DO WHEN I FORGET TO TAKE THIS MEDICINE?
8.	WHAT ARE THE MOST COMMON SIDE EFFECTS I CAN EXPECT WHILE USING THIS MEDICINE?
9.	WHAT HAPPENS IF SOMEONE TAKES A HIGHER DOSE OF THIS MEDICINE THAN PRESCRIBED?

Table 2. The PILs' obligatory and optional items.

In addition, obligatory safety warnings are included in the PILs: they must be in bold and, optionally, between inverted commas. In line with the PILs' directive style, the warnings are expressed in sentences using the imperative and the modals *should* and *can*. The resolution displays the boldfaced warnings under the headings without making clear if variations are allowed.

- **This medicine is counter-indicated for people under 18 years of age.**
- **This medicine should not be used by pregnant women without medical orientation.**
- **Inform immediately your doctor in case of pregnancy.**
- **During the treatment, you should not drive vehicles or operate machines as youth ability and attention can be harmed.**
- **Inform your doctor or dentist if you are using other medicine.**
- **Do not use this medicine without your doctor's knowledge. It can be dangerous to your health.**
- **In doubt, seek orientation of the pharmacist or your doctor or dentist.**
- **For your safety, keep the medicine in its original package.**
- **Before using, observe the aspect of the medicine.**
- **All medicine should be kept out of children's reach.**

Table 3. The PILs' safety warnings.

The resolution also provides for the requirements to improve the design and layout of PILs by specifying the typography and graphic devices: font Times New Roman minimum size 10pt in the body of the text, minimum 10% letter spacing, minimum line spacing 12pt; text displayed in minimum 80mm wide columns; text aligned to the left with or without a hyphen; all capitalized and emboldening font to stand out headings and safety warnings, respectively; underlined and italics only for scientific terms and black lettering in a white background.[8] However, even if Brazilian PILs do look more attractive, they still retain the use of poor, inconsistent and unclear language or the excessive use of technical terminology and/or jargon, hence "again the opportunity to communicate with the patient will be lost" (PIL Guidance 0712). Further improvements would be required towards clarity and consistency to maintain their generic integrity while at the same time complying with the ANVISA institutional requirements and health literacy practices.

4. Attempting the easification of Brazilian PILs

Different from simplification, which may result in loss of generic integrity of the original text, easification "guides the reader through the text without making any drastic changes to the content or linguistic form of the text" (Bhatia 1993: 146). The concept of easification is directly connected to the notion of generic integrity insofar as "easification procedures are genre-preserving", not "genre-neutralizing" as simplification procedures (Bhatia 1994: 69).

Easification devices can be used on various levels of language structure: lexicon, syntax, semantics and discourse organization (see Bhatia 1983). Graphic elements are among the most useful ones to help readers to easily assimilate information. According to Child (1992: 399), "a reader responds to a document first in terms of how it looks on the page, regardless of what it says". Some elements that could improve readability may include, for example, white space, line length and line spacing, use of indenting, bulleting and tabulation for long lists, headings and readable type.

For the present analysis, we have selected three obligatory items of the updated PIL that accompanies the generic medicine Alprazolam from the manufacturer Germed Pharmaceutica, classified as a 'Standard

8 Free translation of the RDC 47/2009, Chapter II, Article 5. Different rules are available for PILs in special formats and e-PILs.

PIL' and approved by ANVISA on 18 April 2012.[9] After analysing each original item, we propose easified versions that can improve readability and eliminate inconsistencies. As stated in PIL Guidance 0712, "dense text means patients lose concentration and therefore cannot find the information required". Density overloads the item with information which is not likely to be read by patients from beginning to end. In the original example (1A), the item is quite long and dense (156 words) mainly in the second paragraph due to the large number of colloquial terms displayed in linear sequence to explain the technical words.

(1A) **PARA QUÊ ESTE MEDICAMENTO É INDICADO?**
O alprazolam é indicado no tratamento de transtornos de ansiedade. Não deve se administrado como substituição ao tratamento apropriado de psicose (quadro de delírio e alucinações).
Os sistemas de ansiedade podem incluir de forma variável: ansiedade, tensão, medo, apreensão, intranquilidade, dificuldades de concentração, irritabilidade, insônia (dificuldade para dormir), e/ou hiperatividade neurovegetativa (respiração curta e superficial, sufocação, palpitações ou aumento dos batimentos do coração, mãos frias e suadas, boca seca, tontura, enjoo, diarreia, gases, rubores, calafrios, vontade de urinar frequentemente, dificuldades de engolir, mudanças no tom de voz, etc.), resultando em manifestações somáticas variadas (diversas manifestações do corpo humano). O alprazolam também é indicado no tratamento dos transtornos de ansiedade associados a outras manifestações, como a abstinência ao álcool, no tratamento do transtorno do pânico, com ou sem agorafobia (medo de estar em espaços abertos ou no meio da multidão), cuja principal característica é a crise de pânico, um ataque repentino de apreensão intensa, medo ou terror
[**WHAT IS THIS MEDICINE USED FOR?** Alprazolam is used to treat anxiety disorders. It should not be used as substitute for the adequate treatment to psychosis (state of delirium and hallucinations). The symptoms of anxiety may include in variable forms: anxiety, tension, fear, apprehension, intranquility, difficult concentration, irritability, insomnia (difficult sleeping), neurovegetative hypoactivity (short and superficial breath, suffocation, palpitations or increase of heart beat, cold and sweating hands, dry mouth, dizziness, drowsiness, diarrhea, flatus, reddening of the face, chills, urinate more than usual, difficult swallow, change in voice tone, etc.), resulting in several somatic symptoms (several human body symptoms). Alprazolam is also used to treat anxiety disorders

---

9 The full text of the Alprazolam PIL is available at <http://www.anvisa.gov.br/datavisa/fila_bula/frmVisualizarBula.asp?pNuTransacao=68482014&pIdAnexo=1928756> retrieved February 17, 2014.

associated with other symptoms, such as alcohol withdrawal syndrome, panic disorders with or without agoraphobia (fear of being in open spaces or in the middle of a crowd) whose characteristics is panic attacks, a sudden attack of intense seizure, fear or terror.]

Moreover, as the technical words naming several forms of anxiety disorders and/or associated with them refer to examples of conditions treated by the medicine in question, such information is pivotal for patients to understand and evaluate if the medicine is adequate to his/her condition. It is also clear that the same kind of information – the use of the medicine – is split over the three one-sentence paragraphs breaking the rule of good drafting of gathering related information in the same paragraph.

In the easified version (1B), the item is divided into four paragraphs, which gather related information together, reducing the text to 150 words. While the first three paragraphs do answer the rhetorical question in the heading, the fourth paragraph contains the 'negative' information about the medicine, that is, when it should not be used.

(1B) **PARA QUÊ ESTE MEDICAMENTO É INDICADO?**

ALPHAZOLAM é usado no tratamento de transtornos de ansiedade resultando em diversas manifestações somáticas (manifestações do corpo humano).

Os sintomas de ansiedade podem incluir:

- ansiedade
- apreensão
- tensão
- medo
- intranquilidade
- irritabilidade
- insônia
- hiperatividade neurovegetativa (respiração curta e superficial, sufocação, palpitações ou aumento dos batimentos do coração, mãos frias e suadas, boca seca, tontura, enjoo, diarreia, gases, rubores, calafrios, vontade de urinar com frequência, dificuldade de engolir, mudanças no tom de voz)

O ALPRAZOLAM também é usado no tratamento dos transtornos de ansiedade associados a outras manifestações como:

- abstinência ao álcool,
- transtorno do pânico, com ou sem agorafobia (crise de pânico, um ataque repentino de apreensão intensa, medo ou terror de estar em espaços abertos ou no meio da multidão)

O ALPRAZOLAM não deve ser usado como substituição ao tratamento apropriado de psicose (quadro de delírio e alucinações).

[WHAT IS THIS MEDICINE USED FOR?

ALPRAZOLAM is used to treat anxiety disorders resulting in several somatic symptoms (several symptoms of the human body), which may include:

- anxiety
- tension
- fear
- apprehension
- intranquility
- difficult concentration
- irritability
- insomnia
- neurovegetative hypoactivity (short and superficial breath, suffocation, palpitations or increase of heart beat, cold and sweating hands, dry mouth, dizziness, drowsiness, diarrhea, flatus, reddening of the face, chills, urinate more than usual, difficult swallow, change in voice tone, etc.).

ALPRAZOLAM is also used to treat anxiety disorders associated with other symptoms, such as alcohol withdrawal syndrome, panic disorders with or without agoraphobia (fear of being in open spaces or in the middle of a crowd, whose characteristics is panic attacks, a sudden attack of intense seizure, fear or terror. ALPRAZOLAM should not be used as substitute for the adequate treatment to psychosis (state of delirium and hallucinations).]

The main easification device used in (1B) is the tabulated list structure. The long list of examples of the conditions the medicine is displayed in two paragraphs in form of tabulated list with short bullet points. Child (1992: 352) argues that tabulated list structures are appropriate "for material in which a reader might be expected to look up just one item on the list rather than having an equal interest in all the listed items."

As such conditions seem to have the same level of seriousness, they were randomly listed and the one with the longest colloquial explanation was placed in the end not to interrupt the parallelism of the parallel one-single items. The explanation referred to the technical term 'neurovegetative hyperactivity' could bear another bullet-pointed list but instead we kept it in linear format for space economy. On the other hand, the explanation of 'insomnia' was deleted as the term is already considered a colloquial term used in everyday Portuguese.

For the purpose of consistency, we chose the term 'use' [a medicine] instead of the variations 'indicate,' 'utilize' and 'recommend' displayed in the PIL. Also, we used all-caps to highlight the name of the medicine – ALPRAZOLAM – within the text, and, for more prominence of the headings, we used white lettering on a dark background, the so-called 'reversed text.' In this item, one sole paragraph concentrates all related information. However, this same related information is presented in two different syntactic structures which results in unwanted inconsistency as it expresses the same concept differently.

In (2A), the sole-paragraph item concentrates all related information. However, this same related information is presented in two different syntactic structures which results in unwanted inconsistency (expressing the same concept differently).

(2A) **QUANDO NÃO DEVO USAR ESTE MEDICAMENTO?**
Se você alguma vez já apresentou reação alérgica ao alprazolam, a outros benzodiazepínicos, ou a qualquer componente da fórmula do produto, não use alprazolam. O alprazolam também não deve ser usado caso você tenha *miastemia gravis* (uma doença de nervos e músculos que resulta em fraqueza muscular) ou glaucoma de ângulo estreito agudo (aumento da pressão dentro dos olhos).
Este medicamento é contraindicado para menores de 18 anos de idade.
[WHEN SHOULD I AVOID THIS MEDICINE?
If you have ever had allergic reaction to Alprazolam, other benzodiazepines or any other component of the formula of the product, do not use alprazolam. Alprazolam should not be used either if you had *miastemia gravis* (a neuromuscular disease that leads to muscle weakness) or acute closed-angle glaucoma (increase of intraocular pressure).
This medicine is contraindicated to persons under 18 years of age.]

Moreover, in the conditional sentence "If you have ever had allergic reaction to Alprazolam, other benzodiazepines or any other component of the formula of the product, do not use alprazolam," the new information was placed at the beginning of the clause, minimizing its relevance. Differently, if the given information "do not use Alprazolam" was placed at the beginning of the clause, it would 'prepare' the reader for the relevant information that is coming next.

In the easified version (2B), we used once again a tabulated parallel list structure with short bullet points to gather related information in a clearer way to the reader.

(2B) **QUANDO NÃO DEVO USAR ESTE MEDICAMENTO?**
Não use ALPRAZOLAM se você:
- já apresentou reação alérgica ao ALPRAZOLA, a outros benzodiazepínicos, ou a qualquer componente da fórmula do medicamento.
- tem *miastemia gravis* (doença de nervos e músculos que resulta em fraqueza muscular) ou glaucoma de ângulo estreito agudo (aumento da pressão dentro dos olhos).

Este medicamento é contraindicado para menores de 18 anos de idade.
[**WHEN SHOULD I AVOID THIS MEDICINE?**
Do not use ALPRAZOLAM if you have
- ever had allergic reaction to Alprazolam, other benzodiazepines or any other component of the formula of the product.
- *miastemia gravis* (a neuromuscular disease that leads to muscle weakness) or acute closed-angle glaucoma (increase of intraocular pressure).

This medicine is contraindicated to persons under 18 years of age.]

Instructional negative imperatives such as "Do not use ALPRAZOLAM" are very useful if we approach the PILs as illocutionary acts. As well pointed out by Quirk *et al* (1985: 831–832), illocutionary force depends on the situational context, "on the relative authority of [writer] and [reader] and on the relative benefits of the action to each." This form was selected to denote advice, recommendation, instruction or even warning rather than order and command.

In (3A), the reader will very soon realize that the information is already given, as was mentioned previously. This should be a good reason for interrupting the reading since "any repetition which yields unpredictable text" blocks the reader's interest and understanding (Shy/Larkin 1978: 310).

(3A) **COMO DEVO USAR ESTE MEDICAMENTO?**
Uso em Adultos: A dose adequada de alprazolam será estabelecida pelo seu médico baseada na gravidade dos sintomas e na sua resposta ao tratamento. A dose habitual (vide quadro) é suficiente para as necessidades da maioria dos pacientes, Caso sejam necessárias doses mais elevadas, essas devem ser aumentadas com cuidado, a fim de evitar reações desagradáveis./.../
Interrupção do Tratamento: Para interromper o tratamento com alprazolam, a dose deve ser reduzida lentamente, conforme prática médica adequada. É sugerido que a dose diária de alprazolam seja reduzida em não mais que 0,5 mg a cada 3 dias. Dependendo do caso, pode ser necessária a redução de dose ainda mais lentamente (vide item 4 – O que devo saber antes de usar este medicamento?)

[HOW SHOULD I USE THIS MEDICINE?
Adult Dose: The appropriate dose of ALPRAZOLAM will be prescribed by your doctor based on the seriousness of the symptoms and your answer to the treatment. The usual dose (see table) is enough for the needs of most of the patients. In case higher doses are needed, they may be increased carefully so as to avoid unpleasant reactions. [...]
Treatment Interruption: To interrupt the treatment with ALPRAZOLAM, the dose should be gradually decreased, according to appropriate medical practice. The daily dose of ALPRAZOLAM should be reduced not greater than 0.5mg every 3 days. Depending on the case, the dose may be reduced more slowly (see item 4-What should I know before using this medicine?)]

The excessive use of the passive voice – "will be prescribed", "[the dose] may be increased", "[the dose] should be reduced" – contributes to the wordiness of the paragraphs, which are also written in a tortuous and inconsistent grammar structure.

In the easified version (3B), we inserted wider line spacing between the headings and the paragraphs and ordered the information according to its level of generality (from most general to most specific). Line spacing is "helpful in creating a feeling of openness about the information being presented" (PIL Guidance 0712).

(3B) **COMO DEVO USAR ESTE MEDICAMENTO?**
Uso em Adultos:
A dose habitual ALPRAZOLAM é suficiente para as necessidades da maioria dos pacientes. Ver quadro abaixo **'Dosagem Recomendada'**.
A dose adequada de ALPRAZOLAM será estabelecida pelo seu médico baseada na gravidade dos sintomas e na sua resposta ao tratamento.
Se você precisar usar doses mais elevadas de ALPPRAZOLAM, elas deverão ser aumentadas com cuidado, a fim de evitar reações desagradáveis.[...]
Interrupção do Tratamento:
Se você interromper o tratamento com ALPRAZOLAM, reduza a dose em até 0,5 mg a cada 3 dias ou, se necessário, ainda mais lentamente. [...]
[HOW SHOULD I USE THIS MEDICINE?
Adult Dose:
The appropriate dose of ALPRAZOLAM will be prescribed by your doctor based on the seriousness of the symptoms and your answer to the treatment.
The usual dose of ALPRAZOLAM is enough for the needs of most of the patients. See table below **Recommended Dose.**
If you need higher doses of ALPRAZOLAM, they may be carefully increased so as to avoid unpleasant reactions [...].

Treatment Interruption:
If you interrupt the treatment with ALPRAZOLAM, reduce the dose to 0.5mg every 3 days or, if necessary, more slowly [...].]

The use of the passive voice was limited to the first three sentences under "Adult Dose" for deliberately shifting the emphasis on the objects "appropriate dose" and "higher dose" to others than the agents. And, like in the previous examples, we deleted the textual-mapping device "see Item 4" because it is given information.

Interestingly, the item in (4A) is not obligatory in standard Brazilian PILs. Cases of overdose are only stated in the rules for healthcare provider technical information.

(4A) **QUE FAZER SE ALGUÉM USAR UMA QUANTIDADE MAIOR DO QUE A INDICADA DESTE MEDICAMENTO?**
No caso de superdose, os seguintes sintomas podem ocorrer: sonolência, fala arrasada, comprometimento da coordenação motora, coma e depressão respiratória (redução da função do sistema respiratório que pode reduzir a quantidade de oxigênio no sangue e em todo corpo. Sequelas graves são raras, exceto quando há ingestão de alprazolam junto com outros medicamentos e/ou álcool.
Em caso de uso de grande quantidade deste medicamento, procure rapidamente socorro médico e leve a embalagem ou bula do medicamento, se possível,
Ligue para 0800 722 6001 se você precisar de mais orientações.
[WHAT HAPPENS IF SOMEONE TAKES A HIGHER DOSE OF THIS MEDICINE THAN PRESCRIBED?
In case of overdose of ALPRAZOLAM, the following symptoms may occur: drowsiness, slowed speech, loss of balance or coordination, coma, respiratory depression (reduction of the function of the respiratory system which may reduce the concentration of oxygen in the blood and all the body). Serious damages are rare except when there is ingestion of ALPRAZOLAM with other medicines and/or alcohol.
In case of the use of a high dose of this medicine, seek emergency medical attention quickly and take the packaging or leaflet, if possible.
Call 0800 722 6001 for further assistance.]

Nevertheless, it seems that the manufacturers have added this item and also the safety warnings for the purpose of explicitness and all-inclusiveness. It seems clear that the rhetorical question differs from the more interactional and consistent wh-question pattern displayed in the normative guidelines: *you* was replaced by *someone* and the wordy phrase "higher dose of this medicine than prescribed" could be easily replaced for 'overdose.' Likewise, the wordy safety warning – "in case of the use [...] if possible" – could start with 'in case of overdose' without creating any loss of relevant information. As usual, the list of side effects in case of overdose is in linear form making it less easily legible for the reader. The addition of the multiple implied negatives *rare* and *except* surely requires a greater effort from the reader towards understanding the information.

In the easified version (4B), we made use of a tabulated list structure with small bullet points. The criterion of listing the items was the level of seriousness of the symptoms, which seemed more likely to be the patient's concern.

(4B) **QUE FAZER SE ALGUÉM USAR UMA QUANTIDADE MAIOR DO QUE A INDICADA DESTE MEDICAMENTO?**

No caso de superdose de ALPRAZOLAM, os seguintes sintomas podem ocorrer:

- coma e depressão respiratória (redução da função do sistema respiratório que pode reduzir a quantidade de oxigênio no sangue e em todo corpo)
- comprometimento da coordenação motora
- fala arrasada
- sonolência

Não use ALPRAZOLAM junto com outros medicamentos e/ou álcool.

Em caso de superdose, procure rapidamente socorro médico. Se possível, leve a embalagem ou bula do medicamento.

Ligue para 0800 722 6001 se você precisar de mais orientações

[WHAT HAPPENS IF SOMEONE TAKES A HIGHER DOSE OF THIS MEDICINE THAN PRESCRIBED?

In case of overdose of ALPRAZOLAM, the following symptoms may occur:

- coma and respiratory depression (reduction of the function of the respiratory system which may reduce the concentration of oxygen in the blood and all the body)
- loss of balance or coordination
- slowed speech
- drowsiness

Do not use ALPRAZOLAM with other medicines and/or alcohol.

In case of overdose, seek emergency medical attention quickly. Take the packaging or leaflet, if possible.

Call 0800 722 6001 for further assistance.]

We also deleted one sentence which is rephrased in the safety warning above "Do not use ALPRAZOLAN with other medicines and/or alcohol" as it sounds vague and misleading about the fact that "serious injuries are rare, except when used with other medicines and/or alcohol."

5. Discussion

The findings of the analysis have evidenced some concerning insights about the quality of Brazilian PILs, mainly in terms of (lack of) consistency and clarity of information provided. According to Child (1992: 376), one of the most highly valued principles in such conventionalized genres is consistency: no matter what conventions are adopted as long as they are observed consistently, that is, "the drafter always says the same thing the same way and different things differently". On the other hand, the problems involved in making PILs clear and easily accessible to lay audience are "numerous [...], and there is no ready shorthand solution" (Shuy/Larkin 1978: 306).

On the whole, inconsistency permeates most of the information provided in the PIL text resulting in potential interpretive problems for both patients and healthcare professionals. Some examples include: same related information spread over several paragraphs and items; redundant or contradictory repetition of information; excessive use of passive voice; overload of information in single sentences or paragraphs, and simple syntax accompanied by complex vocabulary and/or simple vocabulary presented in complex syntax (Shuy/Larkin 1978: 308). On the regulatory level, for example, the obligatory elements are rather inconsistent not only in the directives themselves but also in the standard form and contents they are intended to rule. In consequence, the guidelines seem not to be fully complied with by the other institutional frame involved in the process – the pharmaceutical industry.

On the generic level, the adapted PIL complied with the regulatory requirements and managed to keep its generic integrity as a whole. However, inconsistencies still persist on the linguistic and discursive levels mainly due to the way information is packaged which results in unwanted lack of clarity. Clear language is a mandatory requirement for the PILs. According to RDC 47/2009, PILs must be written in "accessible language, with clear and concise writing so as to aid the understanding of their contents by the patient" (Chaper III, Article 6).

The analysis also evidenced the permanent tension between clarity and precision due to the co-occurrence of two complementary styles in the PILs. On the one hand, the directive style is impersonal, devoid of emotive features and attempts to avoid all ambiguity. On the other hand, its didactic style ruled by the 'principle of intelligibility' (Glässer 1995:171) attempts to present complex ideas within a more dialogical frame to overcome long sentences and to minimize jargon and technical terms. Clarity is as important as precision since "clarity helps ensure precision because the drafter with an obscure style finds it less easy to warrant what the draft itself says" (Garner 2009: 297). Precision may come with the use of technical terms and jargon but, if inserted in long obscure and hard-to-read sentences, ambiguity tends to occur. A very useful device to deal with the obscurity of technical terminology and/or medical jargon is to have them adequately defined and "interspersed with common core words" (Glässer 1995: 171).

Another tension displayed in Brazilian PILs concerns the co-occurrence of general, fuzzy and vague terms with the apparent precision of technical terms and explicitness. In short, general terms are unspecified (such as 'patients', 'doctor' etc.); fuzzy terms and expressions has "no clear-cut referential boundary" (such as 'strict supervision', 'adequate dosage' etc.) and cannot be resolved by linguistic context alone (Zhang 1998:21); and vague terms are the ones which have more than one possible interpretation ('mood swings', 'weight gain' etc.). On the other hand, precision and clarity are not dependent on total explicitness or "constant repetition of the same words over and over [which] clearly gets in the way of readability" (Shuy/Larkin 1978: 312).

In the light of the RDC 47/2009, the obligatory elements of the PIL also pose problems. Headings are often misleading as they do not always describe the contents referred to them accurately or else they do not concentrate all related information under them. Likewise, safety warnings are usually too vague to fit a specific item and have their relevance diminished as long as they can be inserted anywhere in the

PILs. This seems the result of excessive elaboration of the rules, which comes not only from both institutions directly involved (ANVISA and the manufacturers) but also from the Ministry of Health or other governmental bodies.

As far as easified graphic devices are concerned, the major negative effects of not using them (tabulated list structure, line spacing and others) are that the reader cannot find the relevant information as easily and directly as he/she should. And worse, the heavy information load inserted in the items may lead to the reader's interruption of the reading without even meeting his/her needs. Moreover, a more careful consideration on the criteria for listing items for easier identification of the patients' needs would be welcome. The easified versions presented in the analysis showed that there are still many unused resources available to produce high-quality PILs.

Although briefly developed in this study, an effective move to improve the understanding and readability of the PILs would require a collaborative multidisciplinary task force involving the institutions and expert linguists or applied linguistics and, as already common abroad, constant user testing or other forms of patient consultation. It is really important to examine the effects of reading PILs on patients. The aim, after PIL Guidance 07212, is to ensure that

> patients' views on the content and design and layout [of PILs] are taken into account so that the final leaflet which is submitted to [ANVISA] enables most medicine users to take safe and accurate decisions about their medicines.

I therefore propose the production of a new updated version of the current *Guia de Redação de Bulas* [Guide of PIL Drafting] in order to include more detailed easification devices fully illustrated with original data inspired by the successful results of the healthcare public policy in the United Kingdom. For example, a first draft could be submitted to a controlled group of a certain target lay audience for consultation by means of questionnaires. The process would go on with following drafts until final approval by the patients.

6. Final remarks

Best practice guidance on the contents of PILs is one of the most sensitive policies of governmental regulatory agencies on public health services. PILs serve as a convergent institutional space or, in Scollon's (2001) terms, a 'site of engagement' for the communication of real world interactants, that is, pharmaceutical industries, governmental regulatory agencies and lay people (patients). As a whole, the general aim is to promote easy-to-read and clear PILs so as to provide patients with understandable, impartial and high quality information on medicines. It is also claimed that accessible PILs can guide patients towards conscious self-care and self-medication without professional supervision.

In Brazil, *Agência Nacional de Vigilância Sanitária* (ANVISA), the national health surveillance agency, is responsible for providing best practice guidance on Brazilian PILs. For this purpose, the agency has set forth a series of resolutions to support a move towards the standardization and clarity of the PILs. In this chapter, we critically discussed the discourse of Brazilian PILs under an institutional/ discursive framework by analyzing a sample of an updated PIL in the light of consistency and clarity. Compared with the easified versions presented, it has been evidenced that little progress has been made: the language used in Brazilian PILs is still far from being consistent, clear and reader-friendly.

According to ANVISA, only 17% of all Brazilian PILs were adapted according to RDC 47/2009 from 2010 to 2012 due to operational limitations. The implications of the delay are negative for all institutions and actors involved. For the agency, it perpetuates its difficulty to manage the PILs; for the pharmaceutical industry, it is difficult to adapt PILs in a scenario of constant transition between RDCs; and for the population and healthcare professionals, the current PILs fail to guide prescription, administration and rational and safe use of medicines as there are two standards of PILs available on the market nowadays. In addition, few PILs are available electronically (e-Bulas) preventing Brazilian citizens from full and safe access to effective information on medicines.

We claim that Brazilian regulatory agency has to keep on developing projects towards the easification and clarification of the PILs mainly with the aid of expert linguists and applied linguists. There will come a time, we hope, that legislation and/or regulations on medicine and healthcare will involve the collaborative task force of language experts and professional drafters, no more limited to the chambers of jurists, congressmen or bureaucrats. As very little research is conducted in this area, we suggest further studies should include, for example, misunderstandings and interpretive obstacles in PIL communication, and the exploration of further easification procedures to improve the drafting of Brazilian PILs. More practically, the training of PIL drafters directed to both professional and academic audience by expert linguists would surely contribute to create a new class of experts not available in Brazil nowadays.

References

Agar, Michael 1985. Institutional Discourse. *Text Interdisciplinary Journal for the Study of Discourse* 5/3, 147–168.

Bhatia, Vijay K. 1983. Simplification v. Easification. The Case of Legal Texts. *Applied Linguistics* 4/1, 42–54.

Bhatia, Vijay K. 1993. *Analysing Genre: Language Use in Professional Settings*. London: Longman.

Bhatia, Vijay K. 1994. Generic Integrity in Professional Discourse. In Gunnarson, Britt-Louise / Linell, Per / Norberg, Bengt (eds) *Text and Talk in Professional Contexts*. Sweden: Association Suédoise de Linguistique Appliquée, 61–76.

Bhatia, Vijay K. 2004. *Worlds of Written Discourse. A Genre-based View*. New York: Continuum.

Briggs, Charles L. / Bauman, Richard 1992. Genre, Intertextuality, and Social Power. *Journal of Linguistic Anthropology* 2/2, 131–172.

Child, Barbara 1992. *Drafting Legal Documents. Principles and Practices*. St. Paul, Minn.: West Group.

Compêndio de Bulas de Medicamentos- CBM 2005. Ministério da Saúde. Agência de Vigilância Sanitária, Brasília: Anvisa.

Fairclough, Norman 2001. *Discurso e Mudança Social*. Brasília: UnB.

Fage-Butler, Antoinette. 2013. Improving Patient-Information Leaflets: Developing and Applying an Evaluative Model of Patient-Centredness for Text. *Communication & Medicine* 10/2, 105–115.

Garner, Brian A. 2009. *Garner on Language and Writing*. Chicago: American Bar Association.

Gläser, Rosemary 1995. *Linguistic Features and Genre Profiles of Scienfic English*. Frankfurt am Main: Peter Lang.

Halliday, Michael A.K. / Hasan, Ruqaya 1989. *Language, Context, and Text: Aspects of Language in a Social-Semiotic Perspective*. Oxford: Oxford University Press.

Kenny, T., Wilson, R.G., Purves, I.N., Clark, J., Newton, L.D., Neweton, D.P. and Mosel, D.V. 1988. A PIL for Every Ill? Patient Information Leaflets (PILs): A Review of Past, Present and Future Use. *Family Practice* 15/5, 471–179. <http:dx.doi.org/10.1093/fampra/15.5.471>.

Kristeva, Julia 1986. *The Kristeva Reader*. London: Basil Blackwell.

Miller, Carolyn R. 1984. Genre as Social Action. *Quarterly Journal of Speech* 70, 151–167.

Quirk, Randolph / Greenbaum, Sidney / Leech, Geoffrey / Svartvik, Jan 1985. *A Comprehensive Grammar of the English Language*. London: Longman.

Scollon, Ron 2001. *Mediated Discourse: The Nexus of Practice*. London: Routledge.

Shuy, Roger W. / Larkin, Donald L. 1978. Linguistic Consideration in the Simplification/Clarification of Insurance Policy Language. *Discourse Processes* 1, 305–321.

Zhang, Qiao 1998. Fuzziness – Vagueness – Generality – Ambiguity. *Journal of Pragmatics* 29, 13–31.

Rosita Maglie

'Can you Read this Leaflet?': User-friendliness of Patient Information Leaflets in the UK and in Italy*

Notwithstanding the growth of electronically-mediated information, for many people the primary or only source of information about their medicine still remains the patient information leaflet (PIL).[1] The PIL became a legal requirement in 1992 when "the European Commission issued Directive 92/27/EEC on the labeling of medicinal products for human use and on package leaflets" (Graham 2009: 5). As a result, since 1999 all medicines have been supplied with PILs to ensure their secure and effective use. The PIL contains information, in accordance with several legal regulations and standards, produced by the pharmaceutical company. The content and structure of the PIL should be legible, clear and easy to use – therefore it is a legally regulated genre (Askehave/Zethsen 2003) – and should reflect information contained in the Summary of Product Characteristics (SPC).[2]

Like the PIL, the SPC is another document which is produced by the pharmaceutical company; the SPC is used to apply for marketing authorization with the European Medicines Agency (EMA). Unlike the PIL, the SPC is an expert-to-expert text which contains information for healthcare professionals. Composed in English, the SPC uses technical

---

* I would like to thank the Editors of this volume and Professor Sarangi for their constructive comments on an early draft of this chapter. I would also like to thank Max Rankenburg for his help editing the chapter in its various stages.

1 For further information regarding the role of patient information leaflets in an information-rich society, see 'Always Read the Leaflet': getting the best information with every medicine' (2005: 8): <http://www.mhra.gov.uk/home/groups/pla/documents/publication/con2018041.pdf>.

2 Article 63(2) of Directive 2001/83/EC requires that the package leaflet must be written and designed to be clear and understandable, enabling users to act appropriately, when necessary with the help of health professionals. <http://www.mhra.gov.uk/home/groups/pla/documents/websiteresources/con157151.pdf>.

terminology (Nisbeth Jensen/Zethsen 2012: 33). It provides the EMA with a full description of the medicine so that the agency can assess whether the medicine should be authorized. When a pharmaceutical company receives authorization, it produces the English-language PIL, which is intended for a general audience, based on the SPC, which was designed for experts. Considering that the PIL is written in accordance with the SPC, it undergoes a process of intralingual translation[3] as it should be adapted to the new target readership, i.e. the layperson. Then the PIL is translated into the other relevant Member State languages and undergoes another process of translation, i.e. the interlingual translation. Thus, non-English language European PILs are translations as required by Article 63(2) of EU Directive 2001/83/EC according to which the PIL must be available in all the languages of the Member States where the drug is marketed. In addition, the EU Commission has released guidelines for the production of PILs in order to make them "accessible to the general public and [...] ensure appropriate use of the medicine" (Zethsen/Askehave 2010: 98); and EMA has developed a set of templates for the writing of PILs (2010: 98).

Before concluding this background for the present research, I would like to mention one final EU initiative, as it is pertinent to the present analysis. The 'PIL of the month' initiative (Zethsen/Askehave 2010: 99), undertaken by the Medicine and Healthcare Products Regulatory Agency (MHRA) in the UK in 2007, is designed to provide best-practice examples of PILs on its website. Additionally the MHRA has made available a set of quality criteria by which the PILs of the month have been chosen. The quality criteria for PILs provide a numerical score which gives an indication of quality. They are divided into two thematic parts: the first deals with *process indicators* and gives points for involvement of patients in the PIL development, points for evidence that needs of special populations have been catered for, and points for user testing; the second part deals with *leaflet indicators* and gives points for presentation (text readability and ease of navigation)

3 Askehave/Zethsen (2000b: 64–65) advance another label for the intralingual translation process which a PIL undergoes. They call it inter-generic translation, i.e. the translation of a text from one genre into another genre, referring to the fact that PILs should be written in accordance with another genre, i.e. the SPC.

and points for content. Zethsen and Askehave (2010) have found that the published quality criteria on which the selection builds hardly mention linguistic features at all (they only refer to the use of medical jargon). In general Zethsen and Askehave found many positive features and improvements on more traditional solutions, though they also found many features which have a negative impact on user-friendliness. Only one leaflet evaluated in their study was found to demonstrate a real best-practice example, while six leaflets were a mixture of positive and negative features, and three leaflets were far from constituting best-practice approaches from a linguistic point of view. The PIL of the month initiative, and the Zethsen/Askehave study of best practices in UK PILs of the month, suggest the following hypothesis:

- If the UK PIL of the month follows the parameters (e.g. font size, capitals, headlines, lay terms, grouping of side effects, etc.) set out in the quality criteria document, which constitute best practice examples of user-friendliness, the Italian counterpart of the English PIL of the month should do the same.

The initiative and the Zethsen/Askehave study also suggest the following research questions:

- How do the Italian counterparts of the English PILs of the month continue to demonstrate best-practice examples of user-friendliness?
- In what ways does lay-friendliness get 'lost in translation' when PILs cross borders?
- Does lay-friendliness change with the change of the drug category, and if so why?

The chapter is organized as follows. After presenting background information on the PIL, in Section 1 I provide a review of the literature, focusing on three research trends: (1) text analysis studies, (2) studies which draw on consumer consultation and the testing of PILs, and (3) translation-oriented text analysis studies.[4] In the next section I offer

4 As to the division of the literature into different types of studies, I refer to Zethsen/Askehave (2010: 100). I have added the last type in order to better focus my review of research which deals with the PIL.

a description of the data, which consists of a corpus of 65 PILs of the month. A selection of PILs will be analyzed contrastively with their counterparts in the Italian language (i.e. three sets of PILs belonging to three different categories: over-the-counter (OTC) drugs, OTC drugs with medical supervision, and drugs with medical prescription). The last set of PILs is particularly interesting not only in that it addresses another drug category, but insofar as the PILs are parallel texts, direct translations of each other. With the research questions in mind, I then discuss the results, comparing them to previous research and outlining new research pathways and approaches to other genres of medical discourse. I conclude the enquiry on the popularization of medical discourse in the UK and in Italy by providing an account of the degree of differences (greater or lesser) detected across the three categories of drugs investigated, with reference to user-friendliness, norms, ways of conveying information, and presumed level of medical knowledge.

1. Literature review

In close connection with the literature on the accessibility and user-friendliness of PILs, Zethsen and Askehave (2010: 100) distinguish two types of studies:

1. 'text analysis studies', i.e. studies that primarily rely on the researcher's evaluation of text accessibility; and
2. studies which are based on consumer consultation and the testing of PILs – often in 'original' and 'redesigned' forms.

Their distinction is due to the fact that the accessibility of many PILs is "still considered problematic" (Zethsen/Askehave 2010: 102) and type 1 and 2 studies show, with their own peculiar methods of investigation, that "careful consideration and redesign of patient information leaflets tend to result to more user-friendly and accessible leaflets" (2010: 102). This study falls into type 1 study, as it is based on my evaluation of a controversial aspect of text accessibility, that is user-friendliness in British PILs. But it also addresses further aspects of PILs which concern the user-friendliness and accessibility of PILs translated into another Member State language, i.e. Italian. Consequently I suggest to add to the previous ones, a third type of study, namely,

3. translation-oriented text analysis studies, grouping studies that are based on the translation of PILs into the EU languages.

However, several studies of PILs break through barriers as they involve not only one but often two types of studies. This study, as already mentioned above, can be included into type 1, as it investigates lay-friendliness of corpora made up of original PILs, but it also belongs to type 3, as it uses comparable and parallel texts relying on a mixed-method approach composed of corpus and text analysis. On the other hand, Askehave and Zethsen's (2008) study involves both types of studies, i.e. 1 and 2: it deals with another mandatory EU patient information genre, i.e. the European Public Assessment Report (EPAR) summary, and investigates its functionality and readability by identifying a quantity of problematic linguistic areas. Through a questionnaire and a marking exercise, respondents were asked to mark words and passages in the EPAR that they were unable to understand, and to state how specialist language raised significant problems.

Askehave and Zethsen, together with other researchers, have been prolific in the field of PIL studies. Together they have carried out valuable work (2000a, 2003). They have analyzed EU PILs and in particular the passage of information from the Product Summary (PS) to the PIL. By focusing on the common linguistic features found in the PIL which may be hard to understand for a general readership, they list "medical jargon, false friends, officialese, inconsistent terminology, a passive impersonal style, and information-packed sentences" (Askehave/Zethsen 2010: 100). Askehave/Zethsen (2010: 101) cite another study by Clerehan and Buchbinder (2006) that adds other aspects which may hinder PIL accessibility. They note "inconsistent or inappropriate headings, unclear rhetorical functions (e.g. an instruction realized as information), formatting features used randomly, direct/indirect style (thus confusing as to whether the information actually applies to the patient), etc."

Many other studies address the complexity of PIL production and how this influences the final version of the leaflet which, instead of being legible, clear, and easy to use, is not completely user-friendly or readable. Patients in such cases are unable to understand the PIL due to difficult lexis, complex syntax, small font, etc. (Askehave/Zethsen 2000b, 2002, 2003; Dickinson *et al.* 2001; Gal/Prigat 2005; Graham 2009; Harwood/Harrison 2004; Horwitz *et al.* 2009; Nisbeth Jensen 2013; MHRA 2005; Pander Maat/Lentz 2010; Raynor 2007). Specifically, the Pander Maat/Lentz study (2010) can be considered both a type 1 and type 2 study, as it evaluates the usability of three PILs with the aim of improving them while conforming to current EU regulations. These three PILs were tested among 154 potential users. The results reveal that these suffer from usability problems, in particular problems with reference to finding relevant information and comprehension of the information. The authors then revised the leaflets and all three revisions end in "increased localization, comprehension and appreciation" (Pander Maat/Lentz 2010: 118).

Closely connected to type 1 has been the research on PIL and patient empowerment (Aarva/Tampere 2006; Askehave/Zethsen 2010; Askehave *et al.* 2010; Dickinson *et al.* 2003; Johnson 1999; Hall 2006; Larsen/Manderson 2008; Roberts 2006). In particular, Hall's (2006) work warns against the greater availability and transparency of information which is not always a guarantee of empowerment in the hands of laypeople since the empowerment control still remains in the hidden agenda of the powerful (Gotti/Salager-Meyer 2006: 16).

Research on the usability of PILs in languages other than English, which pertains to type 3, continues to report that a large number of PILs are not user-friendly (Askehave/Zethsen 2002, 2003, 2010; Bongaarts 2009; Cacchiani 2006; Nisbeth Jensen/Zethsen 2012; Montalt/ Gonzalez Davies 2007). For instance, Askehave and Zethsen (2003: 40) found that: "the Danish PPIs [patient package inserts, the same as PILs] were more formal and dominated by expert syntax and terms than the English originals". In fact evidence suggests that the translation factor and its complexity is overlooked by the EU since the PIL only needs to be tested in one language, which is usually its original language, that is, English (Raynor 2007, Nisbeth Jensen/Zethsen 2012: 33). The fundamental cause of this user-unfriendliness of the translation products may be found in the PIL translators' qualifications and professional backgrounds (Montalt/Shuttleworth 2012: 18). On this point, Nisbeth Jensen and Zethsen (2012) carried out a study investigating whether any difference exists between Source Text (ST) PIL and Target Text (TT) PIL from pharmaceutical companies that use professional translators and pharmacists, respectively. They show that TT PILs translated by pharmacists overestimate the reader's medical knowledge, and confirm what Bromme *et al.* (2005: 571) claim by quoting them as saying that "there is a good deal of evidence that experts have difficulty in adapting their advice to the information needs of laypersons" (in Nisbeth Jensen/Zethsen 2012: 45).

The present analysis is a type 3 study in that the research question investigates potential dissimilarities in the translation products of PILs. My results are compared with another study by Askehave and Zethsen (2010) which analyzed a corpus consisting of ten PILs of the month, and turn out to be broader in scope as the corpus that I compiled ad-hoc comprises all the PILs of the month and not just a small selection of them. This chapter thus enlarges the aim outlined by Zethsen and Askehave by making a comparison between some of the PILs in PILC with their corresponding counterparts in Italian.

2. PILC: best practices for text readability and ease of navigation

The present study investigates the UK PIL Corpus (PILC; size: 853,291 running words) to determine which linguistic factors contribute to text readability and ease of navigation, drawing on the above literature on PILs which provides evidence that plain language, a user-friendly design, and a clear lay-out improve text comprehension.[5] Of the quality

5 Zethsen and Askehave (2010: 100) recommend Kimble's work (1994–1995: 62–65) for an ad-hoc overview of empirical studies which show how plain language enhances understanding; they also provide a list of linguistic features

criteria used by the MHRA's Commission on Human Medicines Expert Advisory Group on Patient Information to confer the title of PILs of the month, this analysis addresses the involvement of the PIL receiver (i.e. second person pronoun and verbs), the use of lay terms instead of medical jargon (i.e. terminological simplification), and the use of clear and purposeful headlines followed by simple grammatical structures.

2.1 Text readability: the involvement of PIL receiver and terminological simplification

The word list automatically generated in frequency order shows that the texts are reader-oriented. *You* and *your* occur 4,194 and 1,480 respectively. The clustering relationship between a second person pronoun and adjective is quite strong, as they co-occur 908 times in 47 out of the 49 texts; the most frequent pattern is an imperative verb (e.g. *talk to, tell, inform*) + "your doctor if/before you". Such data suggest that advice provided by the PIL (on what to do "if you are pregnant", for instance), insofar as it addresses the reader directly (in the use of the second person), acquires the features of speech rather than of writing (as is the use of the imperative).

As to terminological simplification, in the frequency list the first term to appear refers to the commercial name of a drug, *nicorette* (192 times), which is found in only two texts, and the active ingredient, *methylphenidate* (158 times), which occurs in five texts. The low occurrence of terms and the nature of the terms detected (related to commercial names and active ingredients) cannot be considered a serious obstacle for the reader's full understanding of the PIL. Rather, the low occurrence of terms makes such texts highly divulgatory and readable as they develop a tone similar to that found in a reassuring expert-to-layperson interaction.

---

which boost the accessibility of texts addressed to laypeople. Given the constraints of this chapter, I am only able to deal with a small number of features included in Zethsen and Askehave's list, but think they constitute the correct representation of the most frequent features of the PILC.

2.2. *Ease of navigation: use of headlines followed by simple grammatical structures*

With regard to ease of navigation, the study examines the structure of the English PILs included in the PILC. Their structure is more or less standardized and fixed, usually comprising six important sections (that will be dealt with below), with the exceptions of section 1 (the name of the medicine), section 7 (the Marketing Authorization Holder and Manufacturer), and section 8 (the date of the last revision of the leaflet)[6]. In particular the analysis addresses the use of headers and sub-headings as aids in navigation. Since the most common practice in these PILs is to put at the beginning of the pamphlet a list of numbered headings, this investigation searches for numbers from 1 to 6 – which precede in numerical order each main heading – and then examines their collocates. The introduction to a PIL usually includes a heading that reads "what the medicine is and what it is used for". In particular, the string *what it is used for* occurs twice in 24 out of 60 PILs. It is first included in the list of numbered headings and then it corresponds to the proper heading. The plot for this string shows that it is distributed more or less in the same parts of the 24 texts.

The heading of the contra-indication starts the second section and the searched number + word sequence is *Before*. It occurs 55 times in 28 texts and almost always clusters with *you use/take* + the commercial name of the drug. The third section is on drug dosage and the heading is *how to take/use* + the drug name in 22 texts. In the side-effect section the expression *side effects* is preceded by the adjective *possible* in 23 of the 24 and corresponds to the fourth heading of the PILs. The heading which describes how to store the medicine is generally *how to store* + the drug name, or in some rare cases the gerund of *take* is used followed by *this medicine* or *how* + the drug name + *should be stored.* Only in medicines which help the client to give up smoking does the gerund *taking* collocate with *and disposal* (8 out of 8 times). The sixth and final paragraph gives further information on the drug. The string

6 Sections 1, 7, and 8 are not linguistically significant, since these sections only contain trade names both for drugs and pharmaceutical companies, and numbers, i.e. the PIL revision date.

further information occurs in 40 out of 60 texts proving to be the most frequent and unchanging formula in PILCs.

The practice of starting the leaflet with a list of numbered headings helps the reader become familiar with the leaflet's style and organization. The headlines are clear and purposeful insofar as they use simple, recurring words (e.g. *take, use*) and simple sentence constructions (*wh*-words + to + infinitive/*wh*-words + gerund). If the interaction between functional headings and simple grammatical structures results in a remarkable ease of navigation, the interplay between plain language choices and reader centeredness contributes positively to text readability. Both features are considered best-practice examples in the leaflets.

Concerning section 1, I investigated a selection of Italian PILs in order to verify whether qualities found in the English corpus were duplicated in PILs distributed in Italy. I selected PILs for three drug categories: (a) OTC, (b) OTC after doctor's advice, and (c) with prescription. They were investigated in terms of parameters established in the quality criteria document, such as layout, information distribution and information load (to asses text navigation), lay terminology vs. medical jargon, and second person pronoun and verbs (to test text readability). Each category includes one couple composed of a British PIL with its comparable Italian PIL, as they have in common the same active ingredients, the same name and/or the same drug companies. The last category is comprised of two couples of British and Italian PILs, and includes parallel texts since the Italian texts are the translation of the English ones. As the client's autonomy in drug choice is greater in OTC drugs, I hypothesized that in this category terminological simplification, interaction and user-friendliness would be more important and marked than in the last category of PILs. Additionally, this investigation was carried out contrastively.

3. Over-the-counter drug PILs

In order to address the research hypothesis the following sub-sections will analyze and compare PILs of three different categories in English and in Italian in order to investigate how the British PILs rated so highly according to the Commission on Human Medicines system, and to determine whether the Italian counterparts had linguistic qualities similar to the English PILs. This sub-section starts the analysis with *Vicks Sinex Soother* and the Italian counterpart *Sinex Aloe*[7] which are OTC drugs which you can buy without a prescription. The *Vicks Sinex Soother* PIL was considered the PIL of the month by the Commission on Human Medicines Expert Advisory Group on Patient Information on July 18, 2008. The PIL's clarity and simplicity enable patients to use the medicine safely and efficiently. The Italian counterpart was last approved in March 2009. But does the Italian PIL, released a year after its English counterpart, achieve the clarity of its predecessor?

3.1 Layout, information distribution and information load

At first sight, the English PIL is far more visually engaging than its Italian counterpart. As Montalt and Garcìa Izquierdo observe (oral communication 20 June 2014), the layout of the PIL facilitates text readability and navigation. Accordingly the English PIL frames and highlights sections presenting vital information. Conversely, black print in varying font size is used for the entire text in the Italian PIL. The arrangement of elements, such as paragraph order, also differs. The Italian PIL, unlike its English counterpart, does not begin with a list of numbered headings which would facilitate navigation of the text. The diverse structure of the Italian PIL, assuming that it offers a schema according to readers' expectations, implies that Italian consumers are first of all interested in the active substances in the medicine, and in how the medicine looks. Conversely English patients find this information at the end of the PIL, under a generic heading. The Italian PIL also does not include side effect frequencies, while the English PIL gives details in percentages of

7 The original texts of both PILs are available on the web: the English PIL can be found at <http://www.mhra.gov.uk/Howweregulate/Medicines/Labelspatientinformationleafletsandpackaging/Patientinformationleaflet(PIL)ofthemonth/>, and the Italian PIL in a new revision (April 2012) is now at <http://www.torrinomedica.it/farmaci/schedetecniche/Vicks_Sinex_Aloe_Soluzione_Da_Nebulizzare.asp>.

the probabilities a side effect may occur. On the other hand, the Italian PIL does provide a full and accurate account of all the signs and symptoms the patient might have if using an excessive amount of *Vicks Aloe*, while the English PIL, perhaps to avoid frightening the consumer, states explicitly that in such an event the patient should request a medical check-up. In particular, the English PIL states: "If you use too much *Vicks Sinex Soother* you should contact your doctor or go to a hospital immediately and take the bottle or pack with you". In the Italian PIL we find:

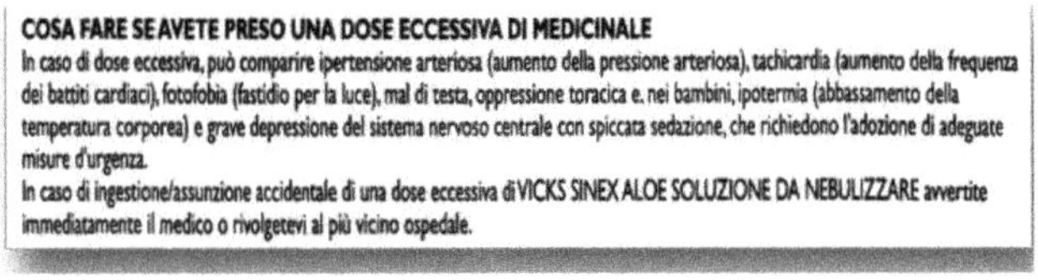

COSA FARE SE AVETE PRESO UNA DOSE ECCESSIVA DI MEDICINALE
In caso di dose eccessiva, può comparire ipertensione arteriosa (aumento della pressione arteriosa), tachicardia (aumento della frequenza dei battiti cardiaci), fotofobia (fastidio per la luce), mal di testa, oppressione toracica e. nei bambini, ipotermia (abbassamento della temperatura corporea) e grave depressione del sistema nervoso centrale con spiccata sedazione, che richiedono l'adozione di adeguate misure d'urgenza.
In caso di ingestione/assunzione accidentale di una dose eccessiva di VICKS SINEX ALOE SOLUZIONE DA NEBULIZZARE avvertite immediatamente il medico o rivolgetevi al più vicino ospedale.

Figure 1. From the *Vicks Aloe* PIL, on the improper use of the medicine.[8]

3.2 Lay terminology vs. jargon

There is a fairly balanced use of common words and technical terms in both PILs. As Figure 1 shows, terminological simplification is achieved by rewording specialist terminology in brackets. However, while the Italian PIL uses brackets coherently, in the case of the technical terms "ipertensione arteriosa (aumento della pressione arteriosa), tachicardia (aumento della frequenza dei battiti cardiaci)", the English PIL sometimes inserts the acronym between brackets – for example, ("monoamine oxidase inhibitors (MAOIs)") – the corresponding simple expression ("sinusitis (inflammation of the passages leading to the nose"),

8 Back translation) **What to do if you have taken too much medicine**. In case of an excessive dose, hypertension (high blood pressure), tachycardia (faster heart rate), photophobia (painful oversensitivity to light), headache, and chest oppression can manifest themselves, and, in children, hypothermia (low body temperature), and serious depression of the nervous system with marked sedation, which need the adoption of urgent measures. In case of accidental swallowing/taking of an excessive dose of *Vicks Sinex Aloe* nebulizer solution immediately inform the doctor or go to the nearest hospital.

or the technical term ("increased eyeball pressure (narrow-angle glaucoma").

3.3 Second person pronoun and verbs

The presence of the personal pronoun *you* (26 occurrences) and of the possessive adjective *your* (20 occurrences) is not only significant but shows how the English PIL addresses the reader through interactive headings: *before you use..., do not use..., if you...* etc. On the other hand, the Italian PIL directly addresses the client in rare occasions. In conformity with Italian grammar norms, second person pronouns never occur. The adjective *vostro/a/e/i* occurs only once ("chiedete consiglio al *vostro* medico o farmacista [ask *your* doctor or pharmacist for advice]"). I searched for *-ate*, *-ete*, and *-ite*, which correspond to the suffixes of verbs in the second person plural and looked for second person singular endings. I found four instances of the verb in the second person plural ending with *-ate*, four instances of *-ete*, and only one of *-ite,* and no occurrence of the verb in the second person singular.

(1) '*-ate*' concordance
1 sul medicinale, pertanto **conserv**ate sia la scatola che il
2 sospettate uno stato di gravidanza o **desider**ate pianificare una maternità.
3 di consultare il medico nel caso **sospett**ate uno stato di gravidanza o
4 consumo di alcol. Se **st**ate usando altri medicinali chiedete

(2) '*-ete*' concordance
1 disturbo si presenta ripetutamente o se **av**ete notato un qualsiasi
2 sue caratteristiche. COSA FARE SE **AV**ETE PRESO UNA DOSE
3 di AUTOMEDICAZIONE che **pot**ete usare per curare disturbi lievi e
4 Se state usando altri medicinale **chied**ete consiglio al vostro medico o

(3) '*-ite*' concordance
1 SOLUZIONE DA NEBULIZZARE **avvert**ite immediatamente il medico o

For headings, the most recurrent titles are drug-oriented. The subject of the heading is usually *Vicks Aloe* ("perchè si usa, quando non deve essere usato, quando può essere usato dopo aver consultato il medico [why it is used, when it cannot be used, when it can be used after having asked the doctor for advice]"). When the subject is not the medicine, the headlines have sentences with generic subjects: with the particle *si* ("quando si usa [when one uses it]"), or the verb in the second person plural ("cosa fare se avete preso una dose eccessiva di medicinale [what to do if you have taken a strong dose of medication]"), or generic titles ("scadenza e conservazione [expiration date and storage]").

The analysis of the first couple of PILs which belong to the category of OTC drugs reveals that the texts differ in the following ways: in information provided, in the level of readability, and in reader involvement. For medicines purchased OTC, face-to-face interaction between the patient and the healthcare professional may be restricted or absent. In this case written information plays a vital role for the safe use of the medicine. Beyond doubt the British PIL is more user-friendly and visually engaging, and the Italian PIL is more medicine-oriented and lacks the visual appeal of its counterpart. In particular, with reference to side effects, the inclusion of frequencies in the English PIL proves to be helpful to readers as it puts the risk in context. On the other hand, the Italian PIL uses a system organ class arrangement for side effects which adopts a logic and presentation that only a healthcare professional can follow. Patients prefer the grouping of side effects in terms of seriousness so that they can understand when to take action and what action should be (on this issue see PIL guidance 0712 final 2012: 5).

4. PILs for OTC drugs taken according to the advice of a doctor or pharmacist

This second sub-section continues the analysis with *Calpol* and *Tachipirina*[9] which are OTC drugs but they may require the direct supervision of a physician. I chose the PILs for *Calpol* and *Tachipirina* because

9 The original texts of both PILs are available on the web: the English PIL can be found at <http://www.mhra.gov.uk/Howweregulate/Medicines/Labelspatientinformationleafletsandpackaging/Patientinformationleaflet(PIL)ofthemonth/>, and the Italian PIL at <http://www.pharmamedix.com/img/pdffogliettiillustrativi/tachipirina_sciroppo_foglietto_illustrativo.pdf>.

they have the same active ingredient, i.e. paracetamol. Both PILs were revised in June 2011.

4.1 *Layout and information distribution*

At the structural level, comparing the Italian PIL for this drug with the English version reveals differences in text choice, font styles, in the use of headings, and in the use of symbols. The English PIL uses a larger font, different color and font type for headings and subheadings, and often incorporates exclamation marks or other informative icons, where as topic-giving and thematizing headings – always a black, bold font – appear in the Italian text (e.g. "indicazioni terapeutiche" [therapeutic indications] versus "what the medicine is for"). Another structural device that helps the reader immediately understand dosage quantities according to age is rendered in the English PIL with a colored table, by the use of icons which catch the reader's attention, and the use of different font sizes and colored headings. The Italian PIL, by comparison, consists of a long list of black-on-white text in a small font, and underscored headings organized in bullet points (Figures 2 and 3).

Children from 3 months to 6 years

Child's age	How much - up to 4 times a day
3-6 months	One 2.5 ml spoonful (small end)
6-24 months	One 5 ml spoonful (large end)
2-4 years	One 5 ml spoonful (large end) and one 2.5 ml spoonful (small end)
4-6 years	Two 5 ml spoonfuls (large end)

- Do not give more than 4 doses in any 24 hour period.
- Leave at least 4 hours between doses.
- Do not give this medicine to your child for more than 3 days without speaking to your doctor or pharmacist.

- Bambini di peso compreso tra 7 e 10 kg (approssimativamente tra i 6 ed i 18 mesi): 5 ml alla volta (corrispondenti a 120 mg di paracetamolo), da ripetere se necessario dopo 6 ore, senza superare le 4 somministrazioni al giorno.

- Bambini di peso compreso tra 21 e 25 kg (approssimativamente tra i 6 ed i 10 anni): 10 ml alla volta (corrispondenti a 240 mg di paracetamolo), da ripetere se necessario dopo 4 ore, senza superare le 6 somministrazioni al giorno.

Figures 2 and 3. Dosage rules in English and Italian PILs.

4.2 *Lay terminology vs. jargon*

The Italian PIL appears to have a highly specific informational purpose, and uses a specialized language which implies communication between equals or near-equals in knowledge and professional role. For example, the term *paracetamol* appears in the Italian PIL but does not appear in the English table. Another example of specialist-to-specialist communication appears in the section addressing the overuse of *Tachipirina*. Here we find language features usually present in specialized texts. For example, the Italian PIL includes:

- Technical terms which are not defined for a general reader (e.g., *transaminasi epatiche, lattico-deidrogenasi, bilirubinemia, protrombina* [liver transaminase; lactic dehydrogenase; bilirubinemia, prothrombin]);
- The use of passive phrases (e.g., *vengono osservati* [are observed]);
- Nominalization, to express concepts related to actions and practices (Maglie 2009) (e.g. *incremento, riduzione, ingestione, ricovero, somministrazione* [increase; lowering; swallowing; admission; administration]);
- Verbs which link nominalizations in thematic position to other nominalizations, or link phrases made of very specialized terms in rhematic positions, lose their role and act as a copula, making sentences longer and longer. For example: "In caso di sovradosaggio il paracetamolo può provocare citolisi epatica che può evolvere verso la necrosi massiva e irreversibile, con conseguente insufficienza epato-cellulare, acidosi metabolica ed encefalopatia, che possono portare al coma e alla morte. [In case of overuse paracemol can cause hepatic cytolysis which can lead to massive and irreversible necrosis, with a consequent epato-cellular deficiency, methabolic acidosis and encephalopatia, which can result in coma and death"].

Conversely, the British PIL simplifies the same section by providing a text which omits information that only a physician would understand and find useful (e.g., "If anyone has too much. Immediate medical advice should be sought in the event of an overdose, even if the child seems well, because of the risk of delayed, serious liver damage").

4.3 Second person pronoun and interpersonal communication

While the English PIL uses a personal and direct tone, the manner of the Italian PIL is detached and impersonal. Describing how to store this medicine, the English PIL states: "Keep the product out of the reach and sight of children [...] Ask *your* pharmacist how to dispose of medicines no longer required." The Italian counterpart to these sentences begins with the infinitive of the verb *keep* which strikes an impersonal note: "*Tenere* il medicinale fuori dalla portata e dalla vista dei bambini. [Keep the product out of the reach and the sight of children]". The PIL then uses the polite third person singular form of the verb *ask*: "*Chieda* al farmacista come eliminare i medicinali che non utilizza più. [Ask the pharmacist how to dispose of medicines no longer used"]. Contrary to the previous Italian PIL, which uses the second person plural to address the reader, here the tone is more detached and formal. Additionally, no personal adjective occurs in this Italian PIL. The word *doctor*, for instance, that in most cases in the English PIL collocates with the personal adjective *your* (in 12 out of 15 cases), in the Italian PIL is preceded by the definite article. In such usage we perceive a lack of emotive language nuance

(4) Chiedete consiglio al **medico** o a farmacista prima di
apprezzabili, consultate il **medico**. Gravidanza e allattamento.
consecutive senza consultare il **medico**. INTERAZIONI
qualsiasi altro farmaco contattare il **medico**. Vedere anche 'Interazioni'.
sotto diretto controllo del **medico**. Guida di veicoli ed utilizzo di
e sotto il diretto controllo **medico**. Durante il trattamento con
immediatamente il **medico** o rivolgersi al più vicino
foglio illustrativo, informare il **medico** o il farmacista. SCADENZA
INTERAZIONI Informare il **medico** o il farmacista se si è
gocce contiene: -sorbitolo: se il **medico** le ha diagnosticato una
contiene: -sorbitolo: se il **medico** le ha diagnosticato una
solo sotto stretto controllo **medico**. Lo stesso vale nei casi di

In the Italian PIL I also found four occurrences of the particle *si*, which functions as a general subject:

(5) aggrava, o se **si** nota la comparsa di un qualsiasi
informare il medico o il farmacista se **si** è recentemente assunto qualsiasi
sciroppo contiene: saccarosio di ciò **si** tenga conto in pazienti diabetici
a carico della madre o del bambino, **si** consiglia di somministrare il

Another way the Italian PIL addresses the reader in general terms is in the use of verbs in the infinitive form: verbs ending with *-are* address a general subject in 30 out of 47 occurrences, in *-ere* in 31 out of the 35 occurrences, and in *-ire* in 2 out of 4.

The analysis of this second group of PILs shows increasing linguistic differences with respect to the first group. In this case, the Italian version of the British PIL is characterized by terminology which addresses a reader, such as a doctor or pharmacist, who has specialized knowledge. The Italian PIL does not provide a best-practice example as it does not promote patient centeredness, which is considered a consistent feature of best-practice examples. As Zethsen/Askehave remark, "[t]he point of departure of the utterances *should* be the patient and his or her immediate situational context and presumed state of knowledge" (2010: 111, my italics). Thus, unlike technical texts which prefer specialized medical terminology, nominalized, objective and passive style with empty verbs, the Italian PILs of OTC drugs taken according to the advice of a doctor or pharmacist should promote user-friendliness by structuring the prose "around a human agent performing actions in a particularized situation" (Killingsworth 1987: 105, quoted in Zethsen/Askehave 2010: 112), i.e. reproducing his or her 'real' ways of doing and acting when s/he suffers from an illness.

5. PILs of Drugs requiring a prescription

The following and final sub-section considers PILs of drugs which require a doctor's prescription. From now on the investigation changes as these couples of PILs are made up of original PILs written in English and their translation into Italian, and it will focus on each section of the PILs, to see better how they differ section by section, and to investigate properly the research question on whether and/or how much of the good work in rendering the PIL informative and lay-friendly is damaged when the PIL is translated (Askehave/Zethsen 2011: 14).

Spiriva and *Spiriva Respimat*[10] are drugs available only with a doctor's prescription. The PILs for *Spiriva* and *Spiriva Respimat* were highly rated by the Commission on Human Medicines Expert Advisory Group on Patient Information on November 5, 2010. The PIL for the Italian counterpart of *Spiriva* was revised in December 2009, and the PIL for the Italian counterpart of *Spiriva Respimat* was revised in December 2010. Of the four texts, the study analyzes the British PILs in order to identify linguistic differences between them. Then it compares these with their Italian counterparts, investigating similarities and differences between the source texts and the target texts. The aim of the investigation is to locate problematic passages and to determine the norms and methods followed by the translator.[11] As Montalt and González Davies have argued,

> Parallel texts are tools which help us to become aware of key aspects of target text production such as tenor, modality, phraseological patterns, prototypical macrostructure and extension of target genre, terminological and stylistic preferences of the client, and so on, and to discover the conventions expected by the readership of a particular genre in a specific context. (2007: 224)

5.1 Section 1: Introduction

Starting from the general information section of these PILs, the study first considers the preferred wordings in both sets of PILs. Prefabricated expressions are identical in the two English PILs but differ in the TTs. Instructions such as "Read all of this leaflet carefully before you start taking this medicine" (see Figure 4) are rendered in the TT with a

---

10 The original texts of both sets of PILs are available on the web: the English PILs can be found at <http://www.mhra.gov.uk/Howweregulate/Medicines/Labels patientinformationleafletsandpackaging/Patientinformationleaflet(PIL)ofthe month/>, and the Italian PILs in a different schematic format at <http://www.torrinomedica.it/farmaci/schedetecniche/Spiriva.asp#P10> and at <http://www.torrinomedica.it/farmaci/schedetecniche/Spiriva_Respimat_Sol_1_Inal_60_D.asp>.

11 As far as typographic conventions are concerned, there is a perfect symmetry between the four PILs: the same background, the same icons, the same black text, the same print size, and the same headings.

shift in tenor and modality ("Legga attentamente questo foglio prima di prendere questo medicinale [Read this leaflet carefully before taking this medicine"], see Fig. 4a). The British PIL uses a far more personal tenor (second person and verb in the imperative) than the one found in the Italian counterpart (third person singular but verb in the imperative). Modality coincides as far as modal verbs are concerned, but in the Italian PILs we notice lexical additions: adverbs such as *mai* [never], *personalmente* [personally], and conjunctions such as *infatti* [indeed] have been used in the interest of increasing clarity.

Read all of this leaflet carefully before you start taking this medicine.
- Keep this leaflet. You may need to read it again.
- If you have any further questions, ask your doctor or pharmacist.
- This medicine has been prescribed for you. Do not pass it on to others. It may harm them, even if their symptoms are the same as yours.
- If any of the side effects gets serious, or if you notice any side effects not listed in this leaflet, please tell your doctor or pharmacist.

Legga attentamente questo foglio prima di iniziare a prendere questo medicinale.
- Conservi questo foglio. Potrebbe aver bisogno di leggerlo di nuovo.
- Se ha qualsiasi dubbio, si rivolga al medico o al farmacista.
- Questo medicinale è stato prescritto per lei personalmente. Non lo dia mai ad altri. Infatti, per altri individui questo medicinale potrebbe essere pericoloso, anche se i loro sintomi sono uguali ai suoi.
- Se uno qualsiasi degli effetti indesiderati si aggrava, o se nota la comparsa di un qualsiasi effetto indesiderato non elencato in questo foglio, informi il medico o il farmacista.

Figures 4 and 4a. Prefabricated expressions.

5.2 Section 2: What x is and what it is used for

The first paragraph 'What *Spiriva/Spiriva Respimat* is and what it is used for' shows some intralingual differences in the two British PILs. "Chronic" – found in the *Spiriva* PIL – was substituted with "long-term" in the *Spiriva Respimat* PIL. Since the *Spiriva Respimat* PIL is the last revised PIL, we can hypothesize that "chronic" was replaced with "long-term" because the latter has a less negative connotation: while "long-term" suggests a prolonged need for drugs, to some readers "chronic" implies a disease which causes suffering, discomfort and pain. Evidence supporting this claim can be found in the Merck Manual Corpus (MMC), where "long-term" occurs 397 times, but only in 13 cases does it occur with "disease" in the R1 position, as it collocates mostly with nouns related to the cure (e.g. use, treatment, therapy, management, hemodialysis etc.) and sometimes indicates positive endings (e.g. improvement, success, benefit).[12] "Chronic," on the other hand, occurs 1,786 times in the MMC and clusters 283 times with "disease" and other words indicating disorders (e.g. infection, failure, hepatitis, leukemia, syndrome).

In the same paragraph we detect some interlingual discontinuities between the British ST and the Italian TT with regard to the disease nomenclature and corresponding acronym. The English "chronic obstructive pulmonary disease (COPD)" appears in Italian as "bronco-pneumopatia cronica ostruttiva (BPCO)". The more informal expression, "pulmonary disease," becomes highly technical in Italian as it is reduced in only one term where the suffix *-patia* indicates disease and the adding of a prefix *bronco-* gives a more precise, detailed and specialized nuance to the term. The acronym does not correspond to the English one, and thus does not follow the standardization process of acronyms. In the last part of the final sentence of the paragraph, "breathing problems" is translated in the singular form and uses a synonym for "problems", i.e., "difficoltà respiratoria" [breathing difficulty]. This expression is followed – as in the STs – by "od altri sintomi" [or other symptoms], which taken together form the subject of the sentence. But in the Italian text the plural subject does not agree with the verb (which is in the third singular form). This mistake is rectified together with the elimination of the euphonious *-d* in the conjunction *o* [or] in the other Italian PIL for *Spiriva Respimat,* which corresponds to the last revised PIL (Figures 5 and 5a).

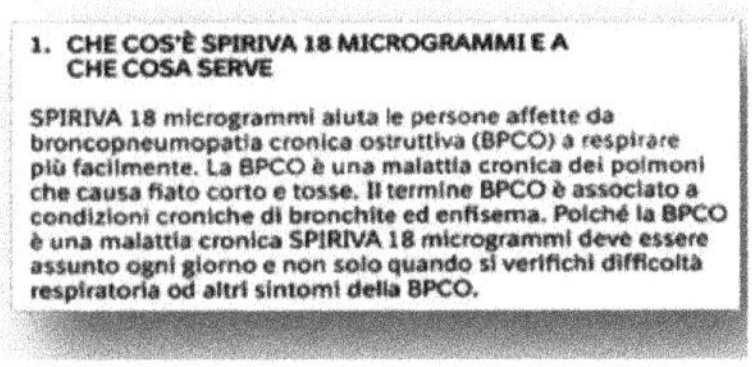
1. CHE COS'È SPIRIVA 18 MICROGRAMMI E A CHE COSA SERVE

SPIRIVA 18 microgrammi aiuta le persone affette da broncopneumopatia cronica ostruttiva (BPCO) a respirare più facilmente. La BPCO è una malattia cronica dei polmoni che causa fiato corto e tosse. Il termine BPCO è associato a condizioni croniche di bronchite ed enfisema. Poiché la BPCO è una malattia cronica SPIRIVA 18 microgrammi deve essere assunto ogni giorno e non solo quando si verifichi difficoltà respiratoria od altri sintomi della BPCO.

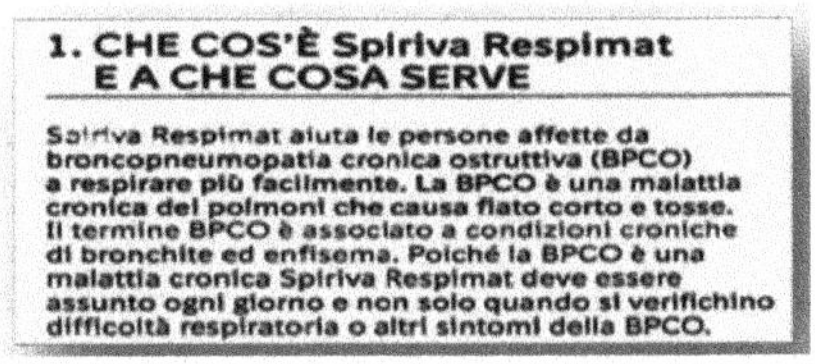
1. CHE COS'È Spiriva Respimat E A CHE COSA SERVE

Spiriva Respimat aiuta le persone affette da broncopneumopatia cronica ostruttiva (BPCO) a respirare più facilmente. La BPCO è una malattia cronica dei polmoni che causa fiato corto e tosse. Il termine BPCO è associato a condizioni croniche di bronchite ed enfisema. Poiché la BPCO è una malattia cronica Spiriva Respimat deve essere assunto ogni giorno e non solo quando si verifichino difficoltà respiratoria o altri sintomi della BPCO.

Figures 5 and 5a. A comparison between the 2009 *Spiriva* PIL and the 2010 *Spiriva Respimat* PIL.

12 The Merck Manual Corpus (MMC) was compiled ad-hoc by the author for her PhD thesis and has been recently updated. The manual can be downloaded from <http://www.merckmanuals.com//mmanual>.

In the second paragraph the two texts coincide but we can notice a case of lexical condensation and density in the Italian PIL which prefers nominalizations (*risposta* [answer], *assunzione* [taking]) to render the passage more context-consistent and technical: "Nel caso di risposta positiva ad una qualsiasi domanda parlarne con il medico prima di iniziare l'assunzione [in case of positive answer to any questions, discuss this with the doctor before the taking of…]". On the other hand, the English text reads "if you answer any of these questions with 'yes' please discuss this with your doctor before taking […]".

In the paragraph following the heading 'Driving and using machines', we can also notice an addition to the *Spiriva Respimat* PIL in English which is lacking in the *Spiriva* PIL. The former includes a sentence (a sort of *caveat* on the part of the pharmaceutical company) which is maintained in the Italian counterpart (see Figures 6, 6a, and 6b). The highly technical structure of the *Spiriva* PIL (nominalization + active voice) is preserved in the TT but changed in the English *Spiriva Respimat* PIL to a more convoluted construction ("In case" + active voice + nominalizations + passive voice).

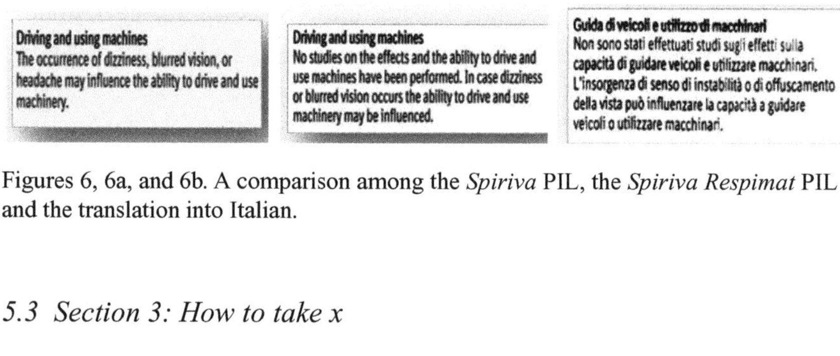
Driving and using machines
The occurrence of dizziness, blurred vision, or headache may influence the ability to drive and use machinery.

Driving and using machines
No studies on the effects and the ability to drive and use machines have been performed. In case dizziness or blurred vision occurs the ability to drive and use machinery may be influenced.

Guida di veicoli e utilizzo di macchinari
Non sono stati effettuati studi sugli effetti sulla capacità di guidare veicoli e utilizzare macchinari. L'insorgenza di senso di instabilità o di offuscamento della vista può influenzare la capacità a guidare veicoli o utilizzare macchinari.

Figures 6, 6a, and 6b. A comparison among the *Spiriva* PIL, the *Spiriva Respimat* PIL and the translation into Italian.

5.3 Section 3: How to take x

The paragraph 'How to Take *Spiriva Respimat*' includes emotive language that is missing in the same paragraph of the *Spiriva* PIL but present in the TTs. The feature is an exception to the rule for this genre, but this is especially the case in the Italian PIL, in which "don't worry" is translated as "non si preoccupi," the polite third person singular form of the verb *preoccupare* [to worry]. Moreover, "Do not take two doses at the same time or on the same day" is translated as usual following the cultural and genre differences of the two PILs (i.e. ST: imperative in the second person vs. TT: indicative in the third person singular) but in the Italian PIL the phrase "per compensare la dimenticanza" [to remedy the omission] is added which, while redundant, emphasizes and clarifies the drug's purpose.

In the paragraph 'Possible side effects', there is a case of translation infelicity. Not only has "clinical trials" (Figure 7) been translated as "dati disponibili" [available data] (Figure 7a), but "according to" (Figure 7) is translated, calquing the English expression, as "in accordo alla" [in accordance with] (Figure 7a); the sentence style is a calque of the English one as well (Figures 7 and 7a). This stylistic infelicity is rendered felicity in the translation of the latest revised *Spiriva Respimat* PIL, where we read not only a faithful translation of "clinical trials" [studi clinici] but also a more accurate rendering of "listed according to frequency" (Figure 7b).

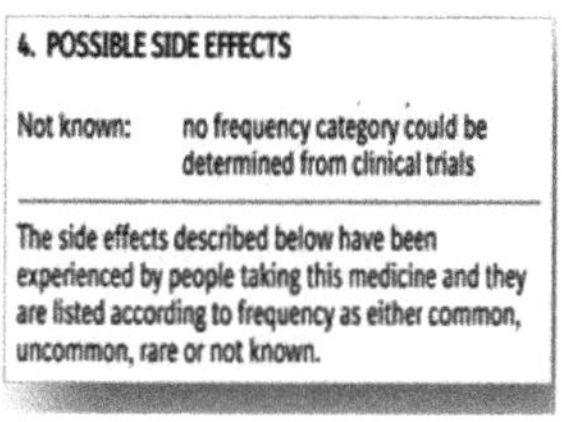
4. POSSIBLE SIDE EFFECTS

Not known: no frequency category could be determined from clinical trials

The side effects described below have been experienced by people taking this medicine and they are listed according to frequency as either common, uncommon, rare or not known.

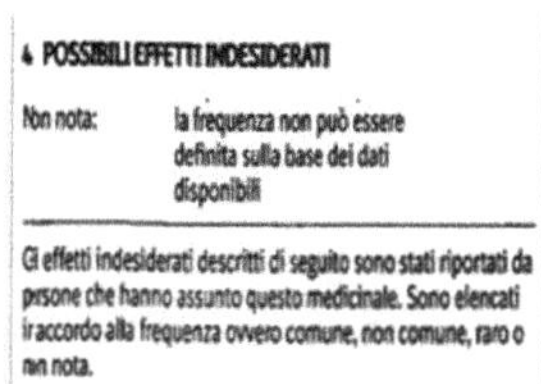
4. POSSIBILI EFFETTI INDESIDERATI

Non nota: la frequenza non può essere definita sulla base dei dati disponibili

Gli effetti indesiderati descritti di seguito sono stati riportati da persone che hanno assunto questo medicinale. Sono elencati in accordo alla frequenza ovvero comune, non comune, raro o non nota.

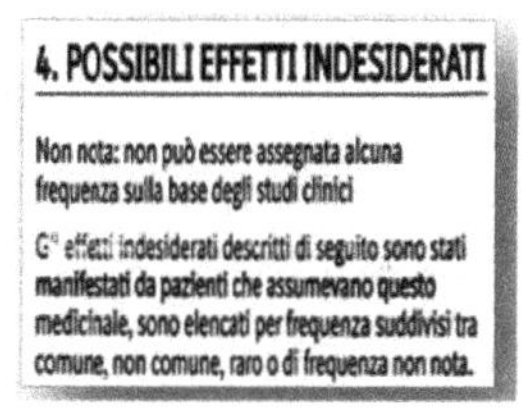
4. POSSIBILI EFFETTI INDESIDERATI

Non nota: non può essere assegnata alcuna frequenza sulla base degli studi clinici

Gli effetti indesiderati descritti di seguito sono stati manifestati da pazienti che assumevano questo medicinale, sono elencati per frequenza suddivisi tra comune, non comune, raro o di frequenza non nota.

Figures 7, 7a, and 7b. Comparison between the ST PIL and its translation in the *Spiriva* PIL and in the *Spiriva Respimat* PIL.

5.4 Section 4: Possible side effects

The long list at the end of the paragraph 'Possible Side Effects' includes examples of terminologisation and de-terminologisation (Montalt/González Davies 2007: 231, 251) in STs and TTs as technical terms are or are not accompanied by explanations. The ST "nettle rash" (urticaria) is rendered in the TT with "orticaria," suggesting that a general Italian readership might be more accustomed to medical terminology than its English counterpart; the ST "depletion of body water" (dehydration) is translated in the TT *Spiriva* PIL only with the term "disidratazione" but in the TT *Spiriva Respimat* PIL – mirroring the ST text – we find "perdita di liquidi del corpo [disidratazione]". This translation is more source- than target-oriented because in everyday Italian *disidratazione* is more common than the expression registered in the PIL.

Generally speaking, a comparison of the characteristics of the original and translated PILs shows they represent highly culture-specific genres. The substantive differences between the PILs could be due to national legal requirements, on the one hand, and different cultural traditions, target readers and assumptions about the intended target readers, on the other.

6. Concluding remarks

With reference to the hypothesis and the research questions pointed out in the introduction to this chapter, the PILC and the four British PILs of the month investigated showed numerous instances of user-friendliness. But diverse cultural backgrounds result in differences between Italian and British PILs at the structural, textual, lexico-semantic and micro-pragmatic levels (in the cases of *Vicks Soother* and *Sinex Aloe*, and of *Calpol* and *Tachipirina*) thus suggesting, as Cacchiani (2006: 37) has argued, "they belong to two closely related subgenres rather than to one single genre". However, new and revised Italian PILs are beginning to follow British PILs (in the cases of *Spiriva* and *Spiriva Respimat*) in clarity and style. The *Spiriva* and *Spiriva Respimat* Italian PILs represent strong textual hybrids, insofar as they closely follow their British counterparts without giving up certain Italian cultural norms associated with this genre. However, from the perspective of translation, the *Spiriva Respimat* PIL represents the most promising format, as lay-friendliness does not get lost in translation. The study thus suggests that the hypothesis was confirmed to a small extent in that only *Spiriva* and *Spiriva Respimat* follow the parameters, set in the quality criteria document, to constitute best practice example of user-friendliness although it also adheres to national cultural patterns associated to this genre.

I anticipated finding in this investigation of PILs greater terminological simplification, and more interaction and user-friendliness in

OTC drug PILs than in doctor's prescription medicine PILs as declared in the last research question. But the evidence invalidates these expectations. First of all, in the British PILs, with the exception of layout, we found a continuum in user-friendliness throughout the three categories studied. But of more significance is the upside-down trend observed in the Italian PILs. Most of the Italian PILs investigated (except for *Spiriva* and *Spiriva Respimat*) use a language more suited to the physician or the pharmacist than to the general reader, thus excluding the patient in the decision-making process related to their health issues.

Clarity and simplicity of expression are important aspects of PIL information architecture – especially of PILs of OTC drugs – that should be improved where the risk of misunderstanding on the part of the reader is likely to come with a cost. The Italian PILs analyzed in this study are not exclusively addressed to the healthcare professional but to the layperson who should have easy access to information which is specifically tailored and relevant to him/her. This study will hopefully be useful for those involved in the design and drafting of PILs who, before submitting PILs to MHRA, should make complex information easy to understand and easy to apply, thereby maximizing the number of people who can use a specific medicine safely and effectively.[13] The English PILs of the month are paragons of readability and user-friendliness as they provide a great deal of examples of good practice which have been investigated in this study mainly in respect of information design (i.e. typography and plain language). Another remedial action that should be taken in Italy is to act in compliance with article 59(3) of Council Directive 2001/83/EC[14] and use questionnaires or other forms of patient consultation to test the leaflet for understanding and usefulness; where problems arise, changes and translations can be further considered. In

13 In this connection the PIL Guidance 0712 Final (2012) advises to present information for healthcare professionals in a separate tear-off portion of the leaflet.

14 "The package leaflet shall reflect the results of consultations with target patient groups to ensure that it is legible, clear and easy to use [...] The results of assessments carried out in cooperation with target patient groups shall also be provided to the competent authority" (Quality Review of Documents human product information template version 8 October 2011, <www.ema.europa.eu/ docs/en_GB/ document_library/Template_or_form/2009/10/WC500004368.pdf)>.

so doing, any reader of the PIL should be able to answer the question "Can you read this leaflet?" with an unequivocal "Yes, I can!"

This analysis has offered great opportunities to study the popularization of medical discourse. Additionally, it has helped us consider an environment in which medical knowledge is produced with patients in mind. Insofar as the target PIL can culturally domesticate the original text by re-contextualizing it to make it accessible or to counterbalance the experts' monologue, it can act as a bridge that crosses the gap between medical practitioners and everyday consumers. Public debate regarding health issues on the Internet and in advertising campaigns is also gaining ground in Italy, even though studies such as this one suggest that the Italian public still has a long way to go in playing an active role in health management.

References

Aarva, Pauliina / Tampere, Marja Pakarinen 2006. Studying the Striving and Opposing Forces in Newspaper Journalism: The Actantial Model of Health Promotion. *Health Promotion International* 21/2, 160–168.

Askehave, Inge / Holmgren, Lise-Lotte / Lassen Inger /Strunck, Jeanne 2010. At styrke patienten I en New Public management warden: En udredning af betydnings-potentialet I begrebet patient empowerment. In Horsbøl Anders / Sørensen Mariann B. (eds) *Sundhedskommunikation i Sygehusvæsenet*, Aalborg: Aalborg University Press, 147–182.

Askehave, Inge / Zethsen, Karen Korning 2000a. The Patient Package Insert for the Future. *Report for the Danish Ministry of Health.* Aarhus: The Aarhus School of Business.

Askehave, Inge / Zethsen, Karen Korning 2000b. Medical Texts Made Simple – Dream or Reality? *Hermes: Journal of Linguistics* 25, 63–74.

Askehave, Inge / Zethsen, Karen Korning 2002. Translating for Laymen. *Perspectives: Studies in Translatology* 10/1, 15–29.

Askehave, Inge / Zethsen, Karen Korning 2003. Communication Barriers in Public Discourse – The Patient Package Insert. *Document Design* 4/1, 23–41.

Askehave, Inge / Zethsen, Karen Korning. 2008. Mandatory Genres: The Case of European Public Assessment Report (EPAR) Summaries. *Text & Talk* 28/2, 167–191.

Askehave, Inge / Zethsen, Karen Korning 2010. 'Check it out' – The Construction of Patient Empowerment in Health Promotion Leaflets. In Garrido, Miguel F. Ruiz / Fortanet-Gómez, Inmaculada / Palmer-Silveira, Juan C. (eds) *English for Academic and Professional Purposes*, Utrecht: Rodopi, 107–122.

Askehave, Inge / Zethsen, Karen Korning 2011. Lost in Translation? When Patient Information Crosses Borders. *European Industrial Pharmacy* December, 14–16.

Bongaarts, Loes J.M. 2009. *Translating Patient Information Leaflets.* Master Thesis, Faculty of Humanities, Universiteit Utrecht.

Bromme, Rainer / Jucks, Regina / Wagner, Thomas 2005. How to Refer to 'Diabetes'?: Language in Online Health Advice. *Applied Cognitive Psychology* 19, 569–586.

Cacchiani, Silvia 2006. Dis/similarities between Patient Information Leaflets in Britain and Italy: Implications for the Translator. *New Voices in Translation Studies* 2, 28–43.

Clerehan, Rosemary / Buchbinder, Rachelle 2006. Toward a More Valid Account of Functional Text Quality: The Case of Patient Information Leaflet. *Text & Talk* 26/1, 39–68.

Dickinson, David / Raynor David K. / Duman, Mark 2001. Patient Information Leaflets for Medicines: Using Consumer Testing to Determine the Most Effective Design. *Patient Education and Counseling* 43, 147–159.

Dickinson, David / Raynor, D.K. Theo / Kennedy, James G. / Bonaccorso, Silvia / Sturchio, Jeffrey L. 2003. What Information do Patients Need about Medicines? *British Medical Journal* 328/7419, 861–864.

Gal, Iddo / Prigat, Ayelet 2005. Why Organizations Continue to Create Patient information Leaflets with Readability and Usability Problems: An Exploratory Study. *Health Education Research* 20/4, 485–493.

Gotti, Maurizio / Salager-Meyer, Françoise (eds) 2006. *Advances in Medical Discourse Analysis: Oral and Written Contexts.* Bern: Peter Lang.

Graham, Jo 2009. Improving Information for Patients: The UK Perspective. *Regulatory Rapporteur* 6/10, 5–9.

Hall, David R. 2006. Medical Leaflets, Empowerment and Disempowerment. In Gotti/Salanger-Meyer (eds), 271–288.

Harwood, A. / Harrison, Jayne E. 2004. How Readable are Orthodontic Patient Information Leaflets? *Journal of Orthodontics* 31, 210–219.

Horwitz, Anna / Reuther, Lene / Andersen, Stig Ejdrup 2009. Patienters vurdering af medicinpakningens indlægssedler. *Ugeskrift for Læger* 171/8, 599–602.

Johnson, Anne 1999. Do Parents Value and Use Written Health Communication? *Neonatal, Paediatric and Child Health Nursing* 2, 3–7.

Killingsworth, M. Jimmie 1987. Guest Editorial: Thingishness and Objectivity in Technical Style. *Journal of Technical Writing and Communication* 17/2, 105–113.

Kimble, Joseph 1994–1995. Answering the Critics of Plain Language. *The Scribes Journal of Legal Writing* 5, 51–85.

Larsen, Eva Ladekjaer / Manderson, Lenore 2008. 'A good spot': Health Promotion Discourse, Healthy Cities and Heterogeneity in Contemporary Denmark. *Health & Place* 15/2, 606–613.

Maglie, Rosita 2009. *Understanding the Language of Medicine.* Roma: Aracne.

Montalt, Vicent / Garcìa Izquierdo, Isabel 2014. Analysing Readability and Legibility of Fact Sheets (FSP) in Spanish in a Real Clinical Setting. Paper presented at CERLIS 2014: *The Language of Medicine: Science, Practice and Academia*, University of Bergamo, 19–21 June 2014.

Montalt, Vicent / Gonzáles, Davies Maria 2007. *Medical Translation Step by Step. Translation Practices Explained.* Manchester: St. Jerome.

Montalt, Vicent / Shuttleworth, Mark (eds) 2012. Translation and Knowledge Mediation in Medical and Health Settings. Special issue of *Linguistica Antverpiensia: Themes in Translation Studies* 11.

Nisbeth Jensen, Matilde 2013. *Translators of Patient Information Leaflets: Translation Experts or Expert Translators? A Mixed Methods Study.* PhD Dissertation. Aarhus: Aarhus University.

Nisbeth Jensen, Matilde / Zethsen, Karen Korning 2012. Translation of Patient Information Leaflets: Trained Translators and Pharmacists-cum-Translators – A Comparison. In Montalt/Shuttleworth (eds), 31–49.

Pander Maat, Henk / Lentz, Leo 2010. Improving the Usability of Patient Information Leaflets. *Patient Education and Counselling* 80/1, 113–119.

Raynor, D.K. Theo 2007. The Importance of Medicines Information for Patients. *Prescriber* 18/2, 60–62.

Roberts, Lisa 2006. First Impressions: An Information Leaflet for Patients Attending a Musculoskeletal Outpatient Department. *Physiotherapy* 92, 179–186.

Zethsen, Karen Korning 2007. Beyond Translation Proper. *TTR (Traduction, Terminologie, Redaction)* 20/1, 281–308.

Zethsen, Karen Korning 2009. Intralingual Translation: An Attempt at Description. *Meta* 54/4, 795–812.

Zethsen, Karen Korning / Askehave, Inger 2010. PIL of the Month: A Study of Best Practice in EU Patient information Leaflets. *Journal of Applied Linguistics and Professional Practice* 7/1, 97–120.

Websites

Directive 2001/83/EC of the European parliament and of the Council of 6 November 2001 on the Community Code Relating to Medicinal products for Human Use: <http://eur-lex.europa.eu/legal-content/EN/ALL/?uri=CELEX:32001L0083>.

Quality criteria for patient information leaflets: <http://www.mhra.gov.uk/home/groups/isinsp/documents/websiteresources/con2032836.pdf>.

MHRA, 2005. 'Always Read the Leaflet' getting the best information with every medicine:<http://www.mhra.gov.uk/home/groups/pl-a/documents/publication/con2018041.pdf>.

Best Practice Guidance on Patient Information Leaflets (or PIL guidance 0712 Final): <http://www.mhra.gov.uk/home/groups/pl-a/documents/websiteresources/con157151.pdf>.

Corpus of 62 PILs of the Month and Annex 1: <http://www.mhra.gov.uk/Howweregulate/Medicines/Labelspatientinformationleafletsandpackaging/Patientinformationleaflet(PIL)ofthemonth/>.

Anna Franca Plastina

Patient (Mis)understanding of Prescription Drug Ads in Social Media: Multimodal Discourse Analysis of eDTCA

1. Introduction

For decades before the 1970s, the promotion of drugs and medical devices was exclusively directed to doctors and "traditionally, the advertising of prescription drugs was limited to medical journals or health care trade publications aimed at physicians" (Hunt 1998: 3). During the 1970s, efforts were made to secure legal rights for patients to be informed about their treatment options. As Donohue (2006: 661) points out, "the pharmaceutical promotion of prescription drugs to consumers was made possible by the rise of consumer-oriented medicine following the social movements for patients' and consumers' rights". While prescription drug advertising became more patient-oriented, patient safety itself continued to be ensured through patient-expert interaction and credible sources (Plastina 2012). On these grounds, efforts were made in the mid-1990s to secure consumer rights in managed care (Rothman 2001). As a result, an exponential growth in direct-to-consumer advertising (DTCA)[1] was witnessed.

The promotion of drugs directed to consumers through television, radio, billboards and print media therefore marked a milestone in the paradigm shift from the traditional provider-centred medical model towards patient-centred medicine. From this point onwards, decision-making would no longer rest in the hands of the physician alone (Sacristán 2013).

1 DTCA is seen as "any promotional effort by a pharmaceutical company to present prescription drug information to the general public in the lay media" in order to better "educate" the lay consumer (Wilkes et al. 2000: 112–113).

By the late 1990s, a more diffuse change was made possible by advances in information technology, which enabled patients to inform themselves and, therefore, to become more involved in medical decision-making (Donohue 2006). Currently, Internet and social media advertising are becoming an increasingly powerful force in medical communication, shaping consumers' attitudes and decisions about prescription drugs. The expanding proliferation of online users searching for health-related information (Ventola 2011) has led DTCA to create its niche within social media environments (Greene/Kesselheim 2010). This phenomenon is strongly influencing the culture of consumer medicine, especially in enabling patients to self-diagnose their health issues.

Due to their interactive nature, current electronic media allow patients/consumers to act as active agents of their medical treatment decisions. This represents a considerable step forward when compared to the role of patients as passive recipients of DTCA through the traditional media. As a result, electronic direct-to-consumer advertising (eDTCA) is gaining ground in the era of consumer medicine, especially due to the increasing popularity of social media. Nevertheless, the ongoing debate between proponents and opponents of this new social phenomenon sheds light on the unprecedented challenges eDTCA is posing to medical communication.

On the one hand, those in favor of eDTCA contend that it is extremely serviceable as it "encourages patients to explore a much wider range of treatment options than simply relying on information from their physicians" (Weinmeyer 2013: 956); those against eDTCA focus on the serious risks it may represent for patients. As proponents, Lee and Crawley (2009: 35) point out that "in addition to fostering a consumer empowerment movement, it promotes the trend of democratizing information". Khosla and Khosla (2011) further underline that eDTCA is beneficial in serving as a health-communication tool to improve informed treatment choices. On the other hand, opponents highlight the numerous risks of this kind of medical communication. For example, Frosch and Grande (2010: 1) warn that eDTCA "promotes inappropriate use of prescription drugs, or diverts consumers from better alternatives", thus deeming that the risks associated with eDTCA outweigh patient benefits. In a different perspective, Liang and Mackey (2011a) argue that eDTCA is used by pharmaceutical companies to market their drugs, while Mackey and Liang (2013) focus on the expanding phenomenon of illicit online drug sellers, who represent a threat to patients' safety. Furthermore, Liang and Mackey (2011b) identify two major factors that pose serious challenges: the regulatory vacuum in which eDTCA is allowed to operate and to transcend geopolitical borders; the escalating use of social media by pharmaceutical companies. Consumers are, in fact, exposed to a wealth of unregulated medical information, also through YouTube-dedicated channels created by pharmaceutical companies. Their increasing investment in multimedia formats of communication is a clear sign that eDTCA is affecting various social aspects of healthcare. Findlay (2001) points out how eDTCA may lead to: a) the development of major consumer awareness of pharmaceutical treatments; b) an increase in the prescription of costly new brand-name drugs over less expensive, but equally effective, over-the-counter drugs; c) the inappropriate clinical use of some drugs; d) a growth in sales revenues; e) a subsequent focus on producing drugs for social health conditions (e.g. baldness, sexual dysfunction), rather than those for more serious life-threatening conditions. All these different socio-economic aspects are, however, commonly tied by eDTCA, i.e., the ways in which communication is shaped and delivered. In this perspective, the current study focuses specifically on the multimodal construction of eDTCA and on its immediate communicative effect on patients. The study's underlying assumption draws upon Wolfe (2002: 524):

> although increased access by patients to accurate, objective information about tests to diagnose and drugs to treat illnesses is an important advance, confusion arises when commercially driven promotional information is represented as educational.

Despite it appearing that "drug advertisements could endanger rather than empower consumers by minimizing risk information and exaggerating benefits" (Brown 2004: 8), this chapter is positioned on the divide between proponents and opponents of eDTCA. The broad purpose is to investigate how this kind of multimodal communication can contribute to patients' understanding, or perhaps, misunderstanding of the risks and benefits of prescription drugs. The investigation is particularly conducted on eDTCA, which is delivered through the popular social medium of YouTube as a current practice performed by several pharmaceutical companies. The subsequent interaction that takes place between pharmaceutical companies as experts, and patients as worldwide consumers is mediated by uploaded eDTCA videos. As this kind of interaction is grounded in a high degree of asymmetric information, providers are expected to promote informative advertising as a valuable means to increase patients' knowledge about the use of prescription drugs. By its very nature, nevertheless, eDTCA is driven by commercial purposes, and choices of semiotic representations are likely directed to persuading consumers of the high quality of prescription drugs. In this light, the study focuses on the interplay between different semiotic systems, and the extent to which these may mislead patients' understanding of eDTCA messages.

2. Basic features of eDTCA

By extending the traditional classification of DTCA (cf. Bradley/Zito 1997) to its electronic counterpart, prescription drug ads can be categorised into three types: health-seeking ads, reminder ads and product-specific ads. Help-seeking ads have the educational purpose of informing consumers about a health condition and its possible treatment without naming specific drugs and being obliged to provide risk information. On the other hand, reminder ads name a specific medication, but do not provide information about its use. Conversely, product-specific ads, which are the most common, present three main features. They: 1) mention the brand of a drug; 2) describe its therapeutic use(s); 3) provide representations of its effectiveness and safety. The inherent danger of prescription drug ads has led the World Health Organization (WHO) to issue *Guidelines for the Regulatory Assessment of Medicinal Products for Use in Self-Medication* which state:

> Advertisements to the general public should help people to make rational decisions on the use of drugs determined to be legally available without a prescription.

> [...] They should not generally be permitted for prescription drugs or to promote drugs for certain serious conditions that can be treated only by qualified health practitioners, for which certain countries have established lists. (2000, 3.2.5.2, comma 14)

The WHO (2007: 8) further announced the decisions taken by one of its working groups: "focusing on current concerns around direct-to-consumer advertising of pharmaceuticals, the group made a unanimous recommendation to prohibit direct-to-consumer advertising". In a similar vein, 22 of the 27 EU member states voted in 2008 against proposed legislation allowing DTCA to provide even limited information to patients (Humphreys 2009). Currently, DTCA is only permitted in the United States and in New Zealand (Silver et al. 2009): in the former country, it is monitored by the Food and Drug Administration (FDA); in the latter, it is regulated under the Medicines Act 1981 and Medicines Regulations 1984. Moreover, "the Food and Drug Administration (FDA) is proposing to amend its regulations concerning direct-to-consumer (DTC) advertisements of prescription drugs" (Federal Register March 29, 2010, vol. 75, n° 29, p. 15376) by adding the following provision:

> in the case of an advertisement for a drug [...] presented directly to consumers in television or radio format and stating the name of the drug and its conditions of use, the major statement relating to side effects and contraindications shall be presented in a *clear*, *conspicuous*, and *neutral* manner [my italics].

What the FDA means by "clear, conspicuous, and neutral manner" is analytically explicated in the same document (p. 15387):

> A major statement is clear, conspicuous, and neutral if: (A) Information is presented in language that is readily understandable by consumers; (B) Audio information is understandable in terms of the volume, articulation, and pacing used; (C) Textual information is placed appropriately and is presented against a contrasting background for sufficient duration and in a size and style of font that allows the information to be read easily; and (D) The advertisement does not include distracting representations (including statements, text, images, or sounds or any combination thereof) that detract from the communication of the major statement.

While the FDA is attempting to set DTCA standards, pharmaceutical companies are pushing into the global market through the electronic medium, thus managing to easily reach consumers in the majority of countries where DTCA is banned. Furthermore, consumers are also currently exposed to unethical or unlawful ads, which may affect them emotionally from the very first time they are viewed. This may induce consumers to fully trust eDTCA information, thus disorienting their understanding of the risks and benefits of prescription drugs (Choi/Lee 2007). As Cho (2000: 230) points out:

> if promotional information is not disclosed as such and is portrayed as educational or as endorsements based on appropriate evaluation criteria, a conflict exists between the interests of the readers or patients and those of the advertisers or the company.

Ultimately, the basic features of unregulated advertising, credibility of information and potential threat to public health are factors operating at the social level of eDTCA discourse. At the discursive level, potential provider-patient conflict may arise due to the type/amount of information communicated to consumers, the semiotic representations of eDTCA discourse, and the manner in which these steer consumers' interpretation of meaning.

3. The case of eDTCA on YouTube

Due to the increasing number of people who access health and drug-related information online, pharmaceutical companies are devoting significant resources to promoting prescription drugs on YouTube. This social medium first emerged as "a key site for the production and distribution of grassroots media" (Jenkins 2006: 274), allowing "easy entry into the community and legitimate engagement even at the periphery" (Chau 2010: 68). Its discourse is characterised by practices of appropriation and remix (Burgess/Green 2009), which make multimodality, or the combination of semiotic modes, one of its key defining features.

The wealth of semiotic resources, which pharmaceutical companies can also potentially use to advertise their products, may *distract* and mislead patients' understanding of the real effects of the products promoted. In this regard, the FDA launched a Distraction Study in 2012 that investigated whether TV and radio ads operate a fair semiotic balance between positive and negative information. This was intended "to ensure that us-er[s] ha[ve] access to a balanced presentation of both risks and benefits of medical products".[2]

In detail, the study explored whether DTCA information is presented in language that is readily understandable by consumers; audio information is understandable in terms of volume, articulation, and pacing; textual information is appropriately placed and presented against a contrasting background for sufficient duration, and in a size and font style that allows for ease of reading. In its Federal Register announcement (March 29, 2010, vol. 75, n° 29, p. 15380), the FDA claimed that:

> When elements of the advertisement such as images, text, graphics or sounds are presented in such a way as to significantly detract from the major statement, consumers are likely to be deterred from attending to and comprehending the risk information being presented.

These concerns, however, have only addressed DTCA in the traditional media, whereas eDTCA in the social media is still a largely unexplored field, both in terms of the wider potential impact on health consumers, and on medical communication. This study makes a contribution to the latter aspect, in the attempt to disclose the semiotic manipulation that is deliberately performed on multimodal texts by pharmaceutical companies for promotional purposes.

3.1 Aim

In the current study, the main principles of the FDA 2010 Federal Register provision and the FDA 2012 Distraction Study are sourced and applied to eDTCA as they help ensure that consumers are not misled

---

2 Public Hearing on Promotion of FDA-Regulated Medical Products Using the Internet and Social Media Tools, Washington, 12–13 November 2009.

or deceived by prescription drug advertising. Based on these principles, the twofold aim of the study is to investigate the manner in which multimodal texts convey risk and benefit information, and the way in which semiotic representations may cause distraction. Two research questions are addressed:

1. Do eDTCA videos present risk and benefit information "in a clear, conspicuous, and neutral manner" with a fair balance between negative and positive information?[3]
2. How may semiotic representations distract, and thus, mislead patients?[4]

3.2 The eDTCA Corpus

A total of twenty-four sample videos were collected from YouTube for the corpus (52 minutes total length; 5,040 words) used in the current study. Sample videos were selected to cover eDTCA of prescription drugs treating three common symptoms, namely, insomnia, high cholesterol and depression. This choice was based on two main reasons. First, as these symptoms affect a wider population, it is likely that these multimodal texts are accessed by a higher number of health consumers worldwide, which can be witnessed by the number of views recorded. Second, these symptoms are increasingly treated by pharmaceutical companies, which appear to be extremely concerned with the promotion of 'lifestyle drugs' (Raven 2004).

Eight sample multimodal texts were chosen for each symptom (see Appendix) to ensure balanced qualitative analysis. To this end, the corpus was purposely small-scaled as multimodal texts are extremely complex, and therefore, require deeper analysis of the different semiotic resources employed to shape meaning.

---

3 Based on the FDA 2010 Federal Register provision.

4 Based on the FDA 2012 Distraction Study.

3.3 Method and Procedure

The methodology adopted was grounded in Multimodal Discourse Analysis (MDA) (e.g. Kress/van Leeuwen 1996; O'Halloran 2004; Kress 2010), as it appears to be extremely suitable to investigate the semiotic elements used within the media-rich environment of YouTube. In this respect, O'Halloran (2004: 1) points out that "the analysis and interpretation of language use is contextualized in conjunction with other semiotic resources which are simultaneously used for the construction of meaning". MDA focuses, in fact, on the "functions and social uses of semiotic systems, the complex interrelations of semiotic systems in social practice" (Hodge/Kress 1988: 1), which in the present case refers to eDTCA. On-screen text and audio information were transcribed, and the phasal shifts of image changes (Thibault 2000) were identified in relation to potential concurrent shifts in the linguistic and audio semiotic representations. MDA was then performed on raw corpus data by introducing the two analytical categories of risk and benefit information, and semiotic distractors with a total of six variables, which were those monitored by the FDA.

In detail, the category of risk and benefit information targeted the manner in which information was conveyed and also the balance between negative (risk) and positive (benefit) information. The independent variables taken into account in this category were three: 1) *understandability of language*: plain language vs. medical jargon; 2) *understandability of risk/benefit audio information*: normal vs. accelerated audio pacing; 3) *fair semiotic balance between risk/benefit information* in terms of time, ease of reading textual information (font size, top/bottom and left/right placement on the screen). According to Kress/van Leeuwen (1996: 193–4), information placed in the upper section of the screen is "the idealized essence of the information [...] its, ostensibly, most salient part"; text placed in the lower section "presents more 'down-to-earth' information", while text is placed in the centre to be noticed first by consumers. Information can further acquire value according to left and right placements, which correspond to the value of Given and New information respectively. Kress/van Leeuwen (1996: 187) point out that "For something to be Given means that it is presented as something the viewer already knows [...] For something to be

New means that it is presented as something which is not yet known [...] to which the viewer must pay special attention".

Moreover, the category of semiotic distractors focused on possible distracting representations, which detract from the communication of the major statement concerning side effects and contraindications of prescription drugs. The three main independent variables which were likely to affect people's understanding of risk information were: 1) *occurrence of superimposed text on audio risk information*: present vs. absent; 2) *emotional tone of visual images*: strong vs. weak tone; 3) *consistency of visual images with written and spoken risk information*: consistent vs. inconsistent.

4. Findings and Discussion

4.1 Risk/benefit information

As for the variable of understandability of language, findings showed that plain language was preponderant in both written and audio semiotic modes (4,441 words; 88.1%) compared to the medical jargon used (599 words; 11.9%) throughout the entire eDTCA corpus (5,040 words). Results from a one-factor ANOVA between the three eDTCA subcorpora (insomnia, high cholesterol and depression) showed no significant variation in the predominant use of plain language ($F=3.1603$, $p<0.063$). On the other hand, medical jargon was used to refer to cases in which the promoted drugs should be avoided, either due to current health conditions (e.g. *chemiosis, MAOIs*, *TTP*) or to other drugs already taken (e.g. *BUvox*, *Thioridazine*). Although medical terms and acronyms were never clearly explained, the ample use of plain consumer-friendly language helped convey information in a *clear* manner.

Nevertheless, the understandability of language was found to be hindered by the understandability of audio information due to the accelerated pace at which risk information was delivered. Understandability of audio information is said to rely on the skill of critical listening, which presupposes two fundamental elements, namely, background knowledge and familiarity with the topic, and the ability of being a skilled listener.[5] Findings thus suggest that audio risk information was extremely speedy (*M*=10.1wps[6]) in that it required consumers to be skilled critical listeners. Accelerated audio pacing was found to be rather high in the case of insomnia (*M*=15.2 wps) and high cholesterol ads (*M*=11.1wps), but significantly lower in depression ads (*M*=4wps). This was probably due to the providers' decision of promoting the 'relaxed' effect of these drugs by using the subtle communicative strategy of reducing word speed, as shown in Example (1) for the prescription antidepressant, *Pristiq*:

(1)	0:36	don't worry about getting any new hobbies or friends
	0:41	you need a prescription antidepressant
	0:46	ahhhhhhh… don't worry about your diet or exercise
	0:50	you just need to be happy… let it go…
	0:56	ahhhhhhh… don't worry about a thing….

Example (1) shows how the voice-over narrator uses a total of 35 words in 20 seconds (*M*=1.75wps) with prolonged interjections (*ahhhhhhhh*) and verbs (*don't worry*) which are repeated to convey the relaxed benefit of the drug, thus drawing consumers' attention to positive audio information.

Furthermore, audio pacing of benefit information was also regulated by a 'semiotic harmony' (Kress 2010) between the visual and audio modes. While risk information was mainly delivered by voice-over narrators, benefit information was always conveyed by the main characters in the videos. In example (2), an attractive healthy lady is in her restaurant, where she talks about the positive effects of *Zetia* in treating high cholesterol:

(2)	0:01	in my restaurant I like to serve what I eat
	0:05	meals that are fresh, healthy and different
	0:06	and when I found out that my cholesterol was still up a little
	0:10	My doctor told me about a different kind
	0:11	of cholesterol medicine: Zetia.
	0:13	We talked about stat as a good option.

---

5 A skilled listener can process information at around 300 to 500 words per minute (Burley-Allen 1982).

6 The acronym stands for 'words per second'.

0:15	Zetia works differently.
0:17	You see stats work mainly with the liver,
0:19	not Zetia.
0:20	It works in the digestive tract like some other medicines,
0:22	but Zetia is unique in the way that it
0:24	helps block the absorption of cholesterol that comes from food…

In the excerpt, audio and visual modes are synchronised for 14 seconds (0.10–0.24; 62 words) to facilitate consumers' understanding of the difference and uniqueness of the promoted medication (*a different kind of cholesterol medicine*, *Zetia works differently*, *Zetia is unique*). By contrast, example (3) indicates the excessive speed at which the voice-over narrator provides risk information regarding the antidepressant drug, *Zoloft*:

(3) 0:36 Zoloft is not for everyone. People taking MAOIs or chemosis shouldn't take Zoloft. Side effects may include dry mouth, insomnia, sexual side effects, diarrhea, nausea and sleepiness. Zoloft is not habit forming. Talk to your doctor about Zoloft.

The excerpt clearly shows that consumers are expected to capture and understand 39 words in one simple second. While the language is plain with the occurrence of only two medical terms: *MAOIs* and *chemosis*, accelerated audio pacing suggests that consumers may experience working memory load, i.e., recalling (if any) background knowledge. In addition, consumers are simultaneously engaged in communication through other semiotic systems, which are likely to induce their inattention to audio risk information. On the whole, audio risk information was delivered in an inconspicuous manner, despite the use of plain language. Inconspicuousness was determined by the asynchrony between the audio and visual semiotic representations, mainly due to the use of voice-over narrators.

The balance between risk and benefit information was also undermined within the linguistic semiotic mode as shown in Table 1.

eDTCA	*Tokens*	*Text Placement*	*Font Size*
1. Rozerem (Insomnia)	Your Dreams Miss You Rozerem Approved in adults with difficulty falling asleep Individual results may vary; By prescription only.	Centre Upper-Centre Upper Right Lower Left	Large Large Large Small
2. Lipitor (Cholesterol)	LIPITOR LIPITOR IS FDA APPROVED TO REDUCE THE RISK OF HEART ATTACK AND STROKE. ALONG WITH DIET, LIPITOR LOWERS BAD CHOLESTEROL 39% TO 60%. Risks factors include: family history of early heart disease, high blood pressure, low good cholesterol, age, and smoking; Average effect depending on dose; Lipitor is one of many treatment options to consider; Available by prescription only.	Centre Upper-Centre Lower Left	Capitals Capitals Small

Table 1. Risk/benefit information: examples of unfair balance in the written mode.

The excerpts in Table 1 clearly show an unfair balance in the display of written risk/benefit information. The first example suggests that consumers' attention is drawn to benefit information (*Approved in adults with difficulty falling asleep*), as it is positioned in the upper right section (New information) in large font size. Conversely, risk information is positioned in the lower left section (Given information) in small font size, suggesting that its value is less salient in the overall composition plan. In addition, risks are generically stated (*Individual results may vary*), leaving consumers with no information about contraindications. The brand name (*Rozerem*) is placed in the upper-centre section of the screen in large characters, and as such, becomes the "ostensibly, most salient part" (Kress/van Leeuwen 1996: 194). The appealing slogan *Your Dreams Miss You* is positioned in the centre in large characters, and thus, immediately attracts the consumer's attention. Benefits are conceptualised in the slogan by engaging consumers (*You*) directly with their dreams, which are personified as suffering from the lack of interpersonal relations with sleepless patients.

In the second example, the brand name (*LIPITOR*) is centrally placed on the screen in capital letters. The essential information in the upper-central section attempts to convince consumers of the benefits, first by building trust in readable capital letters (*LIPITOR IS FDA APPROVED*), and then by making the effort of providing figures, using the same font size (*LIPITOR LOWERS BAD CHOLESTEROL 39% TO 60%*). Conversely, risk information is displayed in small font size in the lower left section, and ambiguously refers to the condition of having high cholesterol (*family history of early heart disease, high blood pressure, low good cholesterol, age, and smoking*), rather than clearly stating possible side-effects (*average effect depending on dose*). In both cases, benefit information was given salience through the main aspects of upper right/centre placement and large/capital font size; risk information was, instead, displayed with less information value by positioning it in the lower left section of the screen in small font size. Finally, findings also revealed an unfair time balance in the display between benefit and risk information as the former (*M*=15secs) outweighed the latter (*M*=5secs). In sum, the eDTCA corpus data revealed how risk information was generally presented, as summarised in Table 2.

Prescription Drug	*Language*	*Main Type of Audio Pacing*	*Text Placement*	*Text Font Size*
INSOMNIA 1. Ambien CR 2. Intermezzo 3. Lunesta 4. Midnite 5. Rozerem 6. Sominex 7. Unisom PM 8. ZzzQuil	PLAIN	ACCELERATED	LOWER LEFT SCREEN SECTION	SMALL

Prescription Drug	*Language*	*Main Type of Audio Pacing*	*Text Placement*	*Text Font Size*
CHOLESTEROL 1. Crestor 2. Lipitor 3. Plavix 4. Simvastatin 5. Trilipix 6. Vytorin 7. Zetia 8. Zocor	PLAIN	ACCELERATED	LOWER LEFT SCREEN SECTION	SMALL
DEPRESSION 1. Abilify 2. Celexa 3. Cymbalta 4. Effexor 5. Paxil 6. Pristiq 7. Wellbutrin 8. Zoloft	PLAIN	NORMAL/SLOW	LOWER LEFT SCREEN SECTION	SMALL
	CLEAR	INCONSPICUOUS	BIASED	UNFAIR

Table 2. Semiotic representation of risk information in the eDTCA corpus.

Findings showed that risk information was mainly presented in clear plain language. This was, however, somewhat obscured by the accelerated pace at which voice-over narration occurred, thus rendering audio risk information inconspicuous and vague. In addition, the manner in which information was conveyed through the written semiotic mode was definitely biased in terms of readability, screen placement and display time. In other words, the linguistic and audio semiotic systems did not engage in semiotic exchanges of meaningful risk information.

4.2 Semiotic distractors

As for the variables in the category of semiotic distractors, findings first showed that superimposed text on risk information was never synchronised with related audio information. Consumers were, in fact, first allowed to view the generic textual information displayed on screen and then to follow the voice-over narrator's vague information. These alternating shifts between superimposed text and aural information was found to disrupt consumers' understanding. The absence of superimposed text on audio risk information was thus seen as an additional obstacle for consumers. Their synchronised mode of complementing risk information would have probably better supported health consumers.

In addition, the emotional tone of visual images was always found to be very strong, thus further detracting from the semiotic representations of side effects and risks. In detail, the tone of visual images was embedded in multimodal narrative texts, which were structured in everyday life narrative settings (visual semiotic mode) with background music (audio semiotic mode), which helps to render the text 'open' (Eco 1989). In these settings, real-life characters tell their stories (linguistic semiotic mode) about health symptoms and assume a 'moral stance' (Ochs/Capps 2001), i.e., an attitude towards what is bad about the health symptoms and what is good about the promoted prescription drug. In this, narratives as semantic-pragmatic resources had a twofold purpose. First, they had a persuasive communicative function in eDT-CA multimodal discourse; second, they supported the strategy of sensory marketing, which according to Krishna (2012: 332), is:

> marketing that engages the consumers' senses and affects their perception, judgment, and behaviour [as] these sensory triggers may result in consumers' self-generation of (desirable) brand attributes, rather than those verbally provided by the advertiser.

Besides relying on multimodal narrative texts, the emotional tone of visual images was also strengthened through the use of semiotic metaphors (Kress 2010), which create new meaning multimodally, as shown in Figure 1. The narrative setting in Figure 1 is a common home kitchen where three characters are gathered around a table, while the fourth is preparing breakfast, as also suggested by the background sound of cutlery, which 'opens' the multimodal text. The consumer's attention is immediately drawn to the visual representation of three uncommon characters who have gathered with the ordinary man (patient) represented on the left. The understanding of the visual metaphor may be difficult for those who are unfamiliar with the cultural context (cf. Feng/O'Halloran 2013). The central character is, in fact, US President Abraham Lincoln who has been waiting for the sleepless patient to resume playing the usual chess game together. The cultural reference here is to Lincoln's well-known addiction to this game, witnessed by his chess sets displayed at the National Museum of American History in Washington, D.C.

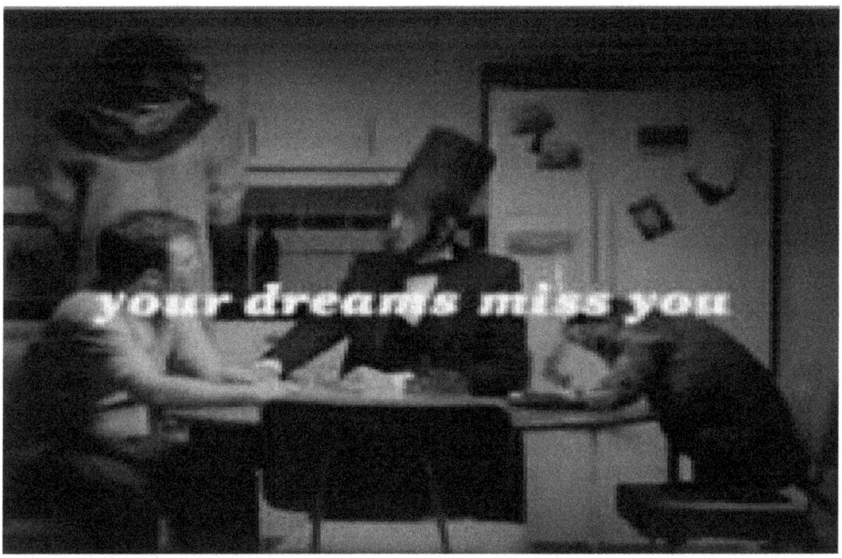

Figure 1. The use of semiotic metaphor for multimodal meaning.

Visual meaning is also intertwined with the superimposed text *Your dreams miss you*. In addition, the beaver next to Lincoln represents both a cultural and a symbolic image. Culturally, it is a semi-aquatic rodent that is found in North America; symbolically, it is known for its nocturnal industriousness. The visual metaphor further interacts with the dialogic narrative between the three characters as shown in Example (4):

(4) [Abraham Lincoln] Hey Sleeping Beauty!
[Patient] Didn't sleep a wink!
[Abraham Lincoln] I know. We've been waiting for you. We have a chess set.
[Beaver] He cheats.
[Abraham Lincoln] Hello honest Abe.
[Beaver] some whatever...
[Abraham Lincoln] We just haven't played for so long.
[Patient] I know, I've just got all this stress at work.
[Abraham Lincoln] It's cool. It happens to a lot of people.
[Patient] Really???!!!!
[Beaver] Absolutely!!
[Abraham Lincoln] We just want you back.
[Patient] Thanks guys!!

In the opening line, Lincoln addresses the patient as *Sleeping Beauty*, and creates a cause-effect mechanism (*didn't sleep a wink-I know, we've been waiting for you; we just haven't played for so long*). This feeds the consumer's desire for a narrative resolution (*It's cool. It happens to a lot of people*; *we just want you back*). Consumers further need to know the cultural context to interpret the way Lincoln addresses the beaver by calling it with his own nickname (*Hello honest Abe*), used for his well-known honesty and integrity. The other character is only visually represented as a deep-sea diver, who personifies the missing dreams the patient is no longer able to dive into. The dull image colours also contribute to constructing the visual metaphorical meaning of sleeplessness.

Despite the semiotic metaphor creating an 'orchestration effect' of different semiotic resources (Kress/van Leeuwen 2001), consumers may be distracted by the surreal visual representation of the characters. Moreover, consumers lacking the cultural background knowledge necessary to grasp the visual metaphor, or those with low literacy skills, will most probably dwell longer on its interpretation, rather than focusing on drug risk information.

Lastly, findings referring to the consistency of visual images with written and spoken risk information showed that visual representations were characterised by the presence of changing events. The phasal shifts between images depicted a change of state in a patient, i.e., from the state of suffering from health disorders to the state of being healthy following drug treatment. This 'type II event' in narration (Hühn 2009) was realised by creating a positive daily context related to a patient who interprets the change of state as shown in Figure 2. The transformational effect of a person represented as a bright light bulb with a sad frowny face into a happy relaxed person who is peacefully sleeping, conveys the meaningful experience of using this prescription drug. The relief that the patient visualizes is inconsistent with the risk information provided by the voice-over narrator: *Intermezzo like most medicines has some risk of dependency. Common side effects are headache, nausea and fatigue.*

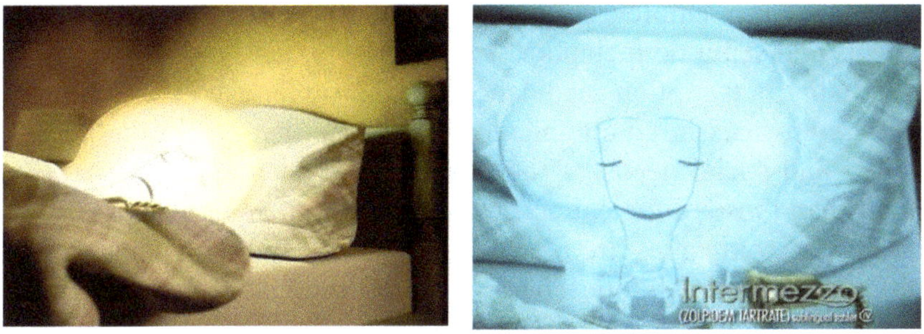

Figure 2. Visual representations of the change of state in the condition of insomnia.

The overall inconsistency found between visual representations and written/spoken risk information was understood to be deliberately misleading, detracting the consumer's attention from being informed about the side-effects in favour of the commercial promotion of the product.

5. Final remarks

In the era of consumer medicine and social media, the proliferation of eDTCA represents a major concern for public health policymakers and patients alike. On their side, pharmaceutical companies are taking advantage of the lack of regulation and access restriction and are investing in YouTube-dedicated channels to reach an increasing number of online health consumers to promote their products. The current study has highlighted how such multimodal discourse may have an immediate communicative effect on patients. Despite the clarity of language used in the prescription drug ads examined, risk information was delivered in an inconspicuous manner through the audio semiotic mode and in a biased manner through the textual mode. Furthermore, a noticeable imbalance between negative and positive information was found both in terms of content and time.

The unsynchronised shifts between audio and linguistic semiotic resources undermined communication dealing with risk information and favoured the predominance of the visual semiotic system. The latter was particularly employed using narrative structures, transformational appeals and semiotic metaphors to capture the consumer's interest. By advertising prescription medications in the same way as other goods, eDTCA engages in communicative processes that "meet the psychological and social needs of the consumer" (David/Greer 2001: 125), rather than those of the patient. Driven by commercial purposes, pharmaceutical companies are actually misleading and deceiving patients through different semiotic distractors, and ultimately, seem to undermine both collective and individual health protection.

References

Bradley, Lynette / Zito, Julie M. 1997. Direct-to-consumer Prescription Drug Advertising. *Medical Care* 35/1, 86–92.

Brown, Bonnie 2004. *Opening the Medicine Cabinet: First Report on Health Aspects of Prescription Drugs. Report of the Standing Committee on Health*. Ottawa, Ontario: House of Commons.

Burgess, Jean / Green, Joshua 2009. *YouTube: Online Video and Participatory Culture*. Cambridge: Polity.

Burley-Allen, Madelyn 1982. *Listening: the Forgotten Skill*. New York: Wiley.

Chau, Clement 2010. YouTube as a Participatory Culture. *New Directions for Youth Development* 128, 65–74.

Cho, Mildred K. 2000. Guidelines for Advertising on Health Web Sites. Who's Guarding the Koop? *Western Journal of Medicine* 172/4, 230–232.

Choi, Sejung M. / Lee, Wei-Na 2007. Understanding the Impact of Direct-to-Consumer (DTC) Pharmaceutical Advertising on Patient-Physician Interactions: Adding the Web to the Mix. *Journal of Advertising* 36/3, 137–149.

David, Sean / Greer David S. 2001. Social Marketing: Application to Medical Education. *Annals of Internal Medicine* 134, 125–127.

Donohue, Julie 2006. A History of Drug Advertising: The Evolving Roles of Consumers and Consumer Protection. *Milbank Quarterly* 84/4, 659–699.

Eco, Umberto 1989. *The Open Work*. Cambridge, MA: Harvard University Press.

Feng, Dezheng / O'Halloran, Kay 2013. The Visual Representation of Metaphor. A Social Semiotic Approach. In Pinar Sanz, Maria Jesus (ed.) *Multimodality and Cognitive Linguistics*. Special issue of *Review of Cognitive Linguistics* 11/2, 320–335.

Findlay, Scott D. 2001. Direct-to-consumer Promotion of Prescription Drugs – Economic Implications for Patients, Payers and Providers. *Pharmacoeconomics* 19, 109–119.

Frosch, Dominick L. / Grande, David 2010. Direct-to-consumer Advertising of Prescription Drugs. *LDI Issue Brief* 15, 1–4.

Greene, Jeremy A. / Kesselheim, Aaron, S. 2010. Pharmaceutical Marketing and the New Social Media. *The New England Journal of Medicine* 363/22, 2087–2089.

Hodge, Robert / Kress, Gunther 1988. *Social Semiotics*. Cambridge, UK: Polity.

Hühn, Peter 2009. Event and Eventfulness. In Hühn, Peter / Pier, John/ Schmid, Wolf/ Schönert, Jörg (eds) *Handbook of Narratology*. Berlin: Walter de Gruyter, 80–97.

Humphreys, Gary 2009. Direct-to-consumer Advertising under Fire. *Bulletin of World Health* 87, 576–577.

Hunt, Michie 1998. *Direct-to-Consumer Advertising of Prescription Drugs*. Washington, DC: The George Washington University.

Jenkins, Henry 2006. *Convergence Culture: Where Old and New Media Collide*. New York: New York University Press.

Khosla, Pratibha / Khosla, Akash 2011. Direct to Consumer Advertising of Prescription Drugs on Internet: A Boon or a Curse. *Indian Journal of Pharmacology* 43/4, 483–484.

Kress, Gunther 2010. *Multimodality: A Social Semiotic Approach to Contemporary Communication*. London: Routledge.

Kress, Gunther / van Leeuwen, Theo 1996. *Reading Images: The Grammar of Visual Design*. London: Routledge.

Kress, Gunther / van Leeuwen, Theo 2001. *Multimodal Discourse: The Modes and Media of Contemporary Communication*. London: Arnold.

Krishna, Aradhna 2012. An Integrative Review of Sensory Marketing: Engaging the Senses to Affect Perception, Judgment and Behavior. *Journal of Consumer Psychology* 22/3, 332–351.

Lee, Sandra S. / Crawley, La V. 2009. Research 2.0: Social Networking and Direct-to-Consumer (DTC) Genomics. *The American Journal of Bioethics* 9/6–7, 35–44.

Liang, Bryan A. / Mackey, Timothy K. 2011a. Prevalence and Global Health Implications of Social Media in Direct-to-Consumer Drug Advertising. *Journal of Medical Internet Research* 13/3, e64. <http://www.jmir.org/2011/3/e64/>.

Liang, Bryan A. / Mackey, Timothy K. 2011b. Direct-to-Consumer Advertising with Interactive Internet Media: Global Regulation and Public Health Issues. *The Journal of the American Medical Association* 305/8, 824–825.

Mackey, Timothy K. / Liang, Bryan A. 2013. Global Reach of Direct-to-Consumer Advertising Using Social Media for Illicit Online Drug Sales. *Journal of Medical Internet Research* 15/5: e105. <www.ncbi.nlm.nih.gov/pmc/articles/PMC3668613/#ref1>.

Ochs, Elinor / Capps, Lisa 2001. *Living Narrative. Creating Lives in Everyday Storytelling*. Cambridge, MA: Harvard University Press.

O'Halloran, Kay L. (ed.) 2004. *Multimodal Discourse Analysis*. London: Continuum.

Plastina, Anna Franca 2012. *Applied Linguistics and Semantic Web Apps: Cases of Mediated Discursive Practices*. Muenchen: Lincom Europa.

Raven, Melissa 2004. Direct-to-Consumer Advertising: Healthy Education or Corporate Spin? *Healthy Skepticism International News* 22/9. <http://www.healthyskepticism.org/news/issue.php?id=5>.

Rothman, David J. 2001. The Origins and Consequences of Patient Autonomy: A 25-Year Retrospective. *Health Care Analysis* 9, 255–264.

Sacristán, José A 2013. Patient-Centered Medicine and Patient-Oriented Research: Improving Health Outcomes for Individual Patients. *BMC Medical Informatics and Decision Making* 13/6. <http://www.biomedcentral.com/1472-6947/13/6>.

Silver, Lawrence S. / Stevens, Robert E. / Loudon, David 2009. Direct-to-Consumer Advertising of Pharmaceuticals: Concepts, Issues, and Research. *Health Marketing Quarterly* 26, 251–8.

Thibault, Paul J. 2000. The Multimodal Transcription of a Television Advertisement: Theory and Practice. In Baldry, Anthony (ed.) *Multimodality and Multimediality in the Distance Learning Age: Papers in English Linguistics*. Campobasso: Palladino, 311–85.

Ventola, C. Lee 2011. Direct-to-Consumer Pharmaceutical Advertising: Therapeutic or Toxic? *Pharmacy and Therapeutics* 36/10, 669–674.

Weinmeyer, Richard 2013. Health Law. Direct-to-Consumer Advertising of Drugs. *Virtual Mentor-American Medical Association Journal of Ethics* 15/11, 954–959.

Wilkes, Michael S. / Bell, Robert A. / Kravitz, Richard L. 2000. Direct-to-Consumer Prescription Drug Advertising: Trends, Impact, and Implications. *Health Affairs* 19/2, 110–128.

Wolfe, Sidney M. 2002. Direct-to-Consumer Advertising – Education or Emotion Promotion? *New England Journal of Medicine* 346/7, 524–526.

World Health Organization 2000. *Guidelines for the Regulatory Assessment of Medicinal Products for Use in Self-Medication.* <http://apps.who.int/medicinedocs/en/d/Js2218e/>.

World Health Organization 2007. How to Get Information from and to End-users (Patients). *WHO Pharmaceuticals Newsletter* 5, 7–10.

Appendix – The eCDTA Corpus

Insomnia
1. Ambien CR <https://www.youtube.com/watch?v=NG1hdWb8yBM>
2. Intermezzo <https://www.youtube.com/watch?v=a5HTLcAOx38>
3. Lunesta <https://www.youtube.com/watch?v=Sl-Pu5xPsMs>
4. Midnite <https://www.youtube.com/watch?v=_h7FvNqj1GQ>
5. Rozerem <https://www.youtube.com/watch?v=wdpOIaGnzvA>
6. Sominex <https://www.youtube.com/watch?v=k-t5oBglXXs>
7. Unisom PM <https://www.youtube.com/watch?v=xDsseSfjwFc>
8. ZzzQuil <https://www.youtube.com/watch?v=qlsREI-cHtk>

High Cholesterol
1. Crestor <https://www.youtube.com/watch?v=-jFKX0bJLfQ>
2. Lipitor <https://www.youtube.com/watch?v=ogyC9rEjxDM>
3. Plavix <https://www.youtube.com/watch?v=sZulydGi65o>
4. Simvastatin <https://www.youtube.com/watch?v=pINMzVw0Nm4>
5. Trilipix <https://www.youtube.com/watch?v=Ro3MQWLhmbA>
6. Vytorin <https://www.youtube.com/watch?v=H6W1-MqmOro>
7. Zetia <https://www.youtube.com/watch?v=iNOsGIypxoM>
8. Zocor <https://www.youtube.com/watch?v=0_3L-uUC-L8>

Depression
1. Abilify <https://www.youtube.com/watch?v=tGymr78FtbU>
2. Celexa <https://www.youtube.com/watch?v=RPPqbfCv-tk>
3. Cymbalta <https://www.youtube.com/watch?v=OTZvnAF7UsA>
4. Effexor <https://www.youtube.com/watch?v=6gSD5bK1Zgo>
5. Paxil <https://www.youtube.com/watch?v=FOgKAkJAn44>
6. Pristiq <https://www.youtube.com/watch?v=0kHNv4a1JdY>
7. Wellbutrin <https://www.youtube.com/watch?v=2ohZdpetU_0>
8. Zoloft <https://www.youtube.com/watch?v=6vfSFXKlnO0>

Girolamo Tessuto

Empowering Patients to Self-Care in Web-mediated Communication: A Multimodal Discourse Analysis

1. Introduction

The last few decades have seen a plethora of discourse-based research studies in the health/medicine and social care domains, emphasizing the growing importance of language and communication. These studies have been informed by conversational, pragmatics, sociolinguistics and other analytical perspectives in different settings (e.g. Sarangi/Roberts 1999; Candlin/Candlin 2002; Sarangi/Clarke 2002; Gwyn 2002; Garzone/Rudvin 2003; Roberts/Sarangi 2005; Gotti/ Salager-Meyer 2006; Heritage/Maynard 2006; Garzone/Sarangi 2007; Iedema 2007; Sarangi 2005; Stivers 2007; Candlin/Sarangi 2011), and have provided a rich set of (quantitative and qualitative) methodological tools for a broader understanding of healthcare discourse. Although such reviewed studies are not exhaustive, they do provide a variety of invaluable and stimulating insights into the construction of health care and its social and professional practices.

However, the World Wide Web is rapidly changing the landscape of health and medical communication, exemplifying a globally-networked, multicultural and multilingual information environment with vast possibilities. Widespread access to healthcare information is increasingly provided over the Web, and numerous publicly and privately-run websites exist to enable diverse users to seek out information about syndromes and diseases, drugs, nutrition, and fitness, by constituting what has been referred to as a growing 'medialized world' of health resources (Richardson 2005: 1). In this world of 'free-for-all' Web health resources, where information utilization by individuals (patients) is likely to address the influences impacting on their health education, the increased public use of healthcare websites supports the idea of "the increased level of patient literacy with ease of access to the health-related websites" (Sarangi 2005: 383), allowing individuals to make more informed health care decisions. Allied to the widespread access to the Web health space is the impact of virtual reality tools offered by the broader term Medicine 2.0 (Eysenbach 2008) or the similar concepts of eHealth 2.0 and Web 2.0 (Giustini 2006; Hughes et al. 2008), where a different set of technologies for use by diverse user groups (patients, caregivers, medical professionals, and other stakeholders in health) generates its applications across health care in general, and has a potential for public health promotion. In this evolutionary framework of electronically available health resources, however, important issues arise as to whether public access to health and medical information contributes to the changing dimensions of the doctor-patient relationship and traditional healthcare settings in general (e.g. Slack 1997; Mooney/Sarangi 2003).

Regardless of these issues, the increased use of healthcare websites runs parallel to the potential advantages of using those sites to deliver self-care and behaviour-change actions by improving the health status of their users. Implicit in these actions is the important role played by the Web-Mediated Communication model, which holds within the inherent properties and characteristics of Web texts, such as hypertextuality (or hypermediality), non-linearity and multimodality (Landow 1992; Bolter 2001). The relevance of this model makes the communication activity via self-care websites a significant subject for research, since it provides the medium in which to disclose a range of semiotic modes (linguistic and visual representations) arising from the rich multimodal nature of those websites. Reliance on these modes therefore provides a common platform for a Multimodal Discourse Analysis (Fairclough/Wodak 1997; Kress/van Leeuwen 2001, 2006; Lemke 2002; Iedema 2003; LeVine/ Scollon 2004; O'Halloran 2004; Garzone 2007; Kress 2010), where the interaction of multimodal semiotic representations contributes to the social practice of meaning making (Fairclough/ Wodak 1997; Kress/van Leeuwen 2001: 21–22; Kress 2010: 79).

Despite a generalised growing awareness of this interaction in the website phenomena, the amount of multimodal analytic work carried out by discourse scholars on self-care websites does seem to have been relatively small until now. To the best of my knowledge, only a few studies are sourced from the UK's NHS information/advice websites, yielding invaluable insights into health care interaction pathways (Mooney/Sarangi 2003), or providing language analyses of healthcare (Grego 2008; Vicentini 2008; Grego/Vicentini 2010, 2011).

In an attempt to address this gap, this study offers a multimodal discourse analytic description of online self-care communication as a dynamic and strategic medium for engaging people in their health. It does so by looking at the linguistic and visual resources used across Web-mediated texts, uncovering the potential meanings created for the social activities and purposes behind those resources. The chapter breaks down as follows. Firstly, the empirical material for corpus-driven analysis is indicated and the research method outlined. Secondly, the key findings of empirical data are analysed and discussed and, thirdly, tentative conclusions are drawn from contextualized material.

2. Material and Method

2.1 The website corpus: audience, content and purpose

The data source for this study comes from the fully-fledged UK-based Self-Care Library website,[1] involving recognised university health research centres and professional health teams in the UK. Besides running on its own, the Library also contributes support to the UK-based College of Medicine non-profit organization website,[2] where it is found in the Knowledge Library menu. This College advocates a whole systems approach across the NHS and contributes to the strength of inter-professional collaboration and practice in health care and medicine by patients, doctors, scientists and others who make up the core of the College itself. The website features as

1 Available at <http://selfcare-library.info>.
2 Available at <http://www.collegeofmedicine.org.uk/home>.

> a not-for-profit online patient resource providing free evidence-based information about health care. In particular [the Library] focuses on self-care treatment options for chronic conditions, as well as providing information for general self care and looking after one's own health and wellbeing. (About Us)

However, the mission disclosure (Our Mission Statement) also addresses other user groups, such as caregivers, health care professionals, and students of self-care approaches. High quality of health information on the site is professionally designed and compiled by medical and healthcare academics and practitioners (About Us: Our Team – Editorial Board), thus being consistent with Silberg et al.'s (1997) criteria for credibility of Internet health sources/authorships.

Although a variety of targeted users are involved in the spectrum of self-care, information search by patients as primary end-users is the most common and influential motive for browsing the website. This rationale readily makes use of the website as a tool for informational communication purposes between expert providers delivering health information for self-care and users seeking such information on the Web. As a reliable informational website, therefore, the Library emphasises the importance of the participants' (providers and users) role and their social ('human-to-system' or 'human-to-documents') interaction/interactivity (McMillan 2002) in the self-care communication process, and leaves out of consideration the use of the site for any advisory or advertising communication purpose. This is overtly addressed by the commonly used Disclaimer and About Us pages, warning users not to employ the site as "a substitute of diagnosis and treatment by an appropriate health care professional", thus representing itself as an information rather than medical-advice source for provider-user interaction. Similarly, the About Us page discloses the site's viewpoint as a "non-commercial resource".

Based on these criteria for corpus building, the Web pages were accessed in the time span of January-February 2014, and stored on a computer, yielding an approximately 158,900 total number of tokens. Stored data were searched automatically via computer for specific linguistic items and frequency, and analyzed through a manual textual reading.

2.2 Methodological framework

Consistent with the call for an integration of mixed methodologies (Sarangi/Candlin 2004), this quantitative and qualitative corpus-based study used a combined framework of theoretical approaches and perspectives in order to study the linguistic and visual modes of communication. To examine the linguistic data, I drew upon Fairclough's (2001) Critical Discourse Analysis (CDA) approach to micro-level *textual* elements (Fairclough 1995: 57), as well as other discourse analysis (DA) perspectives on specific patterns of language use, such as those from the areas of Semantics (Palmer 2001), Appraisal (Martin 2000), or Specialized Discourse (Gotti 2011). Consistent with the CDA interest in exploring how discourse is "socially constitutive as well as socially conditioned" and "discursive practices may have major ideological effects" (Fairclough/Wodak 1997: 258), the goal of this analysis was to reveal the formal properties of the text and the (ideational/ interpersonal/textual) meanings it conveys by establishing role aspects of social identities, social relations and systems of knowledge and beliefs between the participants in the interaction.

To critically examine the visual data, I drew upon the existence of a 'visual code' or 'grammar of visual design' described in Kress and van Leeuwen (2006 [1996]) in their social-semiotic approach to multimodal texts. The analysis of a 'code' in Kress and van Leeuwen's (1996) theory suggests that "[l]ike linguistic structures, visual structures point to particular interpretations of experience and forms of social interactions" (1996: 2). The goal at this level of analysis was to reveal representational, interactive and compositional meanings of visual images proposed in Kress and van Leeuwen's (2006) descriptive framework of multimodality.

By complementing each other in the ongoing analysis of Web-mediated communication, these analytical approaches recursively converge on the social-semiotic aspect of multimodality proposed in Kress and van Leeuwen (2001).[3] These authors (2001: 4–8) consider four domains of practice for analysing multimodal discourse in which

3 In Kress and van Leeuwen's (2001) work, the socially grounded perspective on multimodal texts shares similarities with Kress's (2010) view of multimodality in contemporary communication.

meanings are created: *discourse* (socially constructed knowledge of reality), *design* (semiotic resources to realize discourses), *production* (the actual process of using a medium to create a semiotic message), and *distribution* (how the semiotic message is shared with a larger audience).

3. Results and Discussion

3.1 Content design: an overview

Prior to analysing linguistic and visual modes of communication, it is useful to look briefly at the website design and content, which provide the socio-cultural organization of the current discourse by integrating semiotic resources for meaning making from multiple modes of communication. Glancing at the Home Page of the Self-Care Library website, it is easy to recognize that the central role of Web providers is to appeal to people seeking appropriate information for self care by mouse-over markings of hyperlink clickability. This is visible in the screen shot reported in Figure 1 (Appendix), where an aesthetic rather than cluttered design is utilized, and visual formats such as image maps, fonts, colours, primary navigation menus (About SelfCare, Start the SelfCare Pathway, About the Evidence, Browse Conditions) as well as short and simple texts are employed in a set of horizontally aligned hyperlinks for the surfing public. In addition to the conventional logo signposting the professional achievement of the website and establishing its own social identity, the strategic fit of a specific audience through human images is consistent with the site's rationale of putting the patient first.

When surfing through the website, an aesthetically diversified layout is almost equally apparent, though high amounts of texts are used in lieu of visuals to structure the content of the website for the surfing public/patients, who are most obviously interested in the meanings to be represented. As shown in Figure 2 (Appendix), this content is organized around five vertically aligned browsable pages placed on the left-hand side and presented in the informational/ instructional leaflet genre and labelled as Overview, Make Simple Changes, Buy Something to Try, Attend Classes / Visit Practitioner, and References. To illustrate briefly, the Overview pages describe the symptoms and causes across twelve common long-term conditions in low-risk patients (sleep problems, back pain, migraine, depression, fatigue, sore muscles, headache, IBS, osteoarthritis, menopause, stress and anxiety, period problems), and suggest whether professional advice from doctors or pharmacists should be sought for any such relapsing health condition. At this stage, simplicity of the browser technology allows for more data resources to be added to such pages in a scalable system, and links between relevant health care websites (such as NHS Choices, Royal College of Psychiatrists, Sleep Council) are provided to help in locating specific information. The Make Simple Changes pages explain a variety of behavioural changes and treatments (e.g. diet, exercise, relaxation techniques) that may help the consumer recover from any such health condition, and give each treatment/ therapy a rating for the strength of its Evidence base, its Safety and Costs by including useful graphics at each point in the text. The Buy Something to Try pages include a diverse range of over-the-counter medicines, nutritional supplements and herbal remedies that may be preventative, diagnostic, therapeutic or supportive of self-care actions. Although, at first sight, profiling such a range of products in these pages may stray towards marketing communication purposes of the site, as shown by their message content (e.g. *Vitamins are generally inexpensive and safe if not taken in large amounts / Antihistamines can be bought for relatively low cost from most pharmacies*), the predominant use of the website for informational purposes is readily apparent in these pages, where the focus of producers is simply on product safety and cost-effectiveness to ensure self-care. The Attend Classes / Visit Practitioner pages instruct on how best to use educational health programmes such as yoga, massage, hypnosis, or autogenic training based on research evidence and cost in a hyperlinked environment, and go on to spell out that the user can talk with their nurse or GP if they are unsure about the particular treatment. Finally, the References pages provide research 'conclusions' about the informed treatments through hyperlinked sources of the medical Abstract (Research Article) genre.

3.2 Linguistic mode of communication

Due to space constraints in this study, I will narrow my research findings to the most salient linguistic aspects of the website, and attempt to advance interpretations in line with the digital achievement.

3.2.1 Pronouns

Communication activity via the website builds up relationships that are implicitly claimed by the overwhelming use of *you* personal pronoun (2,772 occurrences) and *your* possessive adjective (1,310). The frequency list drawn up automatically via computer shows that *you* and *your* were the fourth and fifth most occurring content word in the data after the grammatical words *a* (3,151), *to* (3,416) and *the* (4,145), and were much more common than the recurrent pronouns *we* (146), *our* (131) and *us* (58) across the Web pages. *You* was the key discoursal technique used to create *synthetic personalization* (Fairclough 2001), referring to the manipulation of interpersonal meanings and forms for strategic purposes. In the examples below, directly addressing the readers with *you* not only simulates a relationship of "equality, solidarity [and] intimacy" (Fairclough 2001: 52) in a correspondingly 'conversational' relationship, but also individualizes readers as patients in their different roles of individuals, families or others, as is advocated in official self-care policies: [4]

(1) *We* know how important it is that *you* understand where information about *your* health comes from.

(2) *We* are committed to ensuring that *your* information is secure.

By enacting a highly relational discourse value and meaning between interacting producers and readers, synthetic *you* is no less significant in emphasizing the producer's desire to give a 'human face' to social actors as self-care persona. The examples quoted show that the relational value of this type of discourse in the text becomes greater by the possessive case of *you* used as an attribute adjective (*your*), presenting 'synthetic

4 For instance, Department of Health – National Policy and Guidance (*Self Care – A Real Choice: Self Care Support – A Practical Option*, 2005, 2013).

patients' with more 'personalized' care options. The refinement of this seemingly personal relationship is enhanced by text producers representing and constructing communities (academic and professional) and positioning themselves in relation to others (e.g. Fairclough 2003; Fortanet 2003). By personalizing the text, inclusivity of *we* (community-patient) pronoun helps indeed to construct a 'chummy', 'intimate' tone (Wales 1996) between text producers as central, cohesive sources of self-help support and patients, and to similarly ensure that patients feel they are part of a 'joint enterprise' (Quirk et al. 1985), thus creating a favourable impression of shared social identity defined by 'subject positions' (Fairclough 2001).

While the supportive/communal functioning role of the *we* pronoun was the most common choice (112 occurrences) made by text producers, only few pronominal instances (22 occurrences) of the inclusive *we* pronoun achieved other rhetorical effects by making users more receptive to producers' claims:

(3) *We* used a simple rating system for evidence. To decide on the rating for a particular treatment, *we* considered: How much research there was (how many trials) [...].

In these instances, where claims are based on the 'science' behind the evidence and ratings for treatment/therapy, producers seek to convey assurance that 'hard scientific' evidence and ratings are professional credentials that can be trusted by the surfing patients in their informed choice for preventive, therapeutic or supportive self-care actions. Securing ratification of their claims (Latour 1987) therefore serves to anticipate the readers' objections by minimizing the threat to their face. Moreover, other few instances (12) occurred in the About/ Disclaimer pages where the *we* pronoun played an exclusive function, exemplifying that producers were anxious to remove any responsibility mechanism falling upon them (e.g. *However, once you have used these links to leave our site, you should note that we do not have any control over that other website*). In other words, 'we' are all a nice happy community as long as 'you' stay with us, but as soon as 'you' leave, 'we' are no longer with 'you'. The enormous emphasis on binding producers and readers together ('*we* and *you* share alike') therefore suggests a clear sign of engagement with the everyday social action of discourse in the electronic medium, bringing discourse participants into shared understandings, goals and values, and similarly making the health care discourse reciprocal in the Web texts.

Interestingly, synthetic *you* takes a change in direction by the presence of explicit reader reference through the first person singular pronoun *I* (35 occurrences) used across the questionnaire included in the Self-Care Pathway. This can be seen in a set of slides which bring in the patient's ideas and attitudes about self-care by Yes/No answers:

(4) *I* am happy to be touched and massaged. x (yes) x (no)

(5) *I* don't mind taking pills and can usually remember to take them regularly. x (yes) x (no)

By acknowledging the reader's voice temporarily, producers now wish to put their readers firmly in the 'driving seat', and to similarly raise the patient-centred role in health matters. As a conscious choice made by producers, this strategy thus enables self-care information seekers to present affective and interpersonal content in matters of personal preferences, not least because such preferences are electronically stored for later feedback by Web producers. Consequently, the strategy helps to project a patient-situated identity in the online interactive discourse, and to similarly emphasize their own contribution to the self-care options.

3.2.2 Imperatives

The heavy incidence of imperatives (254 occurrences) used throughout the Make Simple Changes pages alone is a clear attempt to direct or instruct readers in some kind of procedural activity. Such is, for instance, instructing health-seekers to attend to some 'Sleep Hygiene Rules' by the use of positive and negative imperatives shown on the right-hand side opposite explanatory and descriptive statements, and marked here as A and B for convenience of use:

(6) Sleep Hygiene Rules

(A)	(B)
Have a consistent bedtime	Your brain and body have their own rhythms of rest and activity. Your brain chemistry and hormone levels vary through the day and night. So having a regular time to sleep and wake can help get you back in synch with your body-clock. This means going to bed regularly, at a time when you are tired. And no matter what sort of sleep you have had, aim to wake at the same time every day, seven days a week. It's best not to make up for a bad night by sleeping in. And if you wake early, rather than lying in bed awake, try to get up and get on with your day. If you establish this sort of strict regime, your body-clock should eventually re-set itself.
Don't cat-nap	A lot of people like an afternoon nap. But sleep scientists say this interferes with night-time sleep. So if you are sleeping badly, don't make up for it by cat-napping in the day, because this will only disturb your sleep rhythm even more. Some elderly people say daytime naps help them sleep better at night, but most insomniacs get a better night's sleep if they give siestas a miss.
Avoid late-night habits	Some people find a very light bedtime snack stops them from waking hungry in the early hours. The traditional hot milky bedtime drink and digestive biscuit may be helpful.
Make your bedroom a restful place	The temperature, light and noise level should be as good as you can make them. Make sure your bed is comfortable: not too hard or soft. If your cat or dog sleeps in your bedroom find it somewhere else if it disturbs you.

As is clear, statements in (B) are used to contextually direct or instruct prospective patients in the adoption of healthy behaviours in (A) by providing them with reasons for action and therefore behavioural change. By serving as cues in such a change, stand-alone imperatives in (A) – sometimes reappearing in (B) – would also naturally be understood as prompting or reminding readers, as it were, that something 'ought to be done' in the particular (speech act) circumstances. However, viewed from the perspective of CDA, text producers take on a privileged position over text receivers since, by using imperatives, they require text receivers to comply with appropriate activities in the resultant interactional structure. In other words, text producers (as expert suppliers of information) exercise their power and control over text receivers (patients). In this context, then, imperatives become an effective tool in the discursive construction of ideology held by text producers, who are able to display their beliefs and values based on their experience and knowledge in the field. Yet, as shown by the contextual cues in (B), the imperative mode in (A) works concertedly with the personalizing (synthetic *you/your*) character of ongoing discourse, so that the examples quoted reveal that the relational value of imperatives serves again to develop solidarity and intimacy in the discourse participants' relations by lowering the pressure on the reader to comply with some procedural action as demanded for by text producers. This, in turn, would seem to provide imperatives in the data with an exhortative rather than a command function, since they work actively to invite patients with heightened awareness to engage in healthy behaviours and recover from health conditions, while at the same time projecting a less authoritative position on the part of text producers.

3.2.3 Questions

Questions occurred in 120 instances across the pages, where they brought readers into the health landscape by driving the argument along:

(7) Are you thinking about eating better, getting more active or fitting in regular relaxation?

(8) So what's most important to you – mind mood and meaning, movement and muscles, or metabolism, diet and medicines?

In a communicative activity where self-care action is the goal, questions specifically invite readers to carry on reading the relevant answers given in sequential units of information across the pages, and are delivered in such a way as to encourage readers to explore problematic health issues that are likely to affect them. Implied in this communicative function of questions is the need to encourage readers in information-based decision making set up by the producer-reader interactional structure, where the 'conversational' talk is part and parcel of the social achievement of the website's goal.

3.2.4 Active/passive voice structure

The greater use of active verb forms (2,634 occurrences) as opposed to the lower use of passive verbs forms (739 occurrences) makes the writing about self-care stronger and more forceful. In our case, where producers of the text aim for the behaviour of the agent (often in the *you* pronoun) to take place in the sentence, active forms conveniently serve to ideologically construct a set of responsibilities for readers as patients, who are thus presented with possible health scenarios and actions to think about and act upon individually:

(9) If you're not properly tired, you may drop off but the sleep you get may not be deep, good-quality sleep, and you could find yourself waking unrefreshed.

(10) Avoid taking the product if you think you may be allergic to any of the ingredients.

Foregrounding readers as patients in the representation of actions or events conveys information about the social relevance of those participants: the more central the patient 'without superior authority', the more likely he or she will be a responsible agent of his/her health in the interactional ('conversational-like') structure of discourse.

3.2.5 Modal auxiliary verbs

Examples 9–10 are also indicative of the heavy weight attached to modalized statements across the Web pages, where the modal verb *can* (1,100) held the lion's share in the data followed in incidence by *may* (520), *will* (370), *should* (287), *might* (240), *could* (79), *have to* (38), *would* (29), and *must* (8). The modal verbs in the corpus reveal the producers' commitment to their propositions, allowing different information to influence the reader's decision or action. In keeping with this discourse function, reference is made first to the producers' commitment to the propositions made around obligation/necessity modals. Although, in the present material, a potential for (deontic) relational authority and power may be concealed by (expert) text producers in obliging text receivers to do certain things, it is conceived that the strong modal claim conveyed by the lower instances of *must* and *have to* necessity/obligation modals is discarded by text producers in favour of the higher occurring (less categorical, weak) *should* semantic profile. Thus, lessening the predictable negative, (expert) authority-based impact of (stronger, more categorical) *must* and *have to* modals by the use of *should* modal marker is helpful to pragmatically establish social relations in the ongoing discourse, while still engaging prospective patients in decision-making:

(11) You *should* consult your medical practitioner if you have any unexplained symptoms of illness or concerns about treatment.

(12) If anxiety or poor sleep are making your life difficult, you *should* see your doctor.

As we can see from the examples quoted, a cue to the social relationships enacted via the text in the discourse is still provided by the synthetic personalization (*you*) invariably occurring with *should* modal followed by the kinds of 'doings' through physical action and speaking and relational verb types (Halliday 2004). As an aside, these examples are also indicative of the communication activity via the informational website intervening between patients and medical practitioners, since patients may postpone getting face-to-face medical care by practitioners until problems that might have been relatively easy to keep in check have become more complicated. Thus, where the information-giving purpose of the website is still the guiding principle for the interactional structure and communication between producers and readers, the effect is that the obligation/necessity modals (*should, must*) function as 'advisives' (Tsui 1994), implying a course of action for the benefit of the readers. Even by means of advisives, however, the producers' belief about their state of knowledge is not downplayed, and has the effect of assigning responsibility to the readers in matters of self-care, or engaging in further medical actions outside the Web.

In the present material, the producers' commitment to their propositions is also revealed by the varying frequencies of *can*, *may*, *might* and *could* modal categories. Whenever health information is given across the Web pages, these modals accommodate only general epistemic statements about what is 'possible' or 'probable', that is, showing that a variety of symptoms and causes across long-term conditions or the availability of over-the-counter medicines/treatments are possible/probable in the relevant circumstances:

(13) A number of good studies have shown that CBT *can* improve sleep problems.

(14) Pain makes it hard to sleep and means that sleep *may* be less refreshing.

(15) Some people are allergic to certain plant families so proceed with care if you think you *might* have an allergy.

(16) Anti-depressant medicines and psychotherapy *could* improve both your mood and your sleep.

By conveying the producers' understanding and representation of reality in authority-marking scheme, these expressive modals thus drive away any relational (deontic) modality from ongoing discourse by those producers. The importance placed on the modal categories in these texts is evident of the consideration of interpersonal meaning of the interactional structure between producers and readers.

3.2.6 Adjectives

The top four adjectives occurring across the pages – *safe* (270), *helpful* (193), *healthy* (113), *good* (121) – are used to refer to physical, mental, or emotional health and well-being. Bearing in mind that the surfing readers are informed about the long-term relapsing health conditions, where demedicalized treatments and deregulated medicines are presented as being satisfactory, 'efficiency' indeed was key in the choice by health-seekers to fill in those condition gaps and remove their health risk. In this framework, therefore, positively connoted adjectives were another important strategy to ensure confidence in the 'efficiency' of those treatments and medicines, since they displayed the producers' attitudinal judgment (Martin 2000) towards those treatments and medicines, and had the potential to evoke similar judgmental responses in readers sharing a particular set of ideological and social values. This way then, positive adjectives enabled text producers to re-construct relapsing conditions as a healthy lifestyle and, just as imperative clauses cultivated such a lifestyle, adjectives served to invite health-seekers to adopt effective behavioural changes such as weight loss, cutting down smoking, doing physical exercise, and so on.

3.2.7 Language register

As has become increasingly clear throughout the description and analysis of the data in the sample, more reader-friendly strategies are used to increase understanding of the health conditions and treatments/therapies being dealt with. This is achieved in ordinary language by including simple and neutral word choice of the NHS semantic entry (e.g. *diet*, *blood pressure*, *pain*, *symptoms*), and by keeping specialized medical terms to a minimum. Where specialist terms did occur, however, they were often accompanied by explanatory sentences (e.g. *Sleep apnoea means having long pauses in breathing during sleep.*). In terms of syntactic arrangement, the use of parataxis prevails over hypotaxis, and in many instances sentences are simply juxtaposed and separated by a full stop. What producers have in mind, therefore, is 'to get the message across' to patient groups who have little or no knowledge of long-term medical conditions and associated treatments. Consequently, texts are realized fluidly across the Web pages resulting in greater patient directness and accessibility to the health care issues explored via the Web, and similarly establishing a common level of shared knowledge and values.

3.2.8 Popularized language

More importantly, these strategies should also be seen through the lens of popularization studies (e.g. Myers 1994, 2003), where the laid back and friendly way of conveying specialized information "involve[s] the transformation of specialized knowledge into 'everyday' or 'lay' knowledge, as well as a recontextualization of scientific discourse" (Calsamiglia/van Dijk 2004: 370). Becoming more 'ordinary' in the ongoing (expert-lay/semi-lay) interactive communication is not just simply a process of simplification of knowledge transfer, but a way of foregrounding people rather than events in a "routinized social activity" (Myers 2003: 267), thus bringing the current discourse closer to the lay reader's everyday experiences (Gotti 2011). Under these circumstances, it is reasonable to believe that the self-care discourse put text producers on a mutual standing with their readers by removing unequal relations likely to arise from their status as expert authors of the Web health pages and their readers. Ensuring that 'all' readers as patients have equal access to public health information therefore suggests a case for the 'democratization' of public discourse (Fairclough 1992) over the Web, where markers that overtly signal relational asymmetries between discourse participants are removed.

3.3 Visual mode of communication

Imagery plays a crucial role in the Home Page alone since, as noted, the Web pages across the site are devoid of images in favour of texts. Figure 1, in fact, illustrates that images of the twelve most common health conditions are placed in the upper side, or 'close up frame' of this Page (Kress/van Leeuwen 2006). These images lead on to other images placed midway down the Home Page.

3.3.1 Top-framed images

In what follows is an analysis of the meanings realized by top-framed images.

3.3.1.1 Representational meaning

As Figure 3 shows, the representational metafunction of those images is revealed in the portrayal of 'thirty-something' upwardly mobile male and female subjects of diverse ethnic origin in various bodily postures. Thus, for instance, the subject in the Migraine image is portrayed with a pained expression, holding her head in her hand. The pain felt in the low back (Back Pain) is a clear depiction of the suffering body, though the image is very much out of a glossy magazine, suggesting that the man is tanned and in good shape. In the Sore Muscles image, the woman seems to be putting on a brave face in spite of the pain. No representation is made of elderly sufferers in those human images, most possibly because discourse producers were aiming to appeal to a younger user-group. The latter would perhaps be more open to the relatively new concept of self-care and eager to engage in Web-supported health care actions, rather than elderly people who might not be using the Web anyway. There is no perceived hint of settings where the subjects might be located, but portrayal of the images is very much individual-focused with the subjects being, as it were, left alone with their disorders. One exception to this 'aloneness' is the depiction of the helping-hands in the osteoarthritis image, which may depend on the fact that osteoarthritis is an age-bound disease and as such requires human closeness and support. This reinforces the suggestion made about younger users/ patients being most likely to be represented on the Home Page, and is therefore in line with the kind of people discourse producers ideologically thought should/might be using the website.

3.3.1.2 Interactive meaning

The 'image act' (Kress/van Leeuwen 2006) of the representations in Figure 3 is what the producers want the viewers to take from it. In this case, the interactive function is enacted by the way human images attract, direct and invoke the desired effect on the specific viewers, namely patients with a vested interest in the topic. In this way the images become objects of thoughtful consideration for those viewers who are already predisposed to the message about reversing long-term conditions. What is more, the focus on individual patients portrayed in the close-up frame of the images allows the viewers to see the face and body of the subjects in full objectivity, and this reasonably makes the interactive scene more personal in meaning by narrowing down the 'social distance' (Kress/ van Leeuwen 2006) between the actors in the images and the viewers. Indeed, the informational load conveyed by those human images is not spared from feelings and emotions being passed on to viewers (Lemke 2002). This is because the visual elements that users as patients are drawn to via the Web are able to communicate data more effectively, and to similarly affect them emotionally in the complex social process of multimedia semiotics.

3.3.1.3 Compositional meaning

The compositional meaning is mainly realized by 'size of frame' and 'colour' of images (Kress/van Leeuwen 2006). As noted earlier, images are marked as clickable when hovered over by a mouse and direct the viewers to informational materials on any one health condition. In this way browsing health conditions becomes subordinate to the placement of images on top position of the Home Page, which makes the information ideologically most significant for discourse producers in their intent to create a personal relationship with viewers. The images appear in large-sized and variously coloured compositions to make them eye catching for viewers, and are laid over in contrast of 'modality background' (Kress/van Leeuwen 2006). In this case, the modality of background allows depicted images to look realistic and to give the clue for coding orientation of health conditions, while colour coherence is used to promote textual cohesion.

3.3.2 Mid-framed images

The producers' desire to showcase the unique informational purpose of the website proceeds with three final human images (Figure 4) placed beneath the twelve images already discussed.

3.3.2.1 Representational, interactive and compositional meanings

Mid-framed images run alongside meaningful texts where three types of (female and male) subjects expressly indicate the intent of the message. In terms of representational features, the images organize the participants into categories. In addition to the 'thirty-something' male sufferer acting as a patient, the values of professionalism and responsibility, which are ideological attributes of doctors and other health practitioners, are depicted in the female healthcare professional image and passed on to patients wishing to reverse their health conditions. Or, depiction of the youngish woman equally seeking care of her childbearing age adds to the physical and emotional care displayed by the daughter's protective hands to the womb of the pregnant woman. What is more, all of the subjects in the textual frames adopt a speech role in *I* pronoun (essentially seeking out health information) and assign to the viewers a complementary role which they wish them to adopt (Halliday 2004). Reasonably, therefore, these images function as a request or 'demand' (Kress/van Leeuwen 2006) for the reader to carry out a particular action or adopt a specific role.

These ways of actively portraying diverse subjects for the viewers through visual as well as (short) textual elements in the image compositions reveal the central role of discourse producers to engage diverse users, whether as patients or health professionals, with self-care information and support.

3.3.3 Culturally unbounded visuals

Following the view that linguistic and non-verbal modalities are bearers of meaning in a particular culture (Baldry/Thibault 2006), it is quite clear that the representational and interactive features of the human images in particular seek to take a predetermined stand in relation to the national (UK) cultural 'usability' of the website, where self-care activities are high on the public agenda of NHS official policies and involve a multicultural, naturalized (white/black) society. However, we should not be adamant in such a narrow view of usability since self-care activities do seem to exert an impact by and within different cultures in English-speaking countries, so that the images above also seek to uncover broader cultural signifiers by emphasizing the wider culturally-neutral infrastructure of the Web.

4. Conclusion

In this chapter, I have reported on the Self-Care Library website as a medic-led, evidence-based repository of patient health care information and risk-removing resource. In presenting a selection of this data set utilized within the content design and organization of the site, I have sought to describe and interpret the ways in which linguistic and visual resources can influence the effectiveness of the site in communicating the desired message by complementing each other to project social meanings multimodally.

The micro-level linguistic data examined from CDA and other DA perspectives have shown the most salient elements of the texts (pronouns, imperatives, questions, active/passive voice, modal verbs, adjectives, register/style) that shape aspects of the social identities, relationships, knowledge and beliefs in the language and discourse of self-care deployed via the Web. In addition to revealing a 'democratizing' style of the discourse to create closer relationships with readers going on the Web, linguistic data reveal that the major strand of self-care discourse is provided by 'conversational', synthetic *you* co-occurring with other grammatically structured features of the texts. Such features are used to construct direct concern and contact with individual readers as patients, who are encouraged to become 'active' agents taking charge of their own physical, mental and emotional health in the communication activity via the Web.

However, reader-patient activation across the website is also linked to the notion of patient empowerment within the UK's healthcare model, and similarly aligns with the CDA's view of language as a socially conditioned process that affects how texts are produced and interpreted. In this framework, in fact, the goal in recent UK policy statements about *self-management*, *self-care*, *self-efficacy*, or other labels, is for individuals as patients to take control of and responsibility for their own health and their interactions with health services so that the individual's potential for health and wellness is maximized. Such priorities by UK policy makers contextualize the elements of social practice that run through self-care discourse via the Web, and similarly develop the notion of readers as patients who are discursively empowered by their sense of 'agency'. Yet, patient empowerment here also becomes a measure of the social trends that are visible in the integration of new communication technologies into healthcare, which enable a variety of Internet users to actively seek out, evaluate and make use of information. In this context, it is no surprise that the role of the website in introducing and engaging readers-patients with self-help informational leaflets becomes central to personal control and therefore empowerment, since it provides the gateway into making informed decisions about illness and behavioural change in the *home* first (the *frontline of self-care* – Self-Care in the NHS Plan 2000, Chapter 1 para. 1.9), and at the same time enables producers to be responsive to the UK's NHS wider framework, which creates a society empowered in its own health.

Just how far the self-care informational website can be a source of personal empowerment will obviously depend on the reader-patient knowledge and skills to assess health-related data and improve the quality of their life. However, the general public's use of the Web for diverse informational purposes (such as online consultations with physicians) is large and growing, and the potential benefit of the informational website in terms of reach, accessibility and cost-effectiveness may provide the first educational step to empowering readers to self-care and to mediating the exchange of information between practitioner and patient.

Like linguistic resources, visual images and the visual processes within them for creating meaning are consistent with the producers' purpose of activating readers as patients, and consequently provide a snapshot of the producers as they stand in the current UK agenda of self-care activities. Besides the compositional meaning, the depiction of the attributes or qualities given to patients in the images (representational meaning) adds to the way images attract the viewer's immediate interest in the depicted subjects (interactive meaning), revealing the producer's level of involvement and interaction with the viewer/patient. Central to the construction of social practice in CDA, the organization of semiotic systems around these three categories of meanings and multimodal representations of knowledge serves to engage the viewers in a relationship with the health 'service' offered by producers, and to similarly establish close connections with those professional actors.

References

Baldry, Anthony / Thibault, Paul 2006. *Multimodal Transcription and Text Analysis. A Multimodal Toolkit and Coursebook.* London: Equinox.

Bolter, David J. 2001. *Writing Space: Computers, Hypertext and the Remediation of Print.* New Jersey: Lawrence Erlbaum.

Calsamiglia, Helena / van Dijk, Teun 2004. Popularization Discourse and Knowledge about the Genome. *Discourse and Society* 15/4, 369–389.

Candlin, Christopher, N. / Candlin, Sally 2002. Discourse, Expertise, and the Management of Health Care Settings. *Research on Language and Social Interaction* 35, 115–137.

Candlin, Christopher N. / Sarangi, Srikant 2011 (eds) *Handbook of Communication in Organisations and Profession.* Berlin: De Gruyter Mouton.

Eysenbach, Gunther 2008. Medicine 2.0: Social Networking, Collaboration, Participation, Apomediation, and Openness. *Journal of Medical Internet Research* 10/3, e22.

Fairclough, Norman 1992. *Discourse and Social Change*. London: Polity.

Fairclough, Norman 1995. *Critical Discourse Analysis: The Critical Study of Language*. London: Longman.

Fairclough, Norman 2001. *Language and Power*. Harlow: Pearson.

Fairclough, Norman 2003. *Analysing Discourse. Textual Analysis for Social Research*. London: Routledge.

Fairclough, Norman / Wodak, Ruth 1997. Critical Discourse Analysis. In van Dijk, Teun A. (ed.), *Discourse as Social Interaction. Discourse Studies: A Multidisciplinary Introduction*, Volume 2. London: Sage, 258–284.

Fortanet, Inmaculada 2003. The Use of *we* in University Lectures: Reference and Function. *English for Special Purposes* 23, 45–66.

Garzone, Giuliana 2007. Genres, Multimodality and the World Wide Web: Theoretical Issues. In Garzone, Giuliana / Poncini, Gina / Catenaccio, Paola (eds) *Multimodality in Corporate Communication: Web Genres and Discursive Identity*. Milano: Franco Angeli, 15–30.

Garzone, Giuliana / Rudvin, Mette (eds) 2003. *Domain-specific English and Language Mediation in a Professional and Institutional Setting*. Milano: Arcipelago.

Garzone, Giuliana / Sarangi, Srikant (eds) 2007. *Discourse, Ideology and Ethics in Specialised Communication*. Bern: Peter Lang.

Giustini, Dean 2006. How Web 2.0 is Changing Medicine: Editorial. *British Medical Journal* 333, 1283–1284.

Gotti, Maurizio [3]2011. *Investigating Specialized Discourse*. Bern: Peter Lang.

Gotti, Maurizio / Salager-Meyer, Francoise (eds) 2006. *Advances in Medical Discourse Analysis: Oral and Written Contexts*. Bern: Peter Lang.

Grego, Kim 2008. Medical English and Institutional Communication: Linguistic Accessibility to Ethically-sensitive Topics in National Health Systems' Websites – UK vs. USA. In Campos Pardillos, Miguel A. / Gómez González-Jover, Adelina (eds) *Proceedings of the 1st International Conference on Language and Health-care*, Instituto Interuniversitario de Lenguas Modernas Aplicadas (IULMA), Universidad de Alicante (Spain), 24–26 October 2007. Alicante: IULMA.

Grego, Kim / Vicentini, Alessandra 2010. Building South African Web Identity: Health Care Information for Citizens vs. Foreigners. In Garzone, Giuliana / Catenaccio, Paola (eds) *Identities Across Media and Modes: Discursive Perspectives*. Bern: Peter Lang.

Grego, Kim / Vicentini, Alessandra 2011. Holiday Dialysis in Italy on the Web: Multidimensional Hybridization in Institutional Healthcare Communication. In Sarangi, Srikant / Polese, Vanda / Caliendo, Giuditta (eds) *Genre(s) on the Move: Hybridization and Discourse Change in Specialized Communication*. Napoli: ESI, 393–406.

Gwyn, Richard 2002. *Communicating Health and Illness*. London: Sage.

Halliday, Michael 2004. *An Introduction to Functional Grammar*, 3rd ed. revised by Christian Matthiessen. London: Edward Arnold.

Heritage, John / Maynard, Douglas (eds) 2006. *Communication in Medical Care: Interaction between Primary Care Physicians and Patients*. Cambridge: Cambridge University Press.

Hughes, Benjamin / Joshi, Indra / Wareham, Jonathan 2008. Health 2.0 and Medicine 2.0: Tensions and Controversies in the Field. *Journal of Medical Internet Research* 10/3, e23.

Iedema, Rick 2003. Multimodality, Resemiotisation: Extending the Analysis of Discourse as Multi-semiotic Practice. *Visual Communication* 2/1, 29–57.

Iedema, Rick (ed.) 2007. *The Discourses of Hospital Communication: Tracing Complexities in Contemporary Health Organisations*. Basingstoke: Palgrave Macmillan.

Kress, Gunther, R. 2010. *Multimodality: A Social Semiotic Approach to Contemporary Communication*. London: Routledge.

Kress, Gunther, R. / van Leeuwen, Theo 2001. *Multimodal Discourse: The Modes and Media of Contemporary Communication*. London: Arnold.

Kress, Gunther, R. / van Leeuwen, Theo 2006 [1996]. *Reading Images: The Grammar of Visual Design*. London: Routledge.

Landow, George 1992. *Hypertext: Convergence of Contemporary Critical Theory and Technology*. Baltimore, MD: Johns Hopkins University Press.

Latour, Bruno 1987. Science in Action: How to Follow Scientists and Engineers through Society. Milton Keynes: Open University Press.

Lemke, Jay 2002. Travels in Hypermodality. *Visual Communication* 1/3, 299–325.

LeVine, Philip / Scollon, Ron 2004. *Discourse and Technology: Multimodal Discourse Analysis*. Washington D.C.: Georgetown University Press.

Martin, James R. 2000. Beyond Exchange: Appraisal Systems in English. In Hunston, Susan / Thompson, Geoffrey (eds) *Evaluation in Texts: Authorial Stance and the Construction of Discourse*. Oxford: Oxford University Press, 142–175.

McMillan, Sally J. 2002. Exploring Models of Interactivity from Multiple Research Traditions: Users, Documents, and Systems. In Lievrouw, Leah / Livingston, Sonia (eds) *Handbook of New Media*. London: Sage, 162–182.

Mooney, Annabelle / Sarangi, Srikant 2003. Click here for Health Information/Advice: Interaction Pathways via the NHS Direct Website. In Crivelli, Benedetta / Rubinelli, Sara (eds) *Televisione, Stampa e Internet tra Medico e Paziente*. Special issue of *Tribuna Medica Ticinese*, 21–27.

Myers, Greg 1994. Narratives of Science and Nature in Popularizing Molecular Genetics. In Coulthard, Malcom (ed.) *Advances in Written Text Analysis*. Routledge: London, 179–190.

Myers, Greg 2003. Discourse Studies of Scientific Popularization: Questioning the Boundaries. *Discourse Studies* 5/2, 265–279.

O'Halloran, Kay L. 2004. *Multimodal Discourse Analysis: Systemic Functional Perspectives*. London: Continuum.

Quirk, Randolph / Greenbaum, Sidney / Leech, Geoffrey / Svartvik, Jan 1985. *A Comprehensive Grammar of the English Language*. Harlow: Longman.

Palmer, Frank R. 2001. *Mood and Modality*. Cambridge: Cambridge University Press.

Richardson, Kay, P. 2005. *Internet Discourse and Health Debates*. New York: Palgrave/Macmillan.

Roberts, Celia / Sarangi, Srikant 2005. Theme-oriented Discourse Analysis of Medical Encounters. *Medical Education* 39, 632–640.

Sarangi, Srikant 2005. The Conditions and Consequences of Professional Discourse Studies. *Journal of Applied Linguistics* 2/3, 371–394.

Sarangi, Srikant / Candlin, Christopher N. 2004. Making Methodology Matter, Editorial. *Journal of Applied Linguistics* 1/2, 101–107.

Sarangi, Srikant / Clarke, Angus 2002. Zones of Expertise and the Management of Uncertainty in Genetics Risk Communication. *Research on Language and Social Interaction* 35/2, 139–171.

Sarangi, Srikant / Roberts, Celia (eds) 1999. *Talk, Work and Institutional Order: Discourse in Medical, Mediation and Management Settings*. Berlin: Mouton de Gruyter.

Silberg, William M. / Lundberg, George D. / Musaccio, Robert A. 1997. Assessing, Controlling, and Assuring the Quality of Medical Information on the Internet: *Caveat Lector et Viewor* – Let the Reader and Viewer Beware. *Journal of the American Medical Association* 277, 1244–1245.

Slack Warner V. 1997. *Cybermedicine: How Computing Empowers Doctors and Patients for Better Health Care*. San Francisco, CA: Jossey-Bass.

Stivers, Tanya 2007. *Prescribing under Pressure: Patient-Physician Conversations and Antibiotics*. Oxford: Oxford University Press.

Tsui, Amy 1994. *English Conversation*. Oxford: Oxford University Press.

Vicentini, Alessandra. 2008. Linguistic Representation of Ethnic Groups in Canadian Healthcare Websites from the Anglophone Perspective: Main and Minor Bilingualism(s). In *Proceedings of the 6th Conference on Communication, Medicine and Ethics* (COMET) 2008. University of the Witwatersrand, Capetown (South Africa), 2–4 July 2008. Power Point Presentation.

Wales, Katie 1996. *Personal Pronouns in Present-Day English*. Cambridge: Cambridge University Press.

Appendix

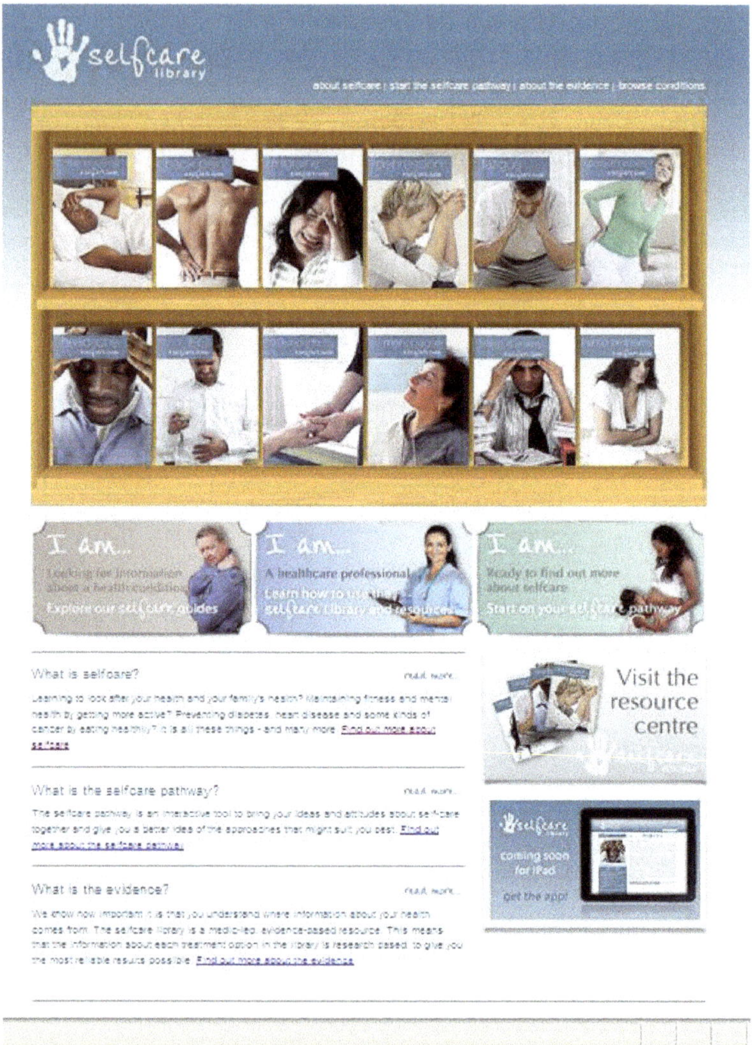

Figure 1. Screen shot of the Self-Care Library Home Page: Conventional Web design features.

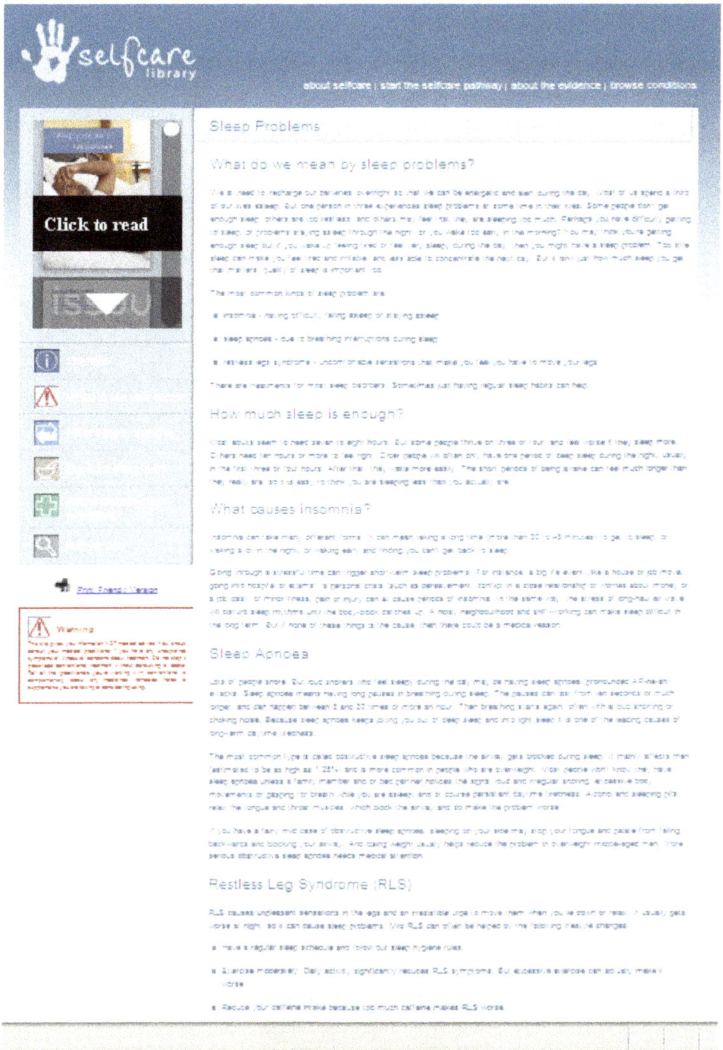

Figure 2. Browsable pages of the Self-Care leaflet.

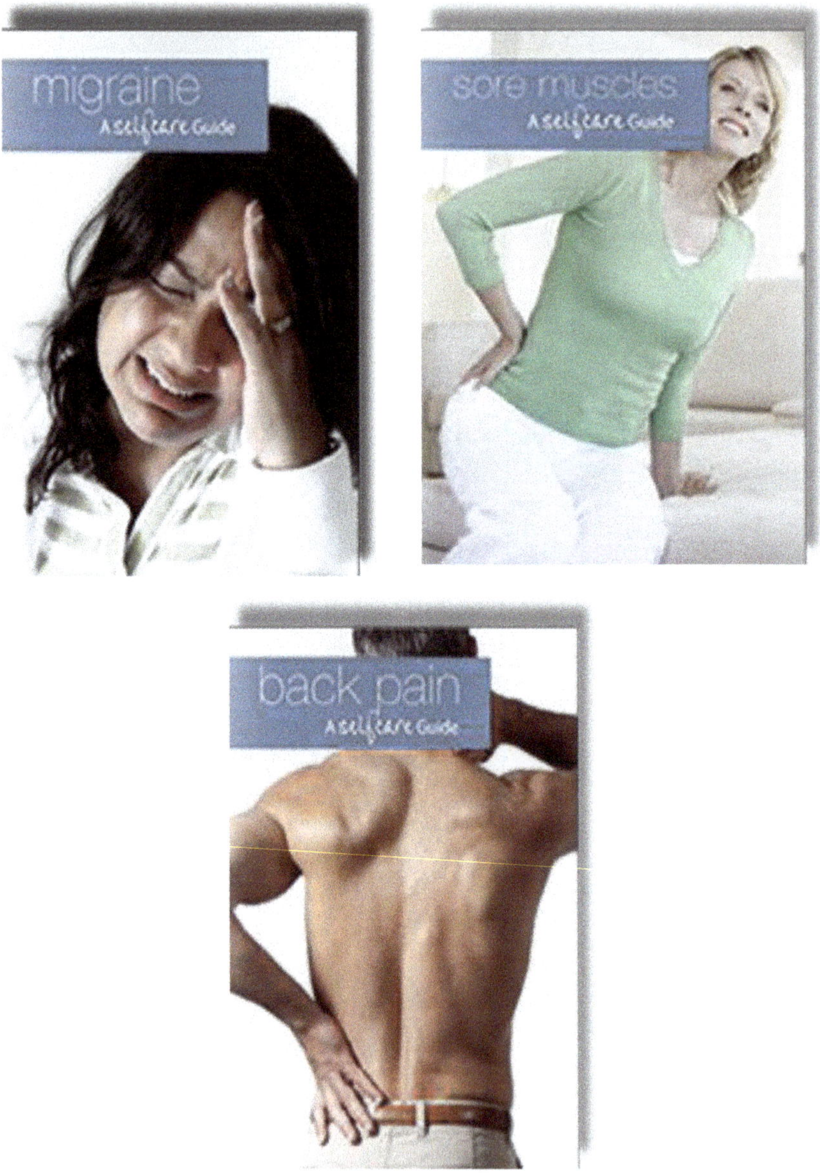

Figure 3. Selected images from Home Page.

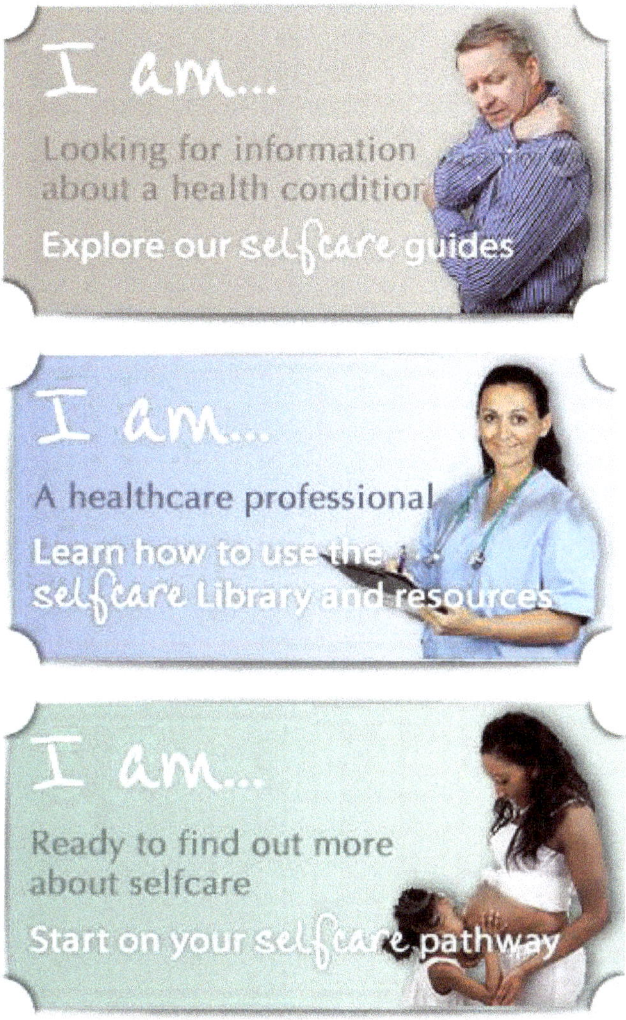
I am...
Looking for information about a health condition
Explore our selfcare guides
I am...
A healthcare professional
Learn how to use the selfcare Library and resources
I am...
Ready to find out more about selfcare
Start on your selfcare pathway

Figure 4. Three final images appearing below the twelve common health conditions.

Communicating Healthcare Information

Judith Turnbull

Living with Diabetes: the Discourse of Medical Information on the Internet for Young People

1. Introduction

Health information is one of the most frequently sought topics on the web. People may search for information before consulting a doctor, look for confirmation of information they have already been given or may even attempt a self-diagnosis online (McMullan 2006: 26). Certainly the Internet brings great benefits in the context of health communication, by stretching out to large numbers of people. But it also has a downside, insofar as patients may feel the amount of information available to be overwhelming, conflicting and confusing. Indeed, online communication is far from simple. First of all, it means one-to-many communication, 'the many' online being an unknown and undefined public coming from a wide range of social, economic and cultural backgrounds, covering all ages with a variety of life experiences and levels of education. They are not a discourse community with a common level of shared knowledge and interests, which makes it more difficult to calibrate the information at a level that is sufficiently simple, without overstepping the mark by dumbing down. Furthermore, the person looking for information has to be multi-literate (Caballero 2008: 15), as he/she will be searching and selecting the information, reading text, interpreting images or watching a video, so it is in no way a passive experience.

This raises the question of health literacy. Whilst health communication can be seen as the strategies and methods used by doctors and health professionals to inform and influence individuals' decisions about health, the other side of the coin is health literacy, which was defined by the World Health Organization in the following way:

> Health literacy […] entails people's knowledge, motivation and competences to access, understand, appraise and apply health information in order to make judgements and take decisions in everyday life concerning health care, disease prevention and health promotion to maintain or improve quality of life during the life course. (World Health Organisation survey: The Solid Facts. Health Literacy, 2013: 4)

The survey also reported on levels of health literacy amongst the general population in Europe and worryingly found:

> Nearly half of all Europeans have inadequate and problematic health literacy skills. (WHO survey: *The Solid Facts. Health Literacy*, 2013: 15)

This makes the task of health professionals all the more difficult to make the online knowledge transfer as simple and effective as possible and all the more important for the well-being of many people. The WHO definition of health literacy specifies four abilities, to access, understand, appraise and apply information, which correspond to the four fundamental and essential phases in health communication, as outlined by Houts *et al* (2006), Delp and Jones (1996) and Michiulette *et al* (1992). They are namely:

- Attracting the attention of the reader;
- Enhancing comprehension;
- Aiding retention and recall;
- Encouraging adherence to the advice.

The communication of health information is similar, in many ways, to science popularizations, because it involves the transfer of knowledge from expert to non-expert and, therefore, requires a simplification that remodels both the content and the language to suit the new target audience. As a result, it is closer to general discourse and the layperson's everyday experiences. However, there is a fundamental difference between the two, which lies in their purpose. Popularizations of science aim to transfer information to broaden the reader's general knowledge, but probably will have no direct effect on his life. In contrast, healthcare information will give practical and pragmatic advice to empower a person, enabling him to understand better his illness in order to manage his condition and even take a more active part in medical decisions.

This study is part of an ongoing research into online medical information for the general public. Previous studies (Turnbull 2013; Turnbull forthcoming) have focused on websites about diabetes, which is a life-long health condition that can affect all ages and requires detailed technical knowledge in order to know how to balance diet, insulin and physical activity and maintain good blood sugar levels on a day-to-day basis. The patient has to be persuaded to adopt a healthy lifestyle to avoid serious, sometimes life-threatening, complications.

The research has so far investigated how technical medical information is communicated to the patient as a non-specialist and in what way the multimodal affordances of the Internet can be exploited to facilitate the process. Much of the content of healthcare information on the Internet has been produced and distributed in a one-way direction; the message is created and controlled in a top-down fashion, from expert to layman. Nowadays websites are using the latest applications and affordances available thanks to web 2.0 to encourage user-to-user conversation, as for example in a forum.

This chapter will continue the research by investigating the sections of the same websites on diabetes that specifically address young children and teenagers, who will probably be competent Internet users and, like their elders, want to search for information about their condition online. Although they will require exactly the same information as adults in order to live with diabetes, they will need to be approached in a way that is appropriate to their age. The study will examine what strategies are used and briefly compare the results with those from the study on the main body of the websites for adults.

2. Data

Of all the websites analysed in the previous studies only two have sections addressed specifically to children and teenagers. The <diabetes.co.uk> is a community website. Its information is provided by diabetes experts, but, above all, by diabetics themselves who share their first-hand knowledge. The sections for young people are called *Kids* and *Teenagers and diabetes*. The other website, <diabetes.org.uk>, is run as a registered charity and works to raise awareness about the condition, collect funds, as well as provide support to sufferers. Its membership includes healthcare professionals, volunteers and diabetics themselves. The sections of interest for this chapter are called *My Life* and *Info for teenagers*. Table 1 summarises the contents of the two websites.

<diabetes.co.uk>	<diabetes.org.uk>
Kids About diabetes Types of diabetes Having fun Out and about	My Life What is diabetes? Me and my diabetes Help and support Fun stuff
Teenagers and diabetes Diabetes at secondary school Diabetes at university Nights out Controlling diabetes Insulin	Info for Teenagers What is diabetes? Me and my diabetes Help and support Fun stuff Get in touch

Table 1. Corpus.

3. Theoretical background

For knowledge transfer to be effective it has to work on two equally important levels – the cognitive and the communicative (Moirand 2003). The cognitive dimension is involved in the actual transmission of information, through descriptions and explanations of states and objects of knowledge, whilst the communicative dimension involves the way writers use language to negotiate the social relationship with their readers.

A number of studies on science popularizations and medical discourse between doctors and patients (Ciapuscio 2003; Gülich 2003; Calsamiglia/van Dijk 2004) have broadly classified the strategies used in this dimension as Illustration and Reformulation, with subcategories in each. Illustration strategies are used to present the knowledge, that is, the verbalization of complex or abstract knowledge to facilitate comprehension. These include definition, exemplification, scenarios and metaphorical language. Reformulation strategies change or modify what has already been said to clarify the meaning and make it more comprehensible. Both are concerned with the concretization of abstract information.

The communicative dimension refers to the rhetorical devices and strategies that can be adopted to create a positive and trusting relationship with the reader. Hyland (2010) and Giannoni (2008) looked at the 'proximity' and 'popularising' features in writing in academic and professional contexts and identified, among others, the following features: personalization, humour, modality, questions, marked lexis and metaphors. Similar devices were found by Adolphs *et al.* (2004) specifically in health communication when health professionals were trying to gain the trust of patients.

The communicative dimension plays a particularly important role in health information because it must, first, be perceived and received as advice and then adhered to. Harvey *et al* (2013) and Adolphs *et al* (2004) pointed out that giving advice is a delicate task, because it can be considered face-threatening in Anglo-Western contexts. The imposition of advice can be mitigated by the use of politeness markers, such as modality, *if* as a logical operator, hedges, vagueness (Adolphs *et al* 2004).

In the case of diabetes there needs to be a strong persuasive force to convince somebody to take on a strict routine of blood testing, diet, carbs counting, medication, injections and so on, especially to avoid some nasty complications that will only become evident to the patient in the future. This will be particularly difficult with young people who may be overwhelmed by the regimen imposed on them (DiMatteo 2004: 340).

A UNICEF publication, *Communicating with Children* (Kolucki / Lemish 2011), stresses the need for communication with children to be age-appropriate and suitable according to the level of conceptual difficulty, but also to the child's stage of behavioural, social and communicative development. It outlines the developmental characteristics of children and suggests different types of interactive communication strategies for the different age groups. In the case of young children who are becoming more independent and responsible for themselves, friends will gradually take a more important role in their lives, although they will still need support of their parents. The study recommends child-centred stories and characters, stories about friendship and strong positive adult and child role models (Kolucki/Lemish 2011: 21). The growing independence of young teenagers means they want to break away from adult authority and therefore positive peer-group behaviours are very important. Humour is considered a useful tool for communication (Kolucki/Lemish 2011: 23). Both age groups need to be able to express their feelings and ideas.

The strategies and devices discussed above are used frequently in the adult sections of the websites (Turnbull 2013, forthcoming). This study will investigate their use in the sections for younger people bearing in mind the different target audiences.

4. Analysis

4.1 Teenagers

Some teenagers may have had diabetes for many years and already be well informed about the technicalities of diabetes. Others who have only recently been diagnosed, will, in any case, be capable of adult-like abstract and logical thinking (Kolucki/Lemish 2011: 23). It is perhaps for these reasons that the explanation of the technical aspects of diabetes is very similar to the sections for adults. The charity website even has a link from the teenagers' section to a video explaining diabetes designed for adults, suggesting that this age group does not require versions that have been simplified further. The similarity between the two sections can be seen in the following extracts from <diabetes.org.uk>.

Teenagers	Adults
Diabetes mellitus (the full name for diabetes) is a common condition in which the amount of glucose (sugar) in the blood is too high because the body is unable to use it properly.	Diabetes is a condition where the amount of glucose in your blood is too high because the body cannot use it properly.
This is because the body's way of converting glucose into energy is not working as it should.	This is because your pancreas doesn't produce any insulin, or not enough insulin, to help glucose enter your body's cells – or the insulin that is produced does not work properly (known as insulin resistance.)
Insulin is a hormone (a chemical messenger) that carefully controls the amount of glucose in your blood. Insulin is made by a gland called the pancreas, which lies just behind the stomach. Glucose from food gives your body energy, and insulin acts as a 'key' to the 'lock' in the cells that need glucose. The cells use glucose as fuel for your body. Glucose comes from the digestion of starchy foods such as bread, rice, potatoes, chapattis, yams and plantain, and from sweet foods.	Insulin is the hormone produced by the pancreas that allows glucose to enter the body's cells, where it is used as fuel for energy so we can work, play and generally live our lives. It is vital for life. Glucose comes from digesting carbohydrate and is also produced by the liver.
When you have diabetes, the glucose in your body is not turned into energy. The glucose stays locked outside the cells, making you feel tired and unwell. This is because your body is not making enough insulin – or none at all.	If you have diabetes, your body cannot make proper use of this glucose so it builds up in the blood and can't be used as fuel.

Table 2. Extracts from *Info for teenagers* and *What is diabetes?* (<diabetes.org.uk>)

Both extracts show many of the strategies outlined in Section 3. Definitions and reformulations of technical terms are more frequent in the teenagers' section, such as *glucose* and *hormone*, and exemplification is used to explain *starchy foods*, whilst some details are omitted (insulin resistance). The metaphor of glucose as *fuel* is used in both extracts. The teenagers' version also uses two other metaphors, insulin as a *chemical messenger* and as a *key*, which are not present in the adults extract, but do appear in other pages and in the video.

The main difficulty of health communication with teenagers lies in engaging with the teenager to persuade him/her to read attentively and with a positive proactive attitude, especially as they may not be well-disposed towards the authority of the website. The same information is obviously given in both websites, with more or less detail, but it is organized in different ways. The charity website gives the basic information about what diabetes is and advice about how to live on a day-to-day basis in separate sections. On the other hand, the community website prefers to start from the point of view of the teenager and incorporates technical information into the discussion of how to manage diabetes in various situations of his academic, family and social life.

(1) Diabetes in teenage years tends to be more difficult than at other points in our life.
We look at different aspects of teenage life from school through to university and night out and give you some practical tips to keep blood sugar levels under good control. (<diabetes.co.uk>)

Communicating with children uses humour as a useful device. It is an important way of creating common ground and a point of contact and in this way can help to bridge the gap between the expert and non-expert, professional and patient, and in this specific case, an adult as a figure of authority and a teenager.

In the midst of a topic that does not really lend itself well to humour, there are some examples of the kind that raise a smile, rather than prompt a burst of laughter. The first two examples appear on the pages to do with injections and food, two areas that cause great concern and worry, so the humour lightens the topic and eases the tension, without diminishing the importance of what is being said.

(2) INJECTIONS
And your point is…?

(3) Your healthy diet doesn't have to be sugar-free – just low in sugar. However, because sweets and sugary drinks cause blood glucose levels to rise quickly, drink low-sugar or sugar-free drinks when you are thirsty. Very sugary foods are bad for your teeth, too – and you don't want falsies too soon, do you? (<diabetes.org.uk>)

The third example may help the reader to recall the technical term *ketoacidosis* as a mnemonic device and hence the problem it refers to.

(4) KETOACIDOSIS
What is that?
You may well ask! Apart from sounding like something straight out of Mary Poppins, it's actually pretty serious. When you have high blood glucose levels (higher than about 15mmol/l) and you are ill, your body may start to produce ketones. (<diabetes.org.uk>)

Although humour is present in the websites, it is not used extensively. The reason may be that it does not want to belittle the importance and seriousness of the advice. Indeed the websites rely on other strategies that can be classified broadly as personalization and, *vice versa*, depersonalization.

As the reader needs to feel the information and advice being given is relevant to him to motivate him in its adherence and to feel involved, strategies are used to attract the reader's attention.

Questions are often used in paragraph headings to organise the information and draw the reader into the topic, first with a general question and then with a more personal reference, the very questions a young diabetic is likely to ask.

(5) TYPE 2 DIABETES
All you need to know
What is Type 2 diabetes?
What does Type 2 diabetes do to me?
Why did *I* get Type 2 diabetes? (<diabetes.org.uk>)

But the two websites generally follow different approaches in their personalization.

The community website shows empathy by often presenting the situations in terms of emotions, how teenagers feel about their condition:

(6) The further we get into our teenage years, the more we want to push diabetes under the carpet. We don't want diabetes to control our lives and that can mean we spend less time looking after our levels. (<diabetes.co.uk>)

(7) Being diagnosed with diabetes will always come as a shock (it's a rare person who isn't shocked to some extent). If you become diagnosed during term time, you may find you need to take some time off school whilst you adjust to your treatment regime. (<diabetes.co.uk>)

Although both these examples refer to emotions, they are expressed in different ways, by using the inclusive *we* and, perhaps rather surprisingly, with a 'personless' gerund form.

The charity website has fewer of these expressions of empathy, but in the subsection *Me and my diabetes*, it gives a very personal perspective on information and advice about living with diabetes, such as *Getting my glucose right?*, *Good to eat*, *At school*, *Away from home*. Given the strong need for teenagers to express their ideas and feelings, readers are invited and encouraged to leave comments.

The comments are written with spelling and grammar mistakes, acronyms, emoticons and typical teenage language, suggesting that it is genuine.

(8) OMG i remember this girl when i was diagnoses that she was like omg stay away from her, you'll catch diabetes. I get so annoyed when people say and do stuff like that. It's an illness that you cant just forget or give away. Us diabetics are stuck with diabetes for life but we still do what we did before. It's a bit annoying and upseting when we cant eat because our sugars are high but in the end if we just eat and eat and dont do anything we could end up seriously ill or even dead !!….- Taylor (<diabetes.org.uk>)

Most comments begin with a declaration of the writer's age and how long they have had diabetes, as if they were giving their credentials for acceptance as part of the discourse community. They then pour forth their emotions and feelings about their condition and how it affects them.

(9) Hi, I'm 14, and I have had diabetes since I was 11. It stinks. I hate it so much because every time I go to the clinic I get told that my long term test is too high but I dot know what to to do :-(I feel that if I tell my mum how I feel, she'll shout and tell me I have to live with it because she has it too but she's always been fine with it! I always get told that I'm doing everything wrong and that either my weight isn't right or I'm eating the wrong foods :-(I just feel that I have no one to talk too and I'm embarrassed to tell everyone at school .–Ciera (<diabetes.org.uk>)

They tell their personal stories, the trials and tribulations of living with diabetes. Negative experiences told by peers may be interpreted and accepted more readily as good advice than warnings or recommendations given directly by professionals or adults.

(10) I was too embarrassed to wear my identity necklace. One day I was trying to get home and I wandered past a pub, well out of it. The police arrived and thought I was drunk and disorderly and then one of them noticed, luckily, that I didn't smell of alcohol. So they took me to the hospital. By that time my blood glucose level was very, very low. Later I realised that, had I been wearing my tag, they would have known so much quicker. Andy, 19.

(<diabetes.org.uk>)

Teenagers can also post their personal stories in a section called *People like me*. As well as being an opportunity for self-reflection, their stories can act as exemplars for other teenagers, when the writer has struggled to follow a rigid regime, but then realises the risks and mends his/her ways. The stories follow Labov/Waletzky's (1987) narrative structure of six stages: abstract, orientation, complicating action, evaluation, result/resolution and coda, as can be seen in the following example:

(11) Emma's wake up call

I was diagnosed with diabetes when I was six. So I have grown up with it most of my life, it was just normal for me. I was used to it. But as I got older, it got harder, a lot harder. […]

Keeping my diabetes under control was hard for me, because I didn't want to. I wanted to be normal, like all my friends, not having to count carbs or judge how much I had eaten. To be carefree and live life the way I wanted. It didn't seem fair to me, and I wasn't going to let it rule my life and the things I wanted to do.

At first I didn't realise the dangers of what I was doing. I wasn't taking my blood sugars as often as I should and just took whatever insulin I thought would cover my food. […]

It wasn't until I was at my annual review and my consultant was horrified with my readings that I came back down to Earth. I was told the dangers and risks of what I had let happen. Stroke, loss of limbs, blindness, and many other complications in day to day life. I was given a wake up call. I decided I had let enough be enough and started to do research on my condition. What I found shell-shocked me and I was horrified at some of the stories posted on the internet.

I realised how stupid I had been and decided to do something about it. Now I'm happier with my condition. I couldn't care less what anybody else thinks because diabetes doesn't affect me as a person. I still don't let it rule my life

and not everything revolves around it, but I have control of it, now at least. I'm living my life the way I would have with the little addition to the side. Diabetes is just part of who I am.
UPDATE
I'm happy to say that since I wrote this I've managed to motivate myself into taking care of myself :) I hope all you guys finding it hard can do the same cos it's scary how much damage you can do if you aren't :(Emma x (<diabetes.org.uk>)

In contrast, although it often shows great empathy with its readers, the online community often resorts to depersonalization to warn about risks. It uses statistics to explain how many teenagers have difficulty in controlling their blood glucose levels:

(12) Getting blood glucose levels under control takes work and, as a teen, it seems to be even harder. Only 1 in 7 teenagers manage to get their long term blood sugar control within the target range (ie an HbA1c value below 7.5%). (<diabetes.co.uk>)

or when advice is being given:

(13) With studying and socialising both important factors at uni, you may find that your diabetes gets left behind. This is not just bad for your health but can also affect other areas such as your motivation, your sleeping pattern and your ability to think clearly.
It's a good idea to commit time each week to reviewing your blood sugar numbers to see if any improvements are needed. (<diabetes.co.uk>)

Although it refers to *your* diabetes, the passive form without the agent depersonalizes and creates a distance from the action, making the statement less threatening. The modal *may* also softens the force of the sentence and the negative inference that they have not been looking after their blood sugars. The expression *It's a good idea* helps to depersonalise the advice and leave the reader with a choice to take up the suggestions.

In another example the argument in favour of testing blood sugar levels frequently is presented in an impersonal way, but it also presents the concession, that *it can seem a real pain*, therefore expressing solidarity and mitigating the imposition.

(14) It can seem a real pain to have to keep testing your blood. Sometimes you *might* feel there's no point because you think you 'know' when your levels are too high or too low. But the way you feel is not always an accurate guide to what's happening inside your body – so it's best to let your testing strips or meter tell you what's really going on. (<diabetes.org.uk>)

4.2 Children

The children's sections of the two websites appear to have many differences not only in relation to the teenager sections, but more significantly between the kids' sections themselves. The approach to communicating with young children is fundamentally different.

Visually the *Kids* section of the community website is exactly the same as the other sections of the website, as far as the layout, colours and structure are concerned. The section is divided into four parts – *About Diabetes*, *Types of Diabetes*, *Having Fun* and *Out and About.* The text on each page about the topic is short, so as not to overload the young reader with too much information at a time. At the bottom of the text there is a box headed *New words to remember*, which highlights approximately five words or expressions, some of which are quite technical, such as 'glucose', 'hypoglycaemia', 'insulin resistance' that need to be understood and learnt by the child. There is also an invitation, *Fancy a quick game*, to play a cowboy game in case he/she has tired of reading. This section is intended to be read by children on their own, with their parents or with their teachers.

In contrast, the <diabetes.org.uk> website's section for young children called *My life* has a completely different layout and colours that distinguish it from the rest of the website, thus marking it out as special. Furthermore, the presentation of the information is made by a group of imaginary friends, cartoon characters who also have diabetes. The reader meets these children on the first page; they are between the ages of six and eleven, therefore peers of the reader. They then go on to give information and advice, sharing their knowledge and experience of diabetes. Although the pages are clearly addressed to young children, the importance of parental support is acknowledged explicitly.

(15) There's lots of info here and you don't have to take it all in at once. But you and Mum and Dad can keep coming back for all the info you need. (<diabetes.org.uk>)

Young children need a simple explanation to understand what is happening in their bodies, because they are still coming to terms with the idea of having diabetes. They also need the technical knowledge in order to begin to manage their condition, at least in part and with the help of their parents.

The community website explains what diabetes is in short sentences as a bulleted list of facts.

(16) Diabetes is linked to digesting food, especially something called carbohydrates.
- When food is digested, something called glucose goes into your blood. Blood is the red stuff that comes out when you cut yourself, and it powers the whole body.
- A type of hormone called Insulin is then released to absorb the leftover glucose.
- If you have type 1 diabetes, your body doesn't produce insulin.
- If you have type 2 diabetes, your body doesn't produce enough insulin.
- Diabetes is a very common condition that affects millions of people.
- Learning about how to manage diabetes is the key to being healthy, fit and strong. (<diabetes.co.uk>)

None of the knowledge transfer strategies mentioned in Section 3, which could have helped illustrate the meaning, is employed. Examples of carbohydrates and some explanation of how insulin works would have been very useful, whereas there is a rather obvious and probably unnecessary explanation of blood. Although it opens with "You may have heard the word diabetes before" and therefore appears to address the child directly, the *you* in the list of statements is generic. The final sentence, which should encourage and persuade the child to take an interest in managing his/her diabetes, is entirely depersonalised by the use of a gerund.

The charity website exploits its multimodal affordances for the technical explanation of diabetes and presents the information in a video. Conceptually, diabetes, like any illness or medical condition, may be difficult for young children to understand, because it is abstract and invisible. A video enables the information to be re-contextualised visually so that a young child can understand more easily.

A Children's Guide to Diabetes shows a little girl lying in bed, trying to go to sleep but is very restless. Suddenly a light in the shape of a ball darts across the room and asks, "What's up?" She explains that she is trying to work out what it means to have Type 1 diabetes. At this point the live action turns into animation as the light takes the little girl into her body and shows her the cells waiting for glucose.

(17) *Light*: Your stomach breaks down carbohydrates from some foods like rice bread and sugar to make glucose and this travels in the bloodstream to your cells.[…] The glucose needs something called insulin to unlock the door to the cells so that it can get in. Your body makes insulin in the pancreas, which is just below your stomach. When you have Type 1 diabetes, your body doesn't make any insulin. It's not because of anything you or your parents or anybody else did. It just happens.[…]
The cells really need glucose.
Little girl: How can we get it to them?
Light: That's where insulin comes in. Because your pancreas doesn't make it anymore, you can give yourself insulin to help the glucose get into the cells so they have all the energy they need.
Little girl: So then it's all OK. (<diabetes.org.uk>)

Examples of the types of food that are converted into glucose are mentioned, whilst the same metaphor found in both the teenager and adult sections is used to explain the function of insulin as a key unlocking the door of the cells to allow the glucose to enter. It also gives a description of the position of the pancreas.

The mixture of live action and animation accompanied by music makes it dynamic, colourful and fun; it also allows the concretization of abstract ideas by 'entering' the body and 'observing' the cells. The personification of the cells, depicted as blue blobs making a wide range of facial expressions, frowning, yawning, makes it more entertaining as they call out:

(18) *Cells*: Glucose, where are you? I'm tired. Time for 40 winks. (<diabetes.org.uk>)

But it also draws a parallel between what is happening to the cells as they feel increasingly tired without glucose and what happens to a child in diabetes, thus facilitating comprehension.

Apart from transferring the basic facts about diabetes, the video also fulfils an important communicative function. Many young children diagnosed with diabetes will have experienced restless nights worrying about their condition and so the video creates empathy with the young viewer. The light is very reassuring and becomes the girl's secret friend.

(19) *Light*: Yes, it's all OK and in fact, it's more than OK. You can do everything just the same as everyone else and of course you get to meet me too! (<diabetes.org.uk>)

As well as understanding diabetes, young children are probably looking for simple straightforward answers to many of their worries, as for example, what they should do if they are having a hypo. Once again, the information given in the two websites is very similar, but the presentation is different. The community website first gives a rather technical definition of a hypo:

(20) A hypo happens when your blood sugar level drops too low (under 4.0 mmols/l on your blood glucose meter). Read this with your parents so you know what the signs of a hypo are. (<diabetes.co.uk>)

It then gives a bulleted list to exemplify how someone feels during a hypo and explains what to do in a gentle, reassuring way. However, this form of presentation may make it difficult to memorize the instructions for instant recall in the case of a hypo.

(21) If you feel low on sugar, have something sugary to eat, such as:
- 3 or 4 glucosetablets
- Some sweets
- A few sugar lumps

You can have a sugary drink but it's easy to drink too much when low so it's often best to stick to sweets and sugar.
Unless you have a hypo just before a meal, it's worth having a little bit of longer acting carbs to stop you going low later on. Longer acting carbs could include crackers or a piece of fruit. (diabetes.co.uk)

In contrast, the charity website presents a similar list of examples of how someone may feel during a hypo and a simple definition.

(22) Hypos happen when there isn't enough glucose (sugar) in your blood. Most people feel a bit strange just before they have a hypo – and these feelings are your body's way of warning you that you're having a hypo. (<diabetes.org.uk>)

It then goes on to give a series of short instructions in the imperative form on what to do. They are presented by Nadeem, one of the imaginary friends, who tells the reader:

(23) Stop whatever you are doing, right away.
If you are with people, tell them what is happening.
Test you blood glucose (sugar).
Eat or drink some fast-acting carbohydrate [...].
Sit down until you feel better. After 15 minutes, test your blood glucose (sugar) again. If it's still low, eat a bit more fast-acting carbohydrate. (<diabetes.org.uk>)

The short and direct form of the imperative should make it easier to recall the information when needed. Each instruction is presented in a separate box to highlight it and is accompanied by an illustration to reinforce the meaning. There is immediately a link to another page explaining what fast-acting carbohydrate is. It does so by listing and illustrating with bright, colourful images of the food types, to attract the attention of the reader and to help recall. Simplification and illustration make the knowledge transfer more effective.

In spite of the age difference, the children's section of the charity website mirrors the section for teenagers, insofar as it invites comments from readers and there is a problem page, in which children may ask questions and receive answers from health professionals. As in the teenage section, their comments start by giving their 'credentials' and then they talk about their personal difficulties as well as feelings and sometimes even give advice.

(24) I have had it for a year and i was on two injections a day until i was high at tea time so i went on 3. I am still on three but now my bloods are lower which is good. At parties you are always going to get cake and sweets but that is ok because if you have type 1 you can always take an injection, so don't be afraid to have fun and sweets because if you go to a party and someone calls you a name u know that your friends will back you up!
Sometimes it does hurt to take an injection, but there is a secret: distract yourself like make a funny voice like i do or remember something funny that has

happened to you or your friends or family! Ok thanks for reading my comment. I hope you enjoyed it.– Erin (<diabetes.org.uk>)

(25) I have had diabetes for six years and I have struggled but I got used to it, so people who have just got diabetes don't be afraid because you will get used to it very soon! – Eleanor (<diabetes.org.uk>)

Unlike the teenager sections, however, humour appears only very occasionally in the websites, using puns as in the following example:

(26) Type 1 diabetes happens partly because of your genes. Not your jeans! When these genes combine with an infection, diabetes can happen. (diabetes.co.uk)

However, there is a very friendly and reassuring tone used throughout by the 'friends':

(27) I get a bit nervous before I go but everyone is always friendly and kind when I get there. (<diabetes.org.uk>)

whilst the community website expresses empathy as it did in the teenager section:

(28) Hypos can sometimes feel quite scary and many happen when you're at school, at home or playing sports (diabetes.co.uk)

5. Discussion and Conclusion

Children are growing up in a world mediated by the Internet and it is only natural that they should be driven by the same motivations as adults to investigate illness and health issues online. At a very young age they are already multi-literate and paediatric health communication must address the child as well as the parents. This is particularly true in the case of a life-long condition like diabetes, where the child not only has to become an expert and take responsibility for managing medication, but also has the necessary first-hand experience as the patient to discuss treatment with his health advisors.

Although the study examined the children's and teenagers' sections in two separate websites for a total of four sections, the intention of the study was not to make a direct comparison between them, but rather to identify the characteristics and strategies used in health communication for young people. During the analysis significant differences emerged in the approaches adopted, which illustrate how delicate and complex the task of health communication is.

It is interesting to note that the same strategies for knowledge transfer found in adult sections, namely definition, exemplification, metaphors and reformulation are used in the teenage websites and also in the children's section of the charity website. The main difference between the kids', teenagers' and adults' sections, as far as the cognitive dimension is concerned, lies understandably in the information load. Fewer details are given for the younger children, but technical terms are introduced for all in order to acquaint the child with the medical language he/she will hear at the doctor's or at the diabetes clinic.

The real differences emerge in the communicative dimension. The community website, perhaps rather surprisingly, adopts a less personal approach, whereas the charity website tries to engage more directly with the reader. This is particularly obvious in the children's pages, where the format and style is not adapted to the young audience. The information remains just that, raw facts that are not contextualised or personalised to make them relevant to the young reader. In contrast, *Me and My Life* in the charity website, as the very name suggests, concentrates on the child, addressing him/her directly and presenting the information through friends. Indeed, it combines many of the elements recommended by *Communicating with children.*

A distinctive feature of the websites is the opportunities given to readers to express their feelings and thoughts. Neubaum and Krämer (2014) point out how personal anecdotes and emotionality play an important role in the persuasiveness of health information in blogs as opposed to official websites. This seems to be true for the younger readers who keenly posted their comments on the charity website, whether it is to unburden themselves, share experiences in order to encourage others or just feel they are not alone. Although it was not included in this part of the study, the community website has a forum with a special section for young children and teenagers that fulfils the same function. However, the fact that the comments in the charity website are posted directly on the pages of information means that two different points of view on the same topic, that of the expert and that of the patients, are presented simultaneously. The 'scientific' and rational, but friendly and reassuring, approach to the condition is placed side by side with the emotional responses. In this way the websites may reach out to the young people and persuade them that they too can manage their diabetes successfully.

References

Adolphs, Svenja / Brown, Brian / Carter, Ronald / Crawford, Paul / Sahota, Opinder 2004. Applying Corpus Linguistics in a Health Care Context. *Journal of Applied Linguistics* 1/1, 9–28.

Caballero, Rosario 2008. Theorizing about Genre and Cybergenre. *Computer Resources for Language Learning* 2, 14–27.

Calsamiglia, Helena / van Dijk, Teun A. 2004. Popularization Discourse and Knowledge about the Genome. *Discourse and Society* 15/4, 369–389.

Ciapuscio, Guiomar 2003. Formulation and Reformulation Procedures in Verbal Interactions between Experts and (Semi-)laypersons. *Discourse Studies* 5/2, 207–233.

Delp, Chris / Jones, Jeffrey 1996. Communicating Information to Patients: the Use of Cartoon Illustrations to Improve Comprehension of Instructions. *Academic Emergency Medicine* 3, 264–270.

DiMatteo, M. Robin 2004.The Role of Effective Communication with Children and their Families in Fostering Adherence to Pediatric Regimens. *Patient Education and Counseling* 55/3, 339–344.

Giannoni, Davide 2008. Popularizing Features in English Journal Editorials. *English for Specific Purposes* 27, 212–232.

Gülich, Elisabeth 2003. Conversational Techniques Used in Transferring Knowledge between Medical Experts and Non-experts. *Discourse Studies* 5/2, 235–263.

Harvey, Kevin / Locher, Miriam / Mullany, Louise 2013. 'Can I be at risk of getting AIDS?' A Linguistic Analysis of two Internet Advice Columns on Sexual Health. *Linguistics Online* 59/2–3, 111–132.

Houts, Peter / Doak, Cecilia / Doak, Leonard / Loscalzo, Matthew 2006. The Role of Pictures in Improving Health Communication: A Review of Research on Attention, Comprehension, Recall and Adherence. *Patient Education and Counseling* 61/2, 173–190.

Hyland, Ken 2010. Constructing Proximity: Relating to Readers in Popular and Professional Science. *English for Academic Purposes* 9/2, 116–127.

Kolucki, Barbara / Lemish, Dafna 2011.*Communicating with Children. Principles and Practices to Nurture, Inspire, Excite, Educate and Heal.* <www.unicef.org/cbsc/files/CwC_Web(2).pdf>.

Labov, William / Waletzky, Joshua 1967. Narrative Analysis: Oral Versions of Personal Experience. In Helms, June (ed.) *Essays on the Verbal and Visual Arts*. Seattle: University of Washington Press, 12–44.

McMullan, Miriam 2006. Patients Using the Internet to Obtain Health Information: How this Affects the Patient-health Professional Relationship. *Patient Education and Counseling* 63/1–2, 24–28.

Michiulette, Robert / Bahnson, Judy / Dignan, Mark / Schroeder, Elissa1992. The Use of Illustrations and Narrative Text Style to Improve Readability of a Health Education Brochure. *Journal of Cancer Education* 7/3, 251–260.

Moirand, Sophie 2003. Communicative and Cognitive Dimensions of Discourse on Science in the French Mass Media. *Discourse Studies* 5/2, 175–206.

Neubaum, German / Krämer, Nicole 2014. Let's Blog About Health! Exploring the Persuasiveness of a Personal HIV Blog Compared to an Institutional HIV Website. *Health Communication*, accessed June 2014. <www.researchgate.net/ Neubaum>.

Turnbull, Judith 2013. *A Linguistic Analysis of English Online. Knowledge Dissemination and the Empowerment of Citizens*. Rome: Universitalia.

Turnbull, Judith (forthcoming). Knowledge Dissemination Online: the Case of Health Information. In Bondi, Marina / Cacchiani, Silvia /

Mazzi, Davide (eds) *The Proceedings of the CLAVIER 14 conference*. Newcastle: Cambridge Scholars Publishing.
World Health Organisation 2013. *The Solid Facts. Health Literacy.* <http://www.euro.who.int/data/assets/pdf_file.3>.

Web sources

<www.diabetes.co.uk>
<www.diabetes.org.uk>

Paola Catenaccio

The Representation of Gambling in Gambling Awareness Campaigns: The Discursive Construction of Addiction

1. Introduction

Over the past three decades, as gambling opportunities have expanded around the world, gambling has received increasing attention on the part of clinicians and researchers. While it is generally acknowledged that not all gambling falls within the definition of a medical condition, pathological gambling was recognized as a psychiatric disorder in the 1980s, when it was included in the influential American Diagnostic and Statistical Manual of Mental Disorders (DSM-III). In the 1990s the DSM-IV significantly reworked the diagnostic criteria, *de facto* sanctioning the inclusion of gambling among chronic and progressive mental illnesses. According to recent research, gambling disorders may affect 0.2–5.3% of adults worldwide, often with a prevalence of comorbidity with mental health, poor learning outcomes and social problems (Ferguson/Couklson/Barnett 2011). Measurement and prevalence vary, but it is undeniable that problem gambling has become a very public concern and, as such, the object of policy intervention, not least in the form of awareness and prevention campaigns, many of which targeted at youths (Byrne *et al.* 2005). At the same time, gambling also represents a source of state income in many countries, resulting in conflicting interests being at play in communication about gambling in general, and warnings about potential gambling addictions in particular.

This chapter investigates the discursive construction of gambling in selected English-language gambling-awareness campaigns recently issued in different countries around the world. The study analyses the communicative strategies deployed in the campaigns with a view to identifying their discursive, rhetorical and linguistic coordinates. The focus of the investigation is on the role played by discourse in the framing of gambling as either a personal problem, a social challenge, or a pathological issue, with the attendant patterns of responsibility attribution and/or pathologization.

The methodological framework adopted is discourse-analytical in focus and relies on a conceptualisation of discourse as social action (Fairclough 2003) which both frames and is framed by social practice. Special attention is paid to the implications of discursive processes both for the social construction of illness and disorder (Conrad/Barker 2010) and for the rhetorical structuring of pathologized self-representation (Rossol 2001).

2. Background

This chapter takes its move from the consideration that the rise of 'problem gambling' as a form of pathological behaviour is a clear example of the way in which illness is socially constructed, and more specifically of the process through which deviant behaviour is medicalized. Discourse plays a key role both in the social construction of illness and in the pathologization of deviance, as it is in and through it that illnesses and pathological behaviours are first constituted and/or identified, and then reinforced and/or contested. In particular, while constant engagement – especially on the part of institutional actors – with medically-oriented discourses of deviance warrants a social perception of problem gambling as an illness, rejection of such discourse denies deviant behaviour pathological status, with far reaching consequences in terms of social acceptance, responsibility attribution, and institutional intervention legitimacy/desirability. While these considerations are common to numerous deviant behaviours where an individual choice component plays a role (such as, for instance, drug abuse, obesity, or smoking), in the case of gambling the scenario is further complicated by the fact that governments are often directly implicated in gambling activities. State and provincial lotteries have been a form of public financing for most of the history of contemporary North America, and starting from the last two decades of the twentieth century state-sponsored, or at least state-sanctioned betting, has become more widespread in many western countries. The de-marginalisation of gambling (a form of socially reprehensible entertainment originally confined to the upper and lower classes), with the attendant growing appeal of betting and gaming among the financially independent and socially influent middle classes, has resulted in a broadening of the public exposed not only to gambling but also to its potential harmful effects, both individually and socially. As a result, the management of the potential problems arising from a larger incidence of gambling habits among the general population has become an issue of concern on the part of those very actors who have contributed to promoting them.

In consequence of the above, public discourses of gambling need to negotiate the contested space between social acceptability and pathological behaviour. This requires the deployment of complex rhetorical and argumentative strategies, which represent the discursive means whereby public perception of gambling is constructed. A discourse-analytical, argumentation-based and rhetorically aware approach to gambling is therefore essential to fully understand the social and ideological implications of gambling discourse, and may help shed light on the discursive processes whereby social acceptability of potentially deviant behaviours is negotiated *vis-à-vis* their medicalization.

2.1 The social construction of illness and the medicalization of deviant behaviours

Over the last few decades the social construction of illness has become a major research perspective in medical sociology. As highlighted by Conrad and Barker in a recent article (2010), among the key findings yielded by this approach to illness and disease is, first, the recognition that "all illnesses are socially constructed at the experiential level, based on how individuals come to understand and live with their illness"; parallel to this is the acknowledgement that "medical knowledge about illness and disease [...] is constructed and developed by claims-makers and interested parties" (and is therefore the object of discursive negotiation); finally, both the social construction of illness and the social construction of knowledge about illness appear to be deeply affected by cultural frameworks (Conrad/Barker 2010: 68). These factors largely determine public attitudes towards illness and, more specifically, towards behaviours and conditions whose pathological nature is uncertain or contested, with important consequences at both the individual and at the societal level.

The medicalization of deviance – of which gambling is a prime example – is an eminent example of social construction of illness. First modelled in a seminal study published in 1980 by Conrad and Schneider, who traced the socio-historical factors involved in the medicalization of deviance and identified the socio-cultural conditions favouring it, it was later shown by Rosecrance (1985) to be suited to be applied to compulsive gambling. Rosecrance's study reconstructs the evolution of the conceptualization of gambling from a morally and legally reprehensible behaviour (a view prevalent up to well into the twentieth century) to an uncontrollable illness. It traces the first fully medicalized conception of gambling to Bergler (1957), who saw gambling as a form of compulsive behaviour determined by a self-destructive desire to punish oneself by rebelling against the rationality of adult authority. Gambling, however, did not gain widespread acceptance as a medical condition until a claims-making group – Gamblers Anonymous – succeeded in fostering the acceptance of a conceptualization of gambling as uncontrollable compulsion, which in turn set the stage for the establishment of a therapeutic regimen capable to control the compulsion (Rosecrance 1985: 278).

A therapy protocol soon followed, developed by a group of psychiatrists linked to Gamblers Anonymous. In this way, medical turf (cf. Conrad/Schneider 1980) was secured, with full institutionalization of gambling as illness achieved in 1980, when it was included in the *Diagnostic and Statistical Manual III* of the American Psychiatric Association.

Rosecrance also predicted that the medical model of compulsive gambling was likely to have a growing influence on the definition of gambling problems (1985: 280), and that – in line with Conrad and Schneider's (1980: 275) observation that "as a particular kind of deviance becomes a middle-class rather than solely a lower-class 'problem', the probability of medicalization increases" – a growing middle-class involvement with the problem was likely to accelerate and consolidate medical approaches.

Thirty years on, Rosecrance's prediction has been by and large confirmed, with gambling addiction featuring extensively in specialized medical publications. However, public discourses of problem gambling appear to be more nuanced in their approaches, displaying varying definitions of problem gambling which, albeit pointing all in the direction of medicalization, bear signs of an ongoing discursive negotiation along the continuum from 'safe gambling' to 'gambling addiction' through interactionally achieved self-diagnosis and the destigmatization of deviance.

3. Materials and research design

The purpose of the study is to investigate the above-mentioned public discourses of gambling as they are instantiated in gambling-awareness communication campaigns on the part of institutional actors. Communication originating in institutions and aimed at the general public was selected as the focus of the investigation as it was deemed particularly suitable to the exploration of the cultural and ideological construction of gambling in society. Institutional communication is particularly influential in the definition of medical conditions or other types of deviance by virtue of the key role it plays in ideology construction: in disseminating dominant discourses, institutional communication naturalizes the ideologies underpinning them, thereby turning them into shared 'truths'. Thus, the view of gambling conveyed in institutional communication exerts a powerful influence on public opinion, especially when such view is disseminated through the media, which heighten and multiply the legitimating effect of institutional sanctioning (Gamson/Modigliani 1989; Lakoff/Ferguson 2006).

As part of the research project, a search was undertaken for gambling awareness campaigns in English promoted by institutional actors at local or state level worldwide. Gambling-related materials posted on institutional websites addressing public health issues were also included in the collection, yielding a sizeable corpus of texts which was, however, largely dishomogeneous due to the varied provenance of the samples. A further difficulty encountered was that gambling campaigns are relatively new and not very frequent, while more consistent (though admittedly probably not quite as effective in terms of public outreach) communication could only be found in dedicated websites.

As mentioned above, the aim of the analysis was to identify the linguistic and rhetorical means whereby gambling comes to be discursively construed as a form of deviance, medical condition, or (ir)responsible behaviour. A preliminary investigation of the materials collected made it possible to isolate three main areas which appeared to play a key role in such construction. The areas related to, respectively, 1) terminological differentiation; 2) interactional co-construction of disease; and 3) normalization of deviant behaviour.

On the basis of these preliminary insights, three campaigns were singled out which were deemed to be representative of the range of approaches detected. The first one consists of a series of press releases issued by the US National Council on Problem Gambling (NCPG) on the occasion of the launch of the National Problem Gambling Awareness Month 2014;[1] the second is a campaign called 'Stop the Chase'[2] issued in the same year by the Canadian Responsible Gambling Council; and the third one is another campaign, this time Australian, launched in the early months of 2014 by the government of Queensland and called 'Gambling too Much?'.[3]

As for the methodology adopted, a mainly qualitative, discourse analytical approach was selected, with specific analytical tools being deployed on an *ad-hoc* basis depending on the type of materials considered. More specifically, the analysis focused on recurrent rhetorical and argumentative strategies, primarily using tools drawn from Argumentation Theory in the pragmadialectic tradition (van Eemeren *et al.* 1993; Van Rees 2006), integrated with other methodological perspectives,

1 The press release corpus is supplemented with further material retrieved from the NCPG website.

2 <http://www.stopthechase.ca/index.html>, last accessed on May 30th, 2014.

3 <http://www.olgr.qld.gov.au/gaming/minimising-harm/gambling-awareness-campaigns/gambling-too-much>, last accessed on May 30th, 2014.

most prominently Evaluation Theory (Hunston/Thompson 2000) and Systemic-Functional Grammar (Halliday 1978).

4. Naming strategies in the conceptualization of gambling and the NCPG

How you call a condition plays a crucial role in identifying it as a disease, as Conrad and Schneider (1985) recognized in attributing to naming a special role in the medicalization process (see also Clarke *et al.* 2003). Indeed, labelling theory (a theory which posits that institutions' reactions to a given behaviour – their labelling of it – plays a crucial role in its definition as deviant or otherwise; cf. Pfhol 1985) is at the heart of their approach. According to Conrad and Schneider, naming, or labelling, is involved at the conceptual level of medicalization, which relies on the use of medical terminology as a form of definitional strategy.

Definitional – and hence terminological – issues are therefore crucial to medicalization. As highlighted by Delfabbro (2013), disorders involving gambling are typically defined as 'pathological gambling', with 'pathological' being a psychiatric term "which refers to the presence of a mental disorder recognised by the DSM-IV" (Delfabbro 2013: 37). This labelling choice frames the gambling-related problem as an illness pertaining to the individual. By contrast, 'problem gambling' – another frequently used term – while often used interchangeably with 'pathological', appears to be typically used in discussions of gambling carried out from within disciplinary fields such as anthropology, sociology and geography, in which the focus is not so much on the individual causes of problem gambling as on the broader social, spatial and cultural factors that contribute to gambling problems (Delfabbro 2013: 73). Other terms used are 'compulsive' and 'excessive', but these are often dispreferred because they only partially or inadequately identify the problem.

Quite apart from the specific implications of the various definitions, the linguistic strategy used to label the illness is interesting in itself, as it indicates a focus on distinguishing between an acceptable form of gambling (typically defined as 'responsible'), and '*pathological* gambling', i.e. a form of gambling which requires medical intervention. The concept of gambling is thus split into two separate concepts: the first one used to define 'fun', socially acceptable gambling, while the second one is used in discussions of problem gambling. This is a strategy shared with other contested fields of institutional intervention located at the crossroads between social acceptability and deviance, such as drinking ('*problem* drinking' vs '*responsible* drinking') and drug use ('*recreational* drugs' vs '*heavy* drugs'), and may therefore be considered a recurring discursive strategy in the definetion of contested illnesses.

This labelling strategy makes it possible first of all to define pathologization as a matter of scale: there is a continuum between responsible gambling and pathological gambling, and it is along this continuum that there is scope for institutional intervention. In addition, by refraining from attributing to the word exclusively negative denotational meanings (as was customary when gambling was considered a 'sin' – cfr. Rosecrance 1985; see above §2.1), it provides the ground for the continued maintenance of gambling as a legitimate individual activity and legal industry.

From a rhetorical perspective, the splitting of the concept of gambling into two separate concepts – 'responsible gambling' and 'pathological/problem gambling' – is a clear example of the use of dissociative techniques to accommodate contradictory positions on the same topic. Insofar as problem gambling must be medicalized without de-legitimating gambling as such, the need arises for a distinction to be made between responsible and pathological gambling which prioritizes one over the other depending on the speaker's standpoint.

Dissociation is one of the two general categories of argument schemes identified by Perelman and Olbrecht-Tyteca (1969) in their taxonomy of argumentative techniques in *The New Rhetoric*. As van Rees (2006: 475) aptly sums up,

> in dissociation the speaker splits up a notion considered by the audience to form a unitary concept into two new notions, one of which comprises the aspects of

> the original notion that the speaker considers real or central (Term II), the other, the aspects that he considers apparent or peripheral (Term I).

Dissociation therefore involves two different speech acts – distinction and definition:

> It involves distinction, because through dissociation a notion that the audience regards as a conceptual unit is split up into two new notions, each comprising part of the original one. And it involves definition, because, as a result, the original term is newly defined and alongside the old one a new term is called into being, receiving a definition of its own (or the old term is replaced by new terms, each with their own definition). (Van Rees 2006: 474)

Because of the double function they serve, dissociative techniques can be used to achieve analytical precision functional to argumentative effectiveness. Additionally, they enable the speaker to reconcile apparently contradictory positions in respect of one and the same notion. Thus, distinguishing between responsible and problem gambling enables the speaker to support the legitimacy of gambling while emphasising its pathological outcomes.

A clear illustration of the way in which dissociative techniques are used in the definition of problem gambling is provided by the opening of one of the press releases issued by the US National Council on Problem Gambling. The text runs as follows:

(1) *Gambling addiction is a public health problem impacting relationships, families, business and communities. The National Council on Problem Gambling highlights National Problem Gambling Awareness Month.*
Washington, DC. Legalised gambling is more readily available now than in any other time in US history: 48 states allow some form of gambling. Although most people gamble for fun and recreation, some can develop a problem that can lead to severe negative consequences. Problem gambling not only causes issues with the gamblers themselves but many other people are affected by an individual's gambling problem, whether they be family members, friends, or even employers. (NCPG press release March 6th, 2014)

The press release assumes an institutionalized medicalization of problem gambling ("gambling addiction is a public health problem"), while at the same time reproducing a general concept of gambling which emphasizes its legitimacy ("legalized gambling is more readily available now than in any other time in US history"). The definition of problem gambling *vis-à-vis* legitimate forms of the activity is arrived at through the use of a concessive structure instrumental to the redefinition process. This structure deploys concession in order to move from a broad, shared concept of gambling as a harmless activity ("most people gamble for fun and recreation") to a narrower one in which gambling is seen as a problem ("some can develop a problem that can lead to severe negative consequences"): thanks to concession, problem gambling is given centrality in the discussion even while legitimate forms of gambling retain their validity. This enables a smooth shift from gambling to *problem* gambling which is instrumental to the medicalization of the latter while leaving the former unaffected (but peripheral in respect of the issue under discussion). This strategy is echoed in many other texts on problem gambling featuring in the corpus, some examples of which are quoted below:

(2) For most people gambling is fun and entertaining, but for some it's a serious problem that continues even after the fun is gone. (Nevada Council on Problem Gambling website)

(3) For many, gambling is a fun activity, but for those who become addicted to gambling, it is a devastating disease. (Californian Council on Problem Gambling website)

The distinction between '*responsible/fun/entertaining*' and '*problem* gambling' can be rhetorically effective, but it is exposed to attempts to associate the two concepts again (in a reverse process aimed at cancelling out the distinction made in the first place). Even though the pathological aspects of gambling are subject to a definition which clearly sets them apart from the more general concept of gambling, the recurrence of the same term in both legitimate and pathological definitions represents a potential source of vagueness, with the negative overtones of problem gambling potentially rubbing off on legitimate gambling practices.

The linguistic structure of the definition heightens the risk that this may happen: the splitting of gambling into two different concepts relies on different premodifications, with the head of the phrase being the same. Of course, it is precisely the premodifying constituents which are key to the definition; in other words, their function is that of classifiers (Halliday/Matthiessen 2004: 319- 321), i.e. of items that "indicate some particular subclass of the thing in question" (2004: 319). However, classifiers are by their very nature a fuzzy category, and it is not uncommon for items occurring in premodifying position to be interpretable as either classifiers or epithets (i.e. words indicating some kind of quality of the following 'Thing'; Halliday/Matthiessen 2004: 319–320). While terminological adequacy rests on the interpretation of the premodifications as classifiers, the fuzziness of the distinction compromises the definitional effectiveness of the two labels. Despite the effort to distinguish between 'responsible gambling' and 'problem gambling', the two expressions continue to share the same syntactic head: this increases the potential for lumping together different gambling behaviours under the same label, thereby erasing the functional differentiation mentioned above.

Probably as a consequence of this, there appears to be a process at work in the discourse of gambling aimed at making the distinction between safe and pathological behaviours even more clear-cut. This is done by replacing the word *gambling* with *gaming* when referring to safe forms of betting, thereby confining the use of *gambling* to contexts in which gambling is a problem. This move appears to be gambling-industry-initiated (even though the gambling industry denies intentionality; cf. Humphreys/Latour 2013) A second press release issued by the National Council on Problem Gambling a week after the one analysed in Example (1) illustrates this process:

(4) **What does responsible gambling mean?**

The National Council on Problem Gambling shares tips for reducing risk of developing gambling disorder.

Washington DC – Mach 17–21 marks the third week of the National Council on Problem Gambling's (NCPG) National Problem Gambling Awareness Month (NPGAM). The goal of the campaign is to raise awareness about *problem gambling* and resources available for help.

According to Keith Whyte, NCPG executive director, *responsible gaming* is essential, ethical, and economical for both individual and the gaming industry. Whyte states, "*Responsible gaming* is the obligation of gambling operators – including lotteries, casinos, and racetracks – to minimize individual and community harm through a formal internal *responsible gaming* program and support for external *problem gambling* services." NGPC calls on all who operate on profit from gambling to dedicate at least one percent of their gambling revenue to *responsible gaming* programs. (NCPG press release March 13th; 2014 emphases added)

In the text above, as in Example (1), the medicalization of problem gambling is taken as a given, and its assumption-based nature signalled through lexical choices ("gambling disorder") which immediately frame the problem as a medical issue. By contrast, safe gambling is referred to as 'gaming'. Thus, the distinction between '*problem*' and '*responsible* gambling' is replaced by the dichotomy 'problem *gambling*' / 'responsible *gaming*', with *gambling* becoming progressively associated with a negative prosody (of a medicalized kind) and *gaming* with a positive one, both words becoming thereby evaluatively charged (Hunston/Thompson 2000). In this way the conceptual distinction between the two aspects of gambling is brought to completion, with the term *gambling* (unspecified) retaining a general meaning, but being progressively relegated in usage to discussions of pathological issues, and *gaming* effectively replacing it in neutral discussions.

Further examples of similar patterns of usage can be found in the policy documents issued by the NCPG. The opening of the "Internet responsible gambling standards" (which appear in a section of the NCPG website devoted to Internet responsible *gaming* standards), issued in 2012, runs as follows:

(5) Gambling has benefits but also has well documented negative consequences. Internet gambling is no exception. It is clear that some who gamble online will develop problems and that these problems are serious. The most ethical and cost-effective response to gambling addiction issues raised by internet gambling is a comprehensive public health strategy [...]. Responsible gaming standards are an important aspect of this approach [...].

NCPG reviewed current internet responsible gaming codes and regulations from around the world (see Appendix A) to guide the development of this standard. The final recommendations in this document flow from our 40 years of experience in problem gambling issues, existing international codes (in particular the Responsible Gambling Council's draft internet gambling standards), empirical evidence and feedback from experts in the field [...]. The NCPG standard is a work in progress as internet gambling-related legislation, regulation and technology continue to evolve rapidly. [...] Analyzing actual player behavior leads to better understanding of gambling and problem gambling.

> It is strongly recommended that operators and regulators consult with experts in the problem gambling field during the development and implementation of internet gambling. Problem gambling, like other diseases of addiction, will likely never be eliminated, but we must make better efforts to mitigate the damage. A portion of all gambling revenue must be dedicated to reduce the social costs of gambling addiction.

The text features an opening concessive structure which distinguishes harmless gambling (peripheral to the discussion) from problem gambling (central to it), and uses the ensuing definition as an explicit premise in an argument in support of the standpoint that Internet gambling standards must be implemented. The definitional strategy deployed in the opening is reinforced in the remainder of the text, where the distinction between 'problem gambling' and 'responsible gaming' is reiterated, with gambling (unspecified) maintaining a neutral connotation.[4] The full institutionalization of problem gambling as a disease is highlighted both at the beginning and at the end of the text, where the pathological nature of this behaviour is taken for granted:

(6) The most ethical and cost-effective response to gambling addiction issues raised by internet gambling is a comprehensive public health strategy that includes prevention, education, treatment, enforcement and research services.

(7) Problem gambling, like other diseases of addiction, will likely never be eliminated, but we must make better efforts to mitigate the damage.

---

4 Further empirical evidence of an ongoing trend towards greater lexical differentiation between gambling and gaming can be found analysing a small corpus of Internet texts retrieved using the Bootcat tool, a software developed for the purpose of aiding in the construction of *ad-hoc* corpora. Using words such as *gambling*, *gaming*, *responsible*, *problem* and *disorder* as seeds to build touples (combinations of words which must occur in a text for it to be selected as part of the corpus), a small corpus (56,769 words) was built. A quick analysis conducted with Wordsmith Tools 4.0 revealed that while the word *gambling* is much more frequent than *gaming* (1,042 occurrences vs 257), the latter collocates more consistently with the adjective *responsible* than with any other qualifier; by contrast, the most frequent collocate of *gambling* is *problem*. While of course not conclusive, evidence found in the corpus suggests that *gaming* is used as an alternative to *gambling* on occasion, and that this use is prevalent in positive prosody, while definitional labels involving the word *gambling* are used in medicalized contexts.

In the first of the two passages, gambling problems are framed in terms of "gambling *addiction*", with the concept being introduced as a given and therefore as something which is not subject to discussion, with a shift in textual make up from argumentation to exposition (Snoeck Henkemans 2001); similarly, in the closing passage the association of problem gambling with "other diseases of *addiction*" reinforces the claim that the pathological nature of the deviance is an accepted truth.

5. The interactional construction of problem gambling as a disease: the 'Stop the Chase' campaign

Another aspect which is crucial to the medicalization of deviance, according to Conrad and Schneider (1985), is its co-construction as a disease in interaction. Typically this involves doctor/patient interaction, and insofar as it relies on persuasion, it may have a substantial argumentative component, as highlighted in a recent volume edited by Rubinelli and Snoeck Henkemans (2012). In the case of problem gambling, however, interactive processes of disease construction do not appear to necessarily involve doctors; in fact, peer interaction has been shown to contribute substantially to the way in which problem gamblers come to recognize themselves as sufferers. Rossol (2001) defines the medicalization of gambling as an interactive achievement, and points out that even compulsive gamblers who seek help rarely define themselves as sufferers upon engaging in counselling, but soon comply with the medicalized definition of problem gambling put forth in interaction by (often non-medical) counsellors, constructing for themselves a new identity as sufferers/patients in need of medical help through discursive alignment with the medicalizing suggestions of the interlocutors.

A similar interactive process of self-identity construction by problem gamblers as disease sufferers is fostered by a campaign promoted in the spring of 2014 by the Canadian Responsible Gambling Council. The campaign website features a grey page upon which a vertical line is shown. The reader is invited to "scroll down to get to the website" (an action which demands his/her interactional cooperation), but the webpage never comes. Instead, further encouragement to continue scrolling appears at regular intervals, in a never-ending cycle. A way out is offered (after long enough scrolling to make one doubt that an exit is possible at all) by a red arrow appearing on the bottom right corner of the page. Clicking on the arrow leads to the actual website, whose textual and discursive articulation revolves around a strategy of progressive self-awareness raising leading to the self-construction of the gambler as sufferer.

The webpage opens with a statement aimed at establishing common ground by making reference to a widely held belief, only to argue that such a truth not always holds:

(8) We have all heard that perseverance pays off. Persist through tough times, shake yourself off when you fall down and keep trying. This works in many areas of life. It does not work when it comes to gambling.

The inclusive *we* placed at the very beginning of the text, combined with the impersonal *you* that immediately follows establishes a neutral ground upon which to build the campaign's persuasive strategy. The entire campaign aims at proving that "perseverance does not work when it comes to gambling", and does so by providing evidence of the negative effects of 'the chase'. A definition of 'the chase' follows:

(9) Chasing losses is when you continue to gamble to try to win back money you've lost. It's a false belief that you are bound to win, so you spend increasingly more money and time gambling despite your increased losses. This is the beginning of more bad things to come.
You say you'll stop gambling when you win big or win back what you've lost. Or you just need to catch up after a bad weekend of losses.
Or maybe you need to change your strategies or your luck. Basically, chasing losses means continuing to bet and increasing the amount of the bet in order to get even.
You really believe that gambling more money is the only way to win back lost money. But it only puts you further and further in the hole. Chasing is a sign that you are losing control of your gambling.
Stop the chase before it starts.

In this text, the neutral, ground-establishing use of interpersonal resources deployed in the opening of the page gives place to a much stronger reader orientation. In a subtle shift from impersonal to personal *you*, the reader is addressed directly, and their rationalizing justifications for continuing gambling are given the lie. This is done by encouraging the reader to apply a strategy which is still of a rationalizing kind, but which recognizes that the positive value of perseverance does not apply to gambling.

The belief that 'perseverance pays off' is the outcome of the application of a pragmatic argumentation scheme (Perelman/Olbrechts Tyteca 1969; Schellens 1987; van Eemeren/Grootendorst 1992; Walton/Reed/Macagno 2008). Pragmatic arguments are built as follows:

> X is desirable
> because it leads to Y
> and Y is desirable

In the case at hand, the argument about perseverance states that

> Perseverance is desirable
> *because* it leads to success
> *and* success is desirable

By contrast, the argument put forth in support of the undesirability of perseverance in gambling starts off from the undesirability of the outcome (consistent failure):

> Perseverance in gambling is undesirable
> *because* it leads to failure
> *and* failure is undesirable

In other words, by showing the undesirability of the outcome, the campaign applies the same principle, reversing its application to demonstrate that the standpoint that perseverance is desirable cannot be defended in the case of gambling. The first step in the strategy of co-construction of problem gambling, therefore, is a rational appeal which acknowledges the reasonability of the counterpart: it does not label the compulsive gambler as a mental illness sufferer, but simply exposes a glitch in his/her rationalising schemes which is further explained in the following sections of the online text. In the next step, rational appeals are replaced by affective appeals, with an emphasis on the negative feelings associated with repeated loss:

(10) The chase doesn't feel good. It's filled with anxiety, frustration, and worry. Gambling doesn't feel the way it did before the chase – when it was a fun night out with friends. It's not fun anymore. It isn't about having a good time. It's about getting even. It's about rationalizing losses: it was the wrong bet, it was the wrong team to back, there wasn't a 'good feeling' about the original bet, 'I should've…' This leads to increasing bets, betting on long shots even with the nagging feeling that you won't win – all in the hopes of a big payoff. The result is more losses than wins, and more frantic bets to win it all back.

The explicit interpersonal engagement of the first section is replaced by a more indirect approach which encourages the reader's self-identification with the predicament described. This discursive strategy mirrors the process of progressive enmeshing which characterizes addiction. Care is taken not to convey blame, even though lack of rationality and loss of control are hinted at (see, for instance, the term *frantic*):

(11) Everyone wins occasionally. Thinking that the very next bet could be a winner makes it difficult to quit. Just one spin could make all your losses go away. Sometimes the desire to win back money makes the original loss seem 'less bad'. It's just a 'losing streak', or the money can be recouped easily. Chasing losses can seem like the logical thing to do. In order to persevere or look good in the eyes of others, gambling can be seen as the only alternative.

In this section, the emphasis on subjective perception persists. At the same time, the fallaciousness of the beliefs spurring disorderly gambling behaviour is indirectly evoked through the use of distancing devices ("chasing losses can *seem* like the logical thing to do"; "gambling can *be seen* as the only alternative) which reduce the truth value of the propositions they frame, thereby opening the door to alternative perspectives. It is noteworthy also that care is taken to maintain shared common ground with the reader by acknowledging the fact that the behaviour of pathological gamblers maintains a kind of apparent rationality. In other words, the reader is not *told* that their behaviour is illogical, but is led to realize its irrationality through a process of self-discovery. The next section brings to conclusion the argumentation strategy developed throughout the text.

(12) Losing doesn't feel good. It's human nature to resent losses and to take it personally. It's understandable that you want to prove to yourself or others that you didn't make the wrong decision. In this case, chasing seems logical to undo the negative. But gambling is not like other areas where perseverance pays off. The more you risk the more you hurt yourself.
Over time, people often borrow money to recoup losses. Continued gambling leads to still more losses and more borrowing. The more money borrowed, the greater the commitment to more gambling to gain enough money to pay off the debt. If you stop chasing, you lose both money and self-esteem.

Again, shared common ground is maintained through reference to the 'logicality' of the addict's behaviour. Such reference is functional to winning his/her cooperation in the co-construction of problem gambling, which is arrived at – finally – through the application of a pragmatic argument which exposes the fallacy of the previous ones.

The closing section of the campaign equates perseverance of the wrong type with loss of control, while emphasising the positive outcomes of persevering in desirable behaviours:

(13) The good news is that the feeling of wanting to chase is your warning signal. Chasing is a sign of losing control, and when the feeling arises it means that it is time to take a break from gambling. Remember, your chance of winning after a loss is no better than before. The best way to avoid chasing is to never break the first rule of gambling: do not gamble more than you can lose. Be honest with yourself. What are the limits that you can live with? How much can you lose so that you can wake up the next day feeling as good as the day before? Set a loss amount that you wouldn't feel bad about losing in a day, and stick to it. Think about another area where you probably know people who are trying to change their behaviours – like trying to losing weight. Yes, that chocolate cake tastes and feels amazing for the couple of minutes you are eating it. However, that enjoyment is short-lived when you realize you are sabotaging those things that are important to you… those things that are worth perseverance.

The text includes advice which suggests that loss of control can be avoided and rational thinking recovered. The problem gambler is not immediately labelled as a pathological subject, but is rather encouraged to self-diagnose his/her problem and ask for help if needed. In line with the strategy of co-construction adopted, the site does not proceed to full medicalization in the same page. Rather, the reader needs to actively decide to move on to the next stage by clicking on another red arrow bearing the words "Need help?". Medicalization, therefore, is not imposed upon the sufferer, but selected by him/her as an act of free will.

6. Shifting the focus: breaking the barrier to self-diagnosis and the 'Gambling Too Much?' campaign

The two campaigns discussed above provide examples of different approaches to the medicalization of problem gambling. While the US NCPG campaign focuses on problem gambling as a public health issue and assumes its pathological nature (with an approach which is institution-initiated and medically oriented), the Canadian campaign is centred on cooperative co-construction of a pathological behaviour located on a cline between rationality and control. Both campaigns acknowledge that problem gamblers may resist pathologization, and indirectly recognize that social stigma may be a contributing factor in their reluctance to seek help, frequently mentioning the possibility of seeking help under conditions of anonymity. Neither, however, explicitly addresses the topic of social stigmatization.

It has been pointed out at the beginning of this chapter (§2) that as part of the process of medicalization, deviant behaviours are reframed as illnesses, thereby moving from morally deplorable conducts to medical conditions worthy of sympathy. Pathologization is therefore closely linked to de-stigmatisation. Indeed, the medicalization process both fosters and is accelerated by de-stigmatization: as a condition ceases to be considered a moral flaw, social acceptance is furthered, which in turns leads sinners-turned-sufferers to seek help. On the contrary, not only the actual persistence of social stigma, but also its perceived endurance represents an obstacle to the voluntary acceptance of one's pathological condition.

It is therefore crucially important for the successful medicalization of gambling that both responsible gambling and problem gambling be normalized, and their perceived deviancy reduced to normalcy, with normalcy being inclusive of pathological behaviours. Such normalization in the service of self-diagnosed medicalization (where applicable) is the objective of an Australian campaign launched in 2014 and called 'Gambling too much?'. The campaign is entrusted to posters featuring tableaux of seemingly carefree everyday life beneath whose surface lurks the menace of gambling addiction. In one of them, a pub scene, two flies exchange the following lines:

(14) "Bet you can't pick the one who's gambling too much?"
"Bet you're right".

Below the dialogue is a caption which states:

(15) They say Aussies will bet on anything. Even two flies climbing up a wall. It's no surprise then that anyone can get it over their head. Maybe it's you? Free and confidential help is available.

The humorous tone of the advertisement belies its serious purpose. The text of the caption frames gambling as a behaviour which is typical of Australian people (a general category to which the addressee belongs), thereby establishing a shared common ground. The risk of problem gambling is seen as a natural consequence ("It's no surprise") of the passion for betting which characterizes the general population. By saying that "anyone" can be affected, the text reinforces the idea that gambling problems are not the result of a flawed character, but are rather the unintended, but nonetheless widespread, consequence of largely innocuous behaviours getting out of control.

The campaign attempts to remove persisting remnants of (perceived) social stigma from gambling addiction by suggesting that nobody is immune. In so doing, it relies on a strategy which is typical of campaigns aimed at promoting social acceptance for mental illnesses, thereby paving the way to the complete medicalization of problem gambling.

Thus, the campaign successfully decouples deviant behaviour from moral/social condemnation – a crucial step in the medicalization of deviance which appears to be here in the process of being accomplished.

7. Conclusions

Problem gambling is a type of deviant behaviour which has been progressively medicalized over the last fifty years. A clear sign of this medicalization is the progressive adoption of disease-related terminology to refer to socially unacceptable aspects of gambling. Labelling of this kind reflects (and at the same time warrants) the adoption of a medicalization-oriented discursive framework for the interpretation of unlicensed gambling behaviour. This is reflected in the wording of many gambling-awareness campaigns (*awareness* having replaced alternative, morally negatively charged labels such as *anti-gambling campaigns*), which focuses on the identification of symptoms of problem gambling and on the need to seek professional assistance, often of a medical kind, to overcome the problem. The linguistic strategies deployed in the labelling of pathological gambling rely on dissociative techniques aimed at differentiating problem gambling from responsible gambling, with a recent discernible trend towards alternative lexicalizations associated with negative and positive prosody respectively (problem gambling vs responsible gaming).

The institutionalization of excessive gambling as a disease appears to be complete in the majority of the gambling awareness materials considered, as illustrated in the analysis of the US NCPG campaign, where the definition of problem gambling is institution-initiated and maintained. Elsewhere, as in the Canadian 'Stop The Chase' campaign, medicalization is interactionally co-constructed with the active contribution of the patient/sufferer. Elsewhere still – and this is the case of the Australian 'Gambling too much?' campaign – issues of social stigma (which must be overcome for the medicalization process to be accomplished) are addressed.

These preliminary findings suggest that there are various stages and strategies in the medicalization of problem gambling, and that all of them are featured in gambling awareness campaigns. In some cases, resistance to full medicalization is discernable. When this is the case, rational arguments are put forth aimed at persuading the potential sufferer of the irrationality of certain gambling behaviours, in a bid to prevent the loss of control which is associated with problem gambling.

Insofar as medicalization implies de-reponsibilization, resistance to it also indicates that greater importance is attributed to individual responsibility. It is also possible that different degrees of medicalization are associated with different treatment policies – whether drug based or counselling oriented. Varying cultural attitudes to medicalization may also be involved. Further investigations focusing on cross-cultural and diachronic differences are needed in order to better understand the phenomenon.

References

Bergler, Edmund 1957. *The Psychology of Gambling.* New York: Hill and Wang.

Byrne, Andrea M. / Dickson, Laurie / Derevensky, Jeffrey L. / Gupta, Rina / Lussier, Isabelle 2005. The Application of Youth Substance Use Media Campaigns to Problem Gambling: A Critical Evaluation. *Journal of Health Communication* 10, 681–700.

Clarke, Adele E. / Shim, Janet K. / Mamo, Laura / Fosket, Jennifer Ruth / Fishman, Jennifer R. 2003. Biomedicalization: Technoscientific Transformations of Health, Illness, and U.S. Biomedicine. *American Sociological Review* 68, 161–94.

Conrad, Peter / Barker, Kristin 2010. The Social Construction of Illness: Key Insights and Policy Implications. *Journal of Health and Social Behavior* 51, 67–79.

Conrad, Peter / Schneider, Joseph 1980. *Deviance and Medicalization.* St. Louis: Mosby.

Delfabbro, Paul 2013. Problem and Pathological Gambling. A Conceptual Review. *The Journal of Gambling Business and Economics* 7/3, 35–53.

Eemeren, Frans H. van / Grootendorst, Rob, Jackson, Sally / Jacobs, Scott 1993. *Reconstructing Argumentative Discourse.* Tuscaloosa: The University of Alabama Press.

Eemeren, Frans H. van / Grootendorst, Rob 1992. *Argumentation, Communication, and Fallacies: A Pragma-dialectical Perspective*. Hillsdale, NJ: Lawrence Erlbaum Associates.

Fairclough, Norman 2003. *Analysing Discourse: Text Analysis for Social Research*. London: Routledge.

Ferguson, Christopher J / Coulson, Mark / Barnett. Jane 2011. A Meta-Analysis of Pathological Gaming Prevalence and Comorbidity with mental Health, Academic and Social Problems. *Journal of Psychiatric Research* 45, 1573–1578.

Gamson, William A. / Modigliani, Andre 1989. Media Discourse and Public Opinion on Nuclear Power: A Constructionist Approach. *American Journal of Sociology* 95/1, 1–37.

Halliday, M.A.K. 1978. *Language as Social Semiotic: The Social Interpretation of Language and Meaning*. Baltimore, MD: University Park Press.

Halliday, M.A.K. / Matthiessen, Christian M.I.M. 2004. *Introduction to Functional Grammar*. 3rd edition. London: Routledge.

Humphreys, Ashlee / Latour, Kathryn 2013. Framing the Game. Assessing the Impact of Cultural Representations on Consumer Perceptions of Legitimacy. *Journal of Consumer Research* 40/4, 773–795.

Hunston, Susan / Thompson, Geoff (eds) 2000. *Evaluation in Text: Authorial Stance and the Construction of Discourse*. Oxford: Oxford University Press.

Lakoff, George / Ferguson, Sam 2006. *The Framing of Immigration*. Berkeley, CA: Rockridge Institute.

Perelman, Chaïm / Olbrechts Tyteca, Lucie 1969. *The New Rhetoric: A Treatise on Argumentation*. Notre Dame: University of Notre Dame Press.

Pfhol, Stephen J. 1985. *Images of Deviance and Social Control: A Sociological History*. New York: McGraw-Hill.

Rees, M.A. van 2006. Strategic Maneuvering with Dissociation. *Argumentation* 7/4, 473–487.

Rosecrance, John 1985. Compulsive Gambling and the Medicalization of Deviance. *Social Problems* 32/3, 275–184.

Rossol, Josh 2001. The Medicalization of Deviance as an Interactive Achievement: the Construction of Compulsive Gambling. *Symbolic Interaction* 24/3, 315–341.

Rubinelli, Sara / Snoeck Henkemans A. Francisca (eds) 2012. *Argumentation and Health*. Special Issue of *Journal of Argumentation in Context* 1/1.

Schellens, Peter Jan 1987. Types of Argument and the Critical Reader. In Eemeren, Frans H. van / Blair, J. Anthony/ Willard, Charles A. / Garssen Bart (eds) *Proceedings of the Sixth Conference of the International Society for the Study of Argumentation*. Amsterdam: Sic Sat, 34–41.

Snoeck Henkemans, A. Francisca 2001. Argumentation, Explanation and Causality. In Sanders, Ted / Schilperoord, Joost / Spooren, Wilbert (eds) *Text Representation: Linguistic and Psycholinguistic Aspects*. Amsterdam: John Benjamins, 231–246.

Walton, Douglas / Reed, Chris / Macagno, Fabrizio 2008. *Argumentation Schemes*. Cambridge: Cambridge University Press.

Miriam Bait

Authority and Solidarity: How Institutional Websites in the US and the UK Communicate Nutritional Guidelines for Children

1. Introduction

The importance of good eating habits throughout life has been widely recognized and promoted in recent decades in developed countries, also as a result of the rapid increase in food-related diseases such as obesity, diabetes, but also eating disorders such as anorexia, bulimia etc. Both private and public organisations have shown interest and concern for nutrition-related communication, increasingly addressing their social and marketing initiatives to specific age groups (Abbott 1977; Featherstone 2007; Scollon 2005). Government agencies may count on the unique position they hold to promote health and sustainable development as they have direct responsibility for key issues that have a major impact on their citizens' lives. Children's health inevitably stands as one of the core issues after it has been acknowledged that childhood obesity, in particular, is rapidly becoming a global phenomenon to the extent that it is called an epidemic by the World Health Organization.[1]

This study will focus on the institutional approaches to discourses connected with food for children, and it will specifically focus on food advice, nutritional tips or dietary guidelines available on the websites of government agencies in the US and the UK. The main purpose of this study is to analyse the communicative strategies adopted by US and UK government agencies and identify salient discursive features deployed to reach a wide audience and impact on the construction of discourses

1 Obesity: preventing and managing the global epidemic, *Report of a WHO Consultation*, WHO Technical Report Series 894, 2000.

concerning children and food; I will also examine possible differences (or similarities) from the two datasets in the way language reflects on this topical issue.

2. Study design

The main points to be investigated are the lexis and phraseology used by institutions in delivering guidelines. Although influenced by local context and concerns, guidelines, in fact, represent a universal opinion-making genre which plays an important role in influencing "social debate, decision-making and other forms of social and political action" (van Dijk 1995: 2). In other words, here the main aim is to establish to what extent public agencies contribute to the interpretation and assessment of scientific findings and to "the formation and change of public opinion" (van Dijk 1995: 2), and to what extent concepts such as 'power' and 'solidarity' act as the main ideological construct which gives meaning and shape to the concept of health.

For this purpose, the texts selected for analysis were taken from the websites of agencies which have shown a major concern for children nutrition. Several departments and agencies of the United States and the United Kingdom have responsibility for various aspects of food production, regulation, safety and consumer protection: in the US, the Department of Health and Human Services (HHS) and the Department of Agriculture (USDA); in the UK, the Department for Education and Skills (DfES), the National Health Service (NHS), the Food Standard Agency (FSA). In particular, concerning the United States, HHS and USDA have published jointly *The Dietary Guidelines* for Americans every five years since 1980. These guidelines provide authoritative advice for people two years and older about how good dietary habits can promote health and reduce risk for major chronic diseases and serve as the basis for Federal food and nutrition education programmes.

The sample under analysis was collected in the period from January 2008 to December 2013. All texts from the sample have been assigned a code (e.g., USDA, FSA) according to their source and appear on the list in the Appendix. The US sample consists of a total of 94,433 words, and the UK sample of a total of 50,140 words. From the methodological point of view, a qualitative approach based on a critical discourse analytical framework was adopted (Fairclough 1989; Hunston/Thompson 2001; Wodak/Meyer 2001), in order to find relevant patterns of use. Particular emphasis was laid on the linguistic choices made by US and UK institutions to inform their citizens about nutrition (Fairclough 1995; Hunston/Thompson 2001; Bhatia 2002).

3. Accountability, visibility, and trust

Institutions have always had to cope with the need to communicate with their citizens adequately and efficiently, but since the 1980s a huge organizational restructuring of Public Administration at national and local level has taken place, with attention given to concepts like productivity, marketization, service orientation, accountability and transparency of actions, and efficiency in policy delivery (Bozeman 1987). This call for greater efficiency and effectiveness is strictly connected with the introduction and development of electronic information and communication technologies (ICTs) in the public sector. Institutional websites represent the basic tools to provide citizens with information and services. In fact, a number of health-promoting campaigns and action-based plans have been implemented to encourage community participation in both countries. Some examples are the healthy weight program *WE CAN!* (an acronym meaning Ways to Enhance Children's Activity & Nutrition)[2] released by different National Institutes of Health, and the *National School Lunch Program*[3] by USDA, in the United States. In the United Kingdom public awareness campaigns have been led by the Government in alliance with the private sector, in the form of 'social marketing' campaigns (Evans *et al.* 2010). For example, Change4Life[4] is an ongoing social marketing campaign established in the UK in 2008

2 See link at: <http://www.nhlbi.nih.gov/health/educational/wecan/>.

3 Cf.: <http://www.fns.usda.gov/nslp/national-school-lunch-program-nslp>.

4 See: <http://www.nhs.uk/change4life/Pages/change-for-life.aspx>.

to create awareness around obesity and developed in conjunction with entities in the public and private sector (e.g. large supermarket chains, food companies, convenience stores). In the following sections, I will explore what communicative strategies have been adopted to foster positive eating choices and develop healthy eating behaviour.

3.1 Textual patterns

Despite the variety of sources, some textual patterns and linguistic conventions emerge as paramount in the samples collected. First of all, to be effective, food tips need to avoid opaque and inaccessible language and be positive, short and simple, as shown by the following examples:

(1) Children need a healthy, balanced diet, which is rich in fruit, vegetables and starchy foods. Just like adults, young children need energy (calories) from food and nutrients such as protein, fat, carbohydrate, vitamins and minerals, to make sure their bodies work properly and can repair themselves. (FSA1)

(2) Your preschooler's normal growth and development also play a big role in their eating habits. Eating healthy can help lead to a healthy weight. (USDA1)

(3) The keys to healthy eating are variety, balance, and moderation. (HHS1)

Since "eating right doesn't have to be complicated",[5] guidelines also include examples of foods and activities that reflect the lifestyle, preferences and culture of the audience:

(4) Remember to include these sorts of foods: milk, cheese, yoghurt, soya beans, tofu and nuts are rich in calcium, which is needed for healthy bones and teeth; at least two portions of fish a week because fish are a good source of protein, vitamins and minerals and they are low in saturated fat. If you choose to give your child packed lunches, it can be a challenge to keep them varied, interesting and healthy. See our tips and menu suggestions […]. (FSA2)

(5) Turn off the TV during meals, and limit children's snacking when watching TV. It is easy to lose track of how much they are eating, especially if the snack is a bag of pretzels instead of a small bowl. […] Serve a vegetable or fruit with every meal and at snack time. (HHS1)

---

5 Link at: <http://www.eatright.org/Public/content.aspx?id=6442473735>.

Then, there is a common structure in the texts consisting basically of two parts: an introductory section featuring short texts and few scientific definitions and the main body text with food selection, providing a conceptual framework for selecting the type and amount of food to meet the specific dietary recommendations for children. In all the samples analysed, the introductory section displays a recurring statement to the effect that good nutrition is important throughout life:

(6) In the big picture, a number of things, in addition to food and physical activity, affect our health. Today's decisions affect our health today, tomorrow, and beyond. [...] Wherever we are in life... whatever the reason... we can prevent many bad health consequences and gain quality time to enjoy things that really matter to us. Whether we are 15, 25, or 65, any time is a good time to start! (HHS 2)

(7) Good health is important for everyone. The Government wants to secure, maintain and improve children's and young people's health [...]. (DfES1)

However, these positive statements are immediately counterbalanced by some 'warnings' which might be either general and soft:

(8) There are no healthy or unhealthy foods, only healthy or unhealthy diets. (NHS1)

or more specific and strong:

(9) Being overweight can increase the risk of getting diseases like diabetes, heart disease and some cancers. (NHS2)

(10) Children are a particularly important focus of the Dietary Guidelines for Americans because of the growing body of evidence documenting the vital role that optimal nutrition plays throughout the lifespan. Approximately 32 percent of children and adolescents ages 2 to 19 years are overweight or obese, with 17 percent of children being obese. In addition, risk factors for adult chronic diseases are increasingly found in younger ages. (HHS3)

The risk of obesity is underlined in both datasets by the frequent use of the terms *overweight* and *obese*. In fact, US texts often resort to the phrase *global childhood obesity epidemic*,[6] used and overused by media after the term was mentioned – together with *Globesity* – by the WHO

---

6 See <http://www.cnpp.usda.gov/DietaryGuidelines>.

in a report dated February 2001. Obesity in general, and child obesity in particular, seems to emerge as a high-profile public issue calling not only for research, but also for acts of the Government. The use of the epidemic as a metaphor is clearly aimed to create a sense of panic, shame and blame that is particularly acute around children. Leaving aside the use of the epidemic as a metaphor, it is a fact that a lifestyle model of disease places obesity among diseases such as heart disease and AIDS, where personal 'choices' and risky behaviours are considered the major causal factors. Politicians are reacting with legislation concerning BMI (Bio Mass Index) report cards, the removal of soft drinks from schools, banning artificial trans fats in restaurant cooking, and requiring fast-food outlets to display the caloric content of each menu item.

As an example of this, President Barack Obama established the first-ever Task Force on Childhood Obesity[7] to develop and implement an inter-agency plan that details a coordinated strategy, with a view to identifying key benchmarks, and outlining an action plan to reduce childhood obesity rate to just five percent by 2030. The White House Task Force is entitled to provide recommendations on four priority areas, which also form the pillars of the First Lady's *Let's Move!* campaign: empowering parents and caregivers: providing healthy food in schools; improving access to healthy, affordable foods; and increasing physical activity.

Turning to the second section of the samples, explanations of nutrients, vitamins and food groups are given, and (quasi-)scientific vocabulary is used to justify a healthy diet and provide explanation for the need of vitamins, nutrients etc., as can be seen in these samples:

(11) Increasing the proportion of fruit that is eaten in the form of whole fruit rather than juice is desirable to increase fiber intake, but it calls for more attention to consuming foods that are high in potassium. The fruit juices most commonly consumed by older children and adults provide more vitamin C, folate, and potassium in portions usually consumed than do the commonly eaten fruits. The recommended intake of fruits and juices achieve an optimal balance. (HHS2)

(12) Children aged 7–10 years old need lots of energy and nutrients because they're still growing. The amount of energy that food and drink contains is measured

---

7 Cf. <http://www.letsmove.gov/white-house-task-force-childhood-obesity-report-president>.

in both kilojoules (kJ) and kilocalories (kcal) and is commonly referred to as calories. A report from 2011 estimated that the average energy requirements for children aged 7–10 years old a day is [...]. (NHS3)

Both samples fully perform a chiefly informative function encouraging consumption of food containing essential nutrients (core food groups) while limiting dietary sodium, fat and added sugar, as can be seen in these examples:

(13) Eating healthy [...] can also help lower the risk of getting some chronic diseases and conditions such as type 2 diabetes, hypertension, certain cancers, and micronutrient deficiencies. (NHS4)

(14) Meat, particularly red meat and fish are rich sources of iron. Pulses (beans and lentils), green vegetables and fortified cereals are also good sources of iron. Iron is needed for healthy blood and research has shown that some children have low intakes of iron, particularly older girls. At least two portions of fish a week because fish are a good source of protein, vitamins and minerals and they are low in saturated fat. Oily fish, such as mackerel, salmon and sardines, also contain omega 3 fatty acids. (FSA3)

The texts promote the value of taking care of the self using a language that is close to general discourse and to the layman's everyday experience (cf. Gotti 2014). As to lexical choices, what can be noticed is the use of explicit evaluative lexis throughout the dataset, mainly in the form of adjectives. The most recurring ones, not surprisingly, are *healthy*, *safe*, *good*, *positive*, *right*, *smart*. Moreover, the use of comparatives, especially *healthier* and *better*, is paramount and this recurrent pattern epitomizes the main message addressed, "feeling better today and staying healthier tomorrow",[8] namely that improvement is always possible in the general living conditions of everybody and of children in particular. Interestingly enough, another element that emerged from a review of both datasets is the frequent use of *fun*, *funny*, *good-tasting*, *great-tasting*, *tasty* and *delicious*:

---

8 See <http://www.health.gov/dietaryguidelines/dga2005/healthieryou/html/chapter1.htm>.

(15) Family Meals: Easy, Tasty, and Healthy! (USDA3)

(16) Tips for Building Tasty, Healthful Lunches (HHS4)

(17) Providing children with nutritious and delicious meals gives them the fuel they need to excel both inside and outside the classroom (NHS5)

It seems that public agencies need to point out explicit characteristics which account not only for a product's health quality, but also for its tastiness and fun. The discussion about taste is interesting since one could infer from these messages that healthy products are not expected to taste good or, even, that they are expected to taste bad. That is why other descriptors are associated with *tasty*, e.g. *delicious*, which, on a taste hierarchy, ranks higher than other taste-related terms.

3.2 Representational level

On the representational level, the institution – the Government – emerges as the main actor in both datasets. However, in the UK texts the institution is presented as the actual doer, as an efficient service-provider which is capable of fully understanding the issues involved in its mission and which is committed to achieving its goals by taking adequate measures and by developing specific plans and projects in close connection with citizens. One could say that disempowered citizens have become empowered customers:

(18) The Government is also setting up the School Food Trust which will bring together caterers, nutritionists, food interest groups, schools and parents. It will play an important role in taking forward the Government's programme for improving school food by giving independent support and advice to schools and parents on how they can improve the standard of school meals and ensure that school food stays high on the education agenda. (DfES2)

(19) The Government wants to secure, maintain and improve children's and young people's health. One of the ways it is doing that is by setting minimum national nutritional standards for lunches for pupils in schools. (DfES3)

As can be seen, the tone is rather neutral, not at all emphatic, which suggests that the informative purpose prevails over other traits. It is an example of 'strategic discourse' (Fairclough 1989) oriented towards instrumental goals, aimed to get results, that is to promote itself, increase its visibility, generate interest and persuade the reader to support its policies.

In the case of the US dataset, terms such as *government* or *administration* are used infrequently. The attention shifts from the service-provider to the community as a result of these and other linguistic choices. Not only do the texts devote considerable attention to the issues of collaboration and partnership; they also provide examples of what Lyons calls 'empathetic discourse' (1977) as they resort, for instance, to the inclusive use of *we* as solidarity builder, as in the following examples:

(20) We have an opportunity to give children the building blocks they need to lead a healthy lifestyle. (HHS5)

(21) We've all had to balance, at one time or another, what children want with what's best for them. (HHS6)

Even the use of *you* is aimed at involving the audience, as the following excerpt points out:

(22) You are not alone. Picky eating is a typical behavior for many preschoolers. (USDA4)

By saying "you are not alone", the writer strengthens his/her solidarity with the reader, reminding readers firstly that children might be behaving in that typical manner and, secondly, that a wider community with similar concerns exists. But who are the addressees of this wealth of suggestions? In both datasets, we find *parents*, *educators*, *doctors* and *child-carers* as the main interlocutors. However, while the UK texts address stakeholders, the US texts refer to a wider audience engaging extended families and friends in the common effort to promote healthier eating, as the following excerpt shows:

(23) As parents, doctors, educators, extended family, or friends – we are all in a position to set good examples.(HHS6)

In American texts the communicative purposes are achieved adopting a style that is also more dialogic as well as colloquial in all texts, as for instance in the following:

(24) What can you do to cope with your preschooler's picky eating? If you don't make it a big deal, it will usually end before school age. Do any of the statements below remind you of your preschooler? "Michael won't eat anything green, just because of the color" "Bananas used to be Matt's favorite food, now he won't even touch them!" (NHS4)

The concepts of personalisation and conversationalisation (Fairclough 1995) are eloquently conveyed by these messages. The topic is personified using quotations that recall 'authentic' experiences of specific persons (including the implied reader). At the same time, the statements are generalised, through the use of *you*, to facilitate acceptance of the message by the audience. Regarding verb moods, imperatives expressing advice, suggestions and recommendations are the most frequent in both datasets. They can be explained by the directive or instructive nature of the content of these texts:

(25) Provide plenty of vegetables
Limit sugar-sweetened beverages
Serve reasonably-sized portions (NHS5)

However, a close analysis has detected some interesting differences between the two datasets as to the roles involved:

(26) Don't forget to give them fruit and vegetables.
Don't give sweet drinks.
Give your toddler foods containing iron
Take care to avoid the following foods [...]. (FSA4)

(27) Let your kids try small portions of food.
Let them learn by serving themselves.
Let your child see that you like it.
Praise their efforts.
Teach them to take small amounts at first.
Reward your child with attention and kind words, not food.
Encourage to help you prepare meals. (USDA5)

We can see from these examples that, on a semantic level, UK institutions do instruct and suggest a distribution of roles which only involves the institution as a provider of guidelines, on the one hand, and parents or care-givers, on the other hand, as the recipients. In this case, children are not allocated a role as the responsibility is considered to rest totally on their parents. Conversely, in the US texts, the choice of *let* to give advice has a semantic structure which includes children as well as parents. Moreover, most verbs (*include*, *consider*, *choose*, *try*, *enjoy*, *savor*, *balance*, *control*, *look for*, *aim for*, *create*, *plan*) are action verbs which insist on the semantic field of practice, experience, learning and discovery. Children are thus constructed as individuals who can decide what to eat, when to eat it and in what quantity. This aspect is codified linguistically, as will be apparent from the following examples, through the use of the modal *may* that in both UK and US datasets is at the top of the frequency list. But when analysing the concordance lines for *may*, one can discover that in the UK dataset the modal is used differently, i.e. to give factual information aimed to provide parents and/or child-carers with useful advice on particular foods or to warn them about possible risks connected with food, such as choking or food contamination:

(28) Vitamin C may help the absorption of iron, so having fruit juice with an iron-rich meal will increase iron absorption. (FSA2)

(29) A chocolate bar on the way home may give you an energy boost, but these snacks are usually the ones that are filled with bad types of fat and sugar. It may damage their teeth. (NHS2)

In the US texts, on the contrary, the focus is on children, and the modal *may* expresses possibility as it is used to refer to situations which are likely to happen and have to be judged as 'normal'. Implicitly, it means that parents are encouraged to consider different options, and children are to be given different choices, as the following statements exemplify:

(30) Your child may be unwilling to try new foods.
Your child may only eat a certain type of food. (USDA6)

Interestingly enough, the only occasion on which US advice becomes really prescriptive is when providing linguistic guidelines as to phrases that help and phrases that hinder. Thus parents have to become aware of phrases that hinder (and more importantly why) and phrases that help (and why):

(31) Avoid phrases that teach your child to eat for approval and love, like, "Eat that for me." Or, "If you do not eat one more bite, I will be mad." This can lead your child to have unhealthy behaviors, attitudes and beliefs about food and

> about themselves. Choose phrases that help your child recognize when he or she is full, like, "Is your stomach telling you that you're full?" "Is your stomach still making its hungry growling noise?" "Has your tummy had enough?" These statements can help prevent overeating. Avoid phrases that encourage kids to ignore signs of fullness, like, "You're such a big girl; you finished all your peas." "Look at your sister. She ate all of her bananas." Or, "You have to take one more bite before you leave the table." Choose phrases that make your child feel like he or she is making the choices, like, "Do you like that?" "Which one is your favorite?" Or, "Everyone likes different foods, don't they?" These statements shift the focus toward the taste of food rather than who was right.[9]

This quotation epitomises the approach as the prescriptive aspect is balanced by personalization that contributes to reducing the distance between institution and citizens. Moreover, parents are often blamed for the poor eating habits of their children and frequently an association between obese mothers and their children is sought. In this case, parents are not blamed. They are not agents. It is just a matter of cause and effect because the focus is on phrases not on persons.

4. Concluding remarks

The present case study has shown the (co-)existence of two poles within institutional discourse, a 'strategic discourse' corresponding to the ideological construct of 'power', oriented towards achieving instrumental goals and targeted at service consumers, and a 'communicative discourse', oriented towards 'solidarity' to create understanding and partnership between participants (Fairclough 1989) by highlighting mutual objectives and common values. More importantly, diet-related claims and nutrition suggestions for better lifestyles contribute to tackling the interplay between health concerns and wider social issues related to this age group.

---

9 Please, cf.: <http://www.eatright.org/kids/article.aspx?id=6442467922>.

References

Abbott, Robert 1977. Food and Nutrition Information. A Study of Sources, Uses and Understanding. *British Food Journal* 99/2, 43–49.

Bhatia, Vijay K. 2002. Professional Discourse: Towards a Multi-dimensional Approach and Shared Practice. In Candlin, Christopher (ed.) *Research and Practice in Professional Discourse*, Hong Kong: City University of Hong Kong Press, 39–60.

Bozeman, Barry 1987. *All Organizations are Public: Bridging Public and Private Organizational Theories*. San Francisco: Jossey-Bass.

Dijk, Teun A. van 1995. Opinions and Ideologies in Editorials. Paper for the 4th International Symposium of Critical Discourse Analysis, Language, Social Life and Critical Thought, Athens, 14–17 December 1995. <http://www.discursos.org/unpublished%20articles/Opinions%20and%20ideologies%20in%20editorials.htm>.

Evans, Douglas W. / Christoffel Katherine K. / Necheles Jonathan W. / Becker Adam B. 2010. Social Marketing as a Childhood Obesity Prevention Strategy. *Obesity* 18, S23–S26.

Fairclough, Norman 1989. *Language and Power*. London: Longman.

Fairclough, Norman 1995. *Critical Discourse Analysis: The Critical Study of Language*. London: Longman.

Featherstone, Mike 2007,*Consumer Culture and Postmodernism*, London: Sage.

Gotti, Maurizio 2014. Reformulation and Recontextualization in Popularization Discourse, *Ibérica* 27, 15–34.

Hunston, Susan / Thompson, Geoff (eds) 2001. *Evaluation in Text*. Oxford: Oxford University Press.

Lyons, John 1977. *Semantics*. vol. 2. Cambridge: Cambridge University Press.

Scollon, Ron 2005. The Discourses of Food in the World System. Toward a Nexus Analysis of a World Problem, *Journal of Language and Politics* 4/3, 465–488.

Wodak Ruth / Meyer, Michael 2001. *Methods of Critical Discourse Analysis*. London: Sage.

Appendix[10]

UK dataset

Food Standards Agency (FSA): <http://www.food.gov.uk/>

FSA1 – <http://www.eatwellscotland.org/agesandstages/children/yrchild/index.html>

FSA2 – <http://www.eatwellscotland.org/agesandstages/children/yrchild/index9a50.html?view=textonly>

FSA3 – <http://www.eatwell.gov.uk/agesandstages/children/yrchild/>

FSA4 – <http://tna.europarchive.org/20110116113217/http://www.food.gov.uk/multimedia/pdfs/feedtoddler0310.pdf>

FSA5 – <http://www.eatwellscotland.org/agesandstages/children/yrchild/index9a50.html?view=textonly>

Department of Education and Skills (DfES):
<https://www.gov.uk/government/organisations/department-for-education>

DfES1 – <http://dera.ioe.ac.uk/6005/1/H01530Nursery.pdf>

DfES2 – <http://www.teachernet.gov.uk>

DfES3 – <http://dera.ioe.ac.uk/6005/1/H01530Nursery.pdf>

National Health Service (NHS):
<http://www.nhs.uk/Pages/HomePage.aspx>

NHS1 – <http://www.wwl.nhs.uk/News/2009/April/catering_award.aspx>

NHS2 – <http://webarchive.nationalarchives.gov.uk/20070807081047/direct.gov.uk/en/YoungPeople/HealthAndRelationships/KeepingHealthy/DG_10030623>

NHS3 – <http://www.nhs.uk/chq/pages/how-many-calories-do-children-need.aspx>

NHS4 – <http://www.cdc.gov/Features/ExpressYourHealth/>

NHS5 – <http://www.nhs.uk/change4life/pages/healthy-lunchbox-picnic.aspx>

US dataset

United States Department of Agriculture (USDA):
<http://www.usda.gov/wps/portal/usda/usdahome>

USDA1 – <http://www.choosemyplate.gov/preschoolers/healthyhabits.html>

USDA2 – <http://www.fns.usda.gov/sites/default/files/Appendices.pdf>

USDA3 – <www.nal.usda.gov/fsn/Loving/FamilyMealsHandout.pdf>

USDA4 – <http://mypyramid.gov/preschoolers/HealthyHabits/PickyEaters/index.html>

USDA5 – <http://www.fns.usda.gov/sites/default/files/Helping_kids_Learn.pdf>

USDA6 – <http://www.choosemyplate.gov/preschoolers/picky-eaters/types.html>

---

10 All websites were accessed on 20/9/2014.

US Department of Health & Human Services (DHHS):
<http://www.hhs.gov>
HHS1 – <http://www.health.gov/dietaryguidelines/dga2005/healthieryou/pdf/Chapter12.pdf>
HHS2 – <http://www.health.gov/dietaryguidelines/dga2005/healthieryou/html/chapter3.html>
HHS3 – <http://health.gov/dietaryguidelines/dga2010/dietaryguidelines2010pdf>
HHS4 – <http://www.fda.gov/downloads/food/ingredientspackaginglabeling/labelingnutrition/ucm410529.pdf>
HHS5 – <http://www.health.gov/dietaryguidelines/dga2005/HealthierYou/contents.htm>
HHS6 – <http://webarchive.library.unt.edu/eot2008/20080916051842/http://www.health.gov/dietaryguidelines/dga2005/healthieryou/html/chapter12.html>

Communicating Research Findings

Ruth Breeze

Media Representations of Scientific Research Findings: From 'stilbenoids raise CAMP expression' to 'red wine protects against illness'

1. Introduction

On 17 September 2013 scientists at the Linus Pauling Institute, Oregon State University, published the results of a laboratory study which showed that two stilbenoid compounds (resveratrol, found in red grapes, and pterostilbene, found in blueberries), when combined with vitamin D, increased the expression of the human cathelicidin antimicrobial peptide (CAMP) gene which plays a role in the innate immune system in humans. On the same day, the communications department of Oregon State University issued an online press release which drew the attention of the British media. The original sober account of laboratory findings is hardly recognisable in the ensuing newspaper stories, which proclaim a dramatic discovery that will have an immediate impact on readers.

This chapter offers a systematic analysis of the transformations made to both the language and the contents of the original paper as they are shaped by media genre conventions, first those of the press release and then those of the three UK newspapers that picked up the story: the *Daily Telegraph*, the *Daily Express*, and the *Mirror*. For the sake of methodological consistency, the Appraisal system will be used (Martin/White 2005), centring on the dimensions of engagement and graduation. These are broadly understood to work together since both influence the alignment between the reader and the various ideas presented in the text. Engagement is a term used to cover the dialogic mechanisms that adjust alignment with the reader, such as monologic assertion or the opening and closing of dialogic space. Graduation operates in parallel to these, since it is present in the up- or down-scaling applied in the different locutions which also influences reader alignment. The chapter will conclude with an assessment of the relevance of this approach in combination with genre theory.

2. Overview of texts

The texts considered here provide an ideal case study to analyse trends in the way scientific news is reproduced in the media today. The original research (Text 1) is a serious empirical research paper focusing on laboratory findings which show that two stilbenoids, that is, compounds present naturally in red grapes and blueberries, may be effective at inducing a gene that fights infection, particularly when used in combination with vitamin D. This research was carried out in laboratory cell cultures, and although it might have applications for those infections that respond to topical medication, such as certain skin infections, it is unlikely to have any immediate application in treating diseases of the rest of the body, since it loses bioavailability on ingestion. The press release (Text 2), published at the same time as the journal article, makes this point clear in a disclaimer attributed to the scientists themselves, positioned immediately after the explanation of the finding, but takes an optimistic slant, stressing the various benefits that the stilbenoid compound has been found to have, and emphasising the need for more research. The three newspaper articles all reproduce many features of the press release, but show evidence of a gradual simplification-sensationalisation process which runs roughly parallel to their position in the market, and which is manifested through various aspects of content and language. For example, in terms of content, the *Daily Telegraph* (Text 3), which is generally considered a serious (broadsheet) newspaper (politically right of centre, with a circulation of half a million copies per day), foregrounds the notion that "red wine" [sic] and "blueberries" boost the body's ability to fight disease, but does include a disclaimer in the last paragraph to remind the reader that the positive results are only found in laboratory cells, which apparently means that it is "too early to say" whether consuming these substances will improve one's health. The *Daily Express* (Text 4) (circulation 0.5 million, right-wing middle-market tabloid) and the *Mirror* (Text 5) (circulation around one million, downmarket tabloid generally associated with the Labour Party) focus on the claim that "red wine and blueberries" (*Daily Express*) or "red grapes and blueberries" (*Mirror*) boost the immune system, and omit the disclaimer altogether. Although the press release and the three news stories are relatively short,[1] in terms of the way they each construct reader alignment they are highly complex, and this is compounded by the fact that they involve at least two different types of claim. It is therefore useful to conduct a systematic analysis, in which a clear distinction is made between the primary claim presented in the original research paper, that stilbenoids boost the immune response of cells in vitro, particularly in combination with vitamin D, and the secondary claim that this will have benefits for human health.

3. Dialogistic resources applied to the two claims

The differences between the way the different texts convey their messages can be seen to operate across two different dimensions of the engagement system: aspects of dialogic positioning considered in combination with the main claims, and aspects of graduation used to modulate these claims. Taken together, both of these dimensions modify the alignment between the reader and the claims in the text. By studying these mechanisms, we should therefore be able to track the way in which the writer acknowledges what prior speakers have said and anticipates the way future readers will respond.

It is important to note that Martin and White (2005: 94) understand engagement and graduation as part of a single system which encompasses

1 The word lengths of the four texts are as follows: Text 2: 495 words; Text 3: 284 words; Text 4: 301 words; Text 5: 211 words.

> all those locutions which provide the means for the authorial voice to position itself with respect to, and hence to 'engage' with the other voices and alternative positions construed as being at play in the current communicative context.

However, to achieve analytical clarity we shall first consider the elements of engagement and graduation separately, before putting them together to draw our overall conclusions.

3.1 Engagement resources

First, let us consider the management of the engagement system within these texts. What Martin and White (2005) term 'engagement' consists of a set of resources that writers use to position themselves with respect to the various propositions they report in the text. It thus covers the monologic or dialogic nature of the assertions made in the text, and the degree of commitment that is expressed to different ideas. As Table 1 illustrates, writers can modulate the way they report information or ideas, in such a way that they either open up space for dialogue (by indicating uncertainty or mentioning other possibilities) or close it down (by endorsing or rejecting a particular view). In doing this, they subtly convey their own position and endeavour to align their readers accordingly. We may look to the original research paper to find the most accurate reflection of the scope and meaning of the two principal types of claim made in the texts, namely, the claim concerning the laboratory findings (LF) and the claim about possible health implications (HI). In Text 1, we are told that the application of stilbenoids with vitamin D "enhanced CAMP gene expression", a statement which is unattributed and unhedged, and can be described using the engagement system (Martin/White 2005: 134, see also Table 1) as an 'assertion' of the laboratory finding, which we shall abbreviate as 'assertion LF'. Regarding the potential health implications (HI), Text 1 explains that these substances "may have the potential to boost the innate immune response", a claim which is expressed as a possibility, and therefore belongs to the class of 'entertain' (henceforth 'entertain HI'). Although these ideas occur several times in the text (in the abstract, and in the results and discussion sections), the nature of the type of claim made for each does not vary: the laboratory finding is asserted, while the health benefits are entertained as an interesting, but remote, possibility.

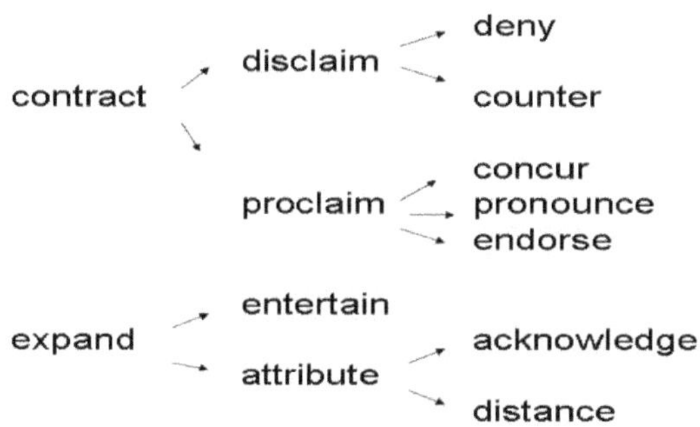

Table 1. The engagement system (from Martin/White 2005: 134).

The titles/headlines of the five texts, shown in Table 2, already provide an indication of which claim is foregrounded in each one. True to genre, the research paper gives the specific finding, providing the degree of scientific detail needed to attract the attention of the professional community. The press release already centres on the aspect that is most likely to interest general readers, namely the potential health impact. Text 3 echoes the headline of text two, only substituting "red grapes" for the potentially more exciting "red wine". Text 4 takes a different line, combining aspects of 'proclaim' (use of *found*, which suggests certainty) with aspects of 'entertain' (*could*). Formally speaking, Text 5 uses 'attribute: acknowledge', in that it states what scientists say, but we might argue that the use of *scientists* actually adds more weight to the statement than might be expected with other types of speaker, and that this attribution functions here as a kind of implied (or 'invoked', in the terminology favoured by Martin/White 2005: 61) endorsement.

Text 1 (research paper): Synergistic induction of human cathelicidin antimicrodial peptide gene expression by vitamin D and stilbenoids. 'assertion LF'
Text 2 (press release): Red grapes, blueberries may enhance immune function. 'entertain HI'
Text 3 (*Daily Telegraph*): Red wine and blueberries could boost immune system. 'entertain HI'
Text 4 (*Daily Express*): Revealed: the secret of living a berry healthy long life. Red wine and blueberries could protect against illness by boosting the immune system, researchers found. 'proclaim: endorse HI'
Text 5 (*Mirror*): Red grapes and blueberries boost immune system, scientists say. 'attribute: acknowledge HI'

Table 2. Titles/headlines of the five texts.

When we analyse the full texts, a clearer pattern begins to emerge. The scientific nature of Text 1 makes its language radically different from that of the other texts. It is clear that the chain of intertextuality truly begins with Text 2, because it is the press release that mediates the information from Text 1 to the newspapers, and the journalists responsible for Texts 3, 4 and 5 relied on Text 2 for their information, rather than Text 1. This analysis therefore centers on the differences that emerge between Texts 2 to 5. As far as the engagement system is concerned, the press release faithfully distinguishes between the laboratory findings, which are either asserted or attributed throughout, and the health impact, which is communicated using features of 'entertain' and 'attribute', sometimes combined. Text 2 thus maintains a careful distinction between what has been discovered in the laboratory, and what impact this might possibly one day have for patients. On the other hand, Text 3 makes no fewer than eight references to the research, always framing it in terms of possible health benefits except in the brief disclaimer provided at the end of the text (see above). In these statements focusing on the health impact, the writer uses 'entertain' ("could protect the body") or 'attribute: acknowledge' ("is thought to have various healthy effects"). It should be noted that a change in the order of information in Text 3 also generates an entirely new claim: a reference to previous studies which have linked one stilbenoid to "fighting cancer and lowering the risk of heart disease" is inserted before the claim that "the new study [...] was the first to clearly show the way in which the compound works with vitamin D to produce this effect". By reordering the information in this way, the strength of this claim, phrased using ‘proclaim: endorse’, is thus associated anaphorically (“this effect”) with two medicinal properties that the original study in no sense addressed. As a result, not only is the claim of health benefits endorsed, rather than entertained – its scope is also greatly magnified.

Text 4, from the *Daily Express*, also blurs the distinction between the laboratory findings and the possible health benefits. Much of the text uses ‘proclaim: endorse’ to emphasise the importance of the laboratory findings, as in the example “experiments showed combining the compounds with vitamin D made them much more potent”, and reserves ‘entertain’ to refer to the health impact on a single occasion. However, near the beginning of the article the writer foregrounds his explanation of the laboratory findings by stating that “scientists have discovered that red grapes and blueberries contain ingredients that work with vitamin D in the body to boost the immune system”. Since the original paper and the press release stress that this actually does not happen “in the body”, this writer is presenting something that belongs only to the realm of speculation as a strong claim (“have discovered”, ‘proclaim: endorse HI’).

The *Mirror* (Text 5) notably avoids hedging altogether except in the subtitle, which contains the phrase “new research has suggested a link”, and conveys meaning almost entirely through a succession of bald assertions and propositions of the ‘proclaim: endorse’ type. Here, too, the ordering of the information in the text leads the reader to understand that stilbenoids with vitamin D hold potential for treating cancer.

To sum up, in terms of engagement, Texts 2 to 5 all show a strong tendency to frame scientific information in terms of its potential health impact, which is natural if we assume that this is the aspect most likely to interest readers (and most likely to ensure future funding). However, they differ in the degree of care that is taken to separate what is certain (the laboratory finding) from what is merely speculation (the possible health impact). The reordering of information and modification of the disclaimer in Text 3, and the omission of any disclaimer in Texts 4 and 5, compound the blurring of truth values and produce a fundamental distortion in the information provided by the sources.

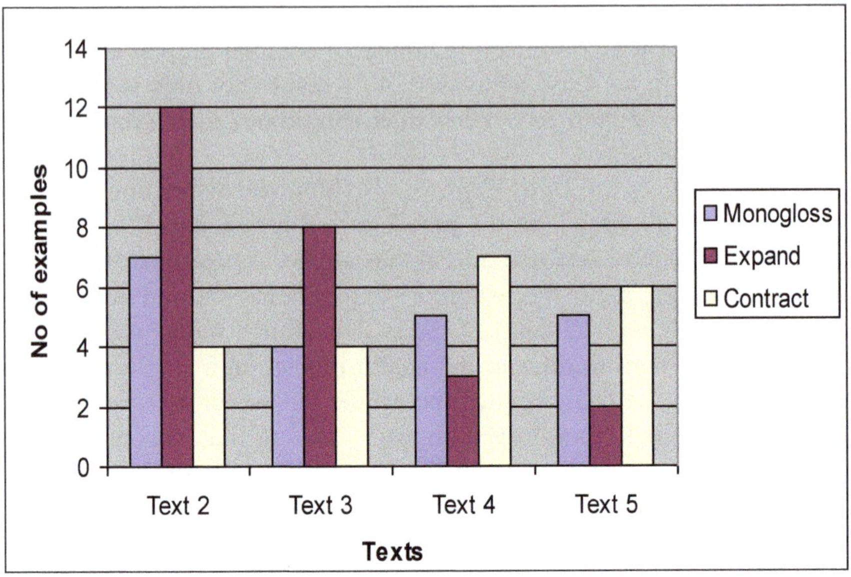

Graph 1. Representation of the number of monoglossic assertions and dialogically expansive or contractive locutions in Texts 2 to 5.

In terms of the engagement system, in simple terms, it is evident that from Texts 2 to 5 there is a decreasing degree of 'entertain' and an increasing proportion of 'contract' and monoglossic assertions (cf. Graph 1). While Text 2 favours 'entertain', particularly in the form of neutral attributions and hedging, Text 3 moves further towards what might be termed an 'assertive' or 'contractive' style. In Texts 4 and 5, monoglossic and contractive assertions outnumber the dialogically expansive moves in the text. These texts tend to accord greater weight to the statements they quote, by fronting them with verbs such as *found*, *showed*, *revealed* or *established* rather than neutral verbs such as *said*, which only occurs twice in each text. This is extremely important in terms of the engagement system, because use of verbs that imply alignment with what is said turns a straightforward attribution into an endorsement (see above, and also Martin/ White 2005: 126). Whereas statements that are simply 'said' are merely held up for the reader's consideration, things that are 'found' or 'shown' are accepted as true by the writer and presented as such to the reader generating a sense of confidence and certainty regarding the truth of the reported material. These subtle shifts in what we might term the engagement repertoire of the texts doubtless reflect aspects of media genre convention. Press releases on scientific issues are supposed not to be misleading, and the more serious newspapers are generally perceived to be more neutral or moderate in the tone of their general reporting. Downmarket newspapers such as the *Daily Express* or, particularly, the *Mirror*, cater for readers who are less familiar with the subtle conventions of academic/scientific reporting. The move from 'entertain' and 'attribute' to 'assert' observed here may well reflect a shift in the underlying paradigms that shape the way news is understood and reported in the different media strata. If we add to this the blurring of the distinction between laboratory findings and health implications, and the absence of any form of disclaimer in the last two texts, we will see that the net result is a considerable erosion of the informational content from the press release.

3.2 Graduation

According to Martin and White (2005: 135), the second important dimension of the engagement system is gradability. We may note that gradability can also be considered part of the attitude system, that is, as influencing values of affect, judgement and appreciation, but the interplay between the two systems falls beyond the scope of the present chapter. Graduation is, in any case, particularly relevant to a study of engagement, in the view of these authors, because it affects the up- and downscaling of the writer's commitment to his/her utterances, and thus has an important role in shaping the dialogic relationship with the reader. For Martin and White (2005: 137), graduation operates across two axes of scalability: grading according to quantity or intensity (grouped together as 'force'), and grading according to prototypicality ('focus') as represented in Table 3. Graduation can be realised on both these axes through 'isolation' (e.g. use of a separate word with a modifying function: "fairly quickly") or 'infusion' (conveyed through one aspect of the meaning of a term: "gushed").

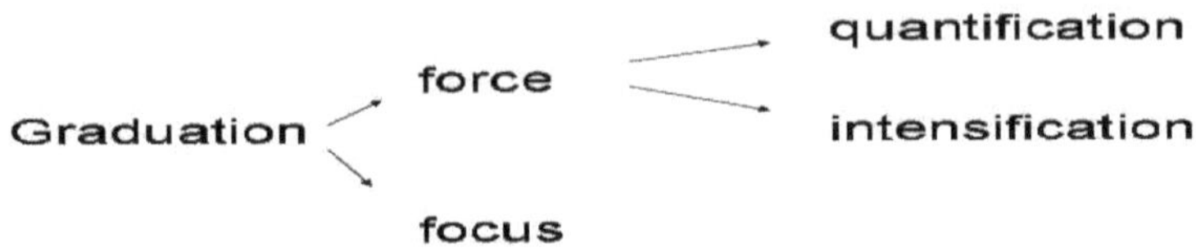

Table 3. Graduation: force and focus (from Martin/White 2005: 141).

In the sample of texts considered here, there was little evidence of 'focus', but 'force' was found to be an important factor. It is not surprising that the density of 'force' elements was much greater in all four media texts than in the original scientific paper. Text 1 included a few items that could be interpreted as aspects of intensification, such as "for the first time" (abstract), "the discovery [...] is intriguing" (discussion), and "interestingly" (discussion). The writers' use of evaluative resources is quite characteristic of scientific texts, in that it is sparingly applied and operates within the range of 'appreciation: reaction' (Martin/White 2005: 56). As Hyland (2000), among others, has discussed, scientific writers write primarily for the discourse community of their fellow scientists, and to be taken seriously there, it would be risky for them to overstate their case. Texts 2 to 5 were all composed within a very different paradigm, that of the media, where writers do not appear to be constrained in this way. All four media texts contain a considerable number of locutions in which features of graduation can be observed. We can make a clear distinction between three particular places in which such elements are present in Texts 2 to 5: 1) in one high-profile direct quotation attributed to the head of the research team, which is echoed in all four texts; 2) in various other instances of reported speech that are blended into the text with more general attributions to 'the scientists'; and 3) in assertions made by the writer. We shall consider these separately, because the nature of the up-scaling (in this case) is obviously rather different, in dialogic terms, if it is inserted as a quotation, or if it is asserted in the writer's own voice.

First, the comment presented as a direct quotation from the head of the research team has a particularly marked status, since it is the only one attributed to a named person, and the only one labelled as a direct quotation by the use of quotation marks: "Out of the hundreds of compounds, just these two popped right out. Their synergy with vitamin D was significant and intriguing. It's a pretty interesting interaction." This quotation is presented in complete form in Texts 2, 3 and 4, and in a curtailed form in Text 5, accompanied by the name and affiliation of the scientist in all cases. The dramatisation of the discovery using the verb *popped out* engages a metaphor of animation which can be regarded as an intensification through infusion (cf. Martin/White 2005: 143–4), functioning within the text to reinforce the impact of the discovery. We may note that the three adjectives that follow closely on one another (*significant, intriguing, interesting*), conveying elements of reaction and valuation, could also be seen as an instantiation of intensification through repetition which adds to the impact of this quotation.

Secondly, the other attributed comments reported in the texts are presented in a less striking way: the absence of quotation marks means that they tend to blend into the background text. The press release contains various non-marked quotations from 'scientists' or 'researchers' containing locutions such as "the first to show", "play a key role", "especially important", "a strong link", and "considerably more biological impact". These quotations are characterized by the frequent use of intensifiers and comparatives, which appear to reflect aspects of intensification by up-scaling or infusion, in the sense understood by Martin and White (2005: 153–4). In the Appraisal system, up-scaling is regarded as a tool used by the writer to convey greater commitment to the position or proposition being advanced, and thereby to align the reader to a shared value position

In another section, the writer refers to "dozens of studies for a range of possible benefits", thus engaging the principle of quantification (Martin/White 2005: 152–3), which is often used in parallel to intensification as a means of aligning the reader towards a shared position. Interestingly, though, in Text 2, it is common to find a blend of intensified assertions with hedges: thus Text 2 states "it appears that combining these compounds [...] has considerably more biological impact". In a sense, the writer of Text 2 seems to be sailing close to the wind: he or she uses a considerable degree of up-scaling, but generally either hedges this by using a modal verb, or attributes the assertion to someone else. In Text 3, the pattern is similar but less varied, with various up-scaling or intensifying locutions attributed to 'researchers', still sometimes accompanied by hedges such as *linked to* and *suggests*. On the other hand, Texts 4 and 5 also use intensification in statements attributed to 'researchers', but endorse them with verbs such as *revealed* or *established* (see above), thus engineering strong reader alignment with these up-scaled assertions. Altogether, Texts 4 and 5 present the scientific findings and their health implications with a high degree of certainty, aligning the reader to accept the truth of the various findings. Although these texts often lift material directly from the press release, they imbue it with greater certainty.

One extract from the texts serves to illustrate these tendencies. The press release presents the information carefully, though with up-scaling in the form of an intensified comparative, fronting it with the verb *appear*: "It appears that combining these compounds with vitamin D has considerably more biological impact than any of them would separately". Text 3 first entertains the same idea using *appear* and intensification through infusion (*boost, fight*), stating that "the two compounds appeared to work with vitamin D to increase the activity of a gene […] which helps boost the body's ability to fight disease"; but almost immediately after this, the information is reformulated in a dialogically contractive way: "the new study […] was the first to clearly show the way in which the compound works with vitamin D to produce this effect". Text 4 opts for dialogic contraction plus intensification from the outset, stating that the "lab experiments showed combining the compounds with vitamin D made them much more potent" (Text 4). Text 5 presents a simplified version which is also intensified and contractive: "scientists […] found that combining blueberry and red grape stilbenoids with vitamin D made them much more potent" (Text 5).

Finally, the writer him/herself takes responsibility for those statements in the text which are bald assertions, neither hedged nor attributed to any other speaker. Interestingly, Text 2 contains very few assertions of this kind, since most of the ideas put forward in the article are attributed to 'researchers' and 'scientists'. Those which are unattributed are either brief accounts of the laboratory findings or explanations concerning the scientific background. The latter, in particular, show a strong degree of force through both intensification ("unique", "importance") and quantification ("millions of years"). In Text 3, the writer's voice follows a similar pattern, presenting the account of the experiment and findings succinctly as fact, with occasional mild intensification ("stood out"). Text 4 has a higher proportion of monoglossic assertions, used to explain the scientific background ("the stilbenoid in red grapes is resveratrol") and to convey the main findings ("blueberries give the body's immune system a boost"). These are often subject to a high degree of intensification: "when the system goes awry, it can trigger inflammation, responsible for deadly and debilitating conditions".

Even when the information is presented with a certain degree of hedging, the writer uses considerable infusion and quantification, surely intended to secure reader alignment. Examples such as "compounds that harness the health-boosting power of certain fruits could be the key to avoiding a host of chronic health problems" combine metaphor with a rhetoric of quantification that engages the notion of a threat to the reader. Lastly, although Text 5 has a headline and subtitle which belong to the 'entertain' category (using "scientists say" and "research [...] has suggested"), the body of the text operates almost entirely through monoglossic assertions and dialogic contraction. The unattributed statements contain considerable intensification: "the innate immune response is especially important for fending off bacteria, which are increasingly becoming resistant to antibiotics". Locutions such as this draw on a rhetoric of animation and play on readers' fears, as has been widely studied in the bibliography (Fowler 1991).

Although Martin and White (2005: 64–67) discuss metaphor mainly in the context of attitude, the function of metaphor obviously overlaps with the figurative realisations of up- and down-scaling associated with graduation. If we look at the text in terms of dialogue, metaphor is used to sway the reader in one direction or another. In the particular case studied here, the most frequent metaphor is the one which has been variously described as a 'combat' or 'violence' metaphor (Semino 2008), which is characteristically used to explain the relationship between patients or health care professionals, on the one hand, and disease, on the other. Although some consider this to be a dead metaphor, even within the narrow confines of this small sample it can be seen to be both pervasive and generative. Text 2 already draws on this metaphor in a rather conventionalised way ("fighting cancer", "combat bacterial infection"), as does Text 3, but Texts 4 and 5 go further, dramatising scientific research as a struggle between the forces of good and evil: scientists "harness health-boosting power" in order to "fight infections", tackle "debilitating and deadly conditions", "fight cancer" and "fend off bacteria". Once again, what begins in a more moderate form in the press release is communicated in a more direct, dramatic style in the newspaper articles, and the more popular the newspaper, the stronger this tendency is.

4. Discussion

The five texts in this study illustrate the transformations that scientific information can undergo in its transition from academia to the mass media. Of course, it is common knowledge that newspapers, particularly tabloid newspapers, both simplify and sensationalise their subject matter, and if that were the only conclusion, this chapter would contribute nothing new. The aim of this research, however, was to do rather more than this. First, the purpose was to establish, in a principled way, exactly what the discursive manifestations of this 'sensationalising' process are. Second, my aim was to assess the usefulness of the engagement framework proposed by Martin and White (2005) in revealing how the writer undertakes a dialogue with prior texts and anticipates how readers will respond to the propositions involved.

Regarding the first of these aims, it is clear that there is a gradual shift in both engagement and graduation from Text 2 to Text 5. Text 2 combines features of scientific writing (maintaining the important distinction between laboratory findings and health impact, using hedging, and applying a high frequency of attribution) with features more characteristic of journalism (narrative, high-impact direct quotation, rhetoric of quantity, intensity, metaphor). In Text 3, journalistic features predominate, but there is still some distinction between what is / may be / is said to be, attribution to sources, and a (modified) disclaimer. Texts 4 and 5 omit the disclaimer and present most of the information as fact. Importantly, they blur laboratory findings with health implications, presenting the latter as fact. Moreover, they have a 'saturated' style with a high degree of infusion. In terms of reader alignment, we might observe that while Text 2 and, to some extent Text 3, are written for readers with some critical awareness of the nature of scientific progress and an eye for strict truthfulness, Texts 4 and 5 assume a compliant, uncritical reader who would not appreciate finely tuned modulation of the epistemic system. It is interesting, too, that all these texts, from the press release onwards, instantiate a high degree of intensification. The writers of the press release know that rhetorical resources have to be brought into play to attract media attention, but they are careful not to sacrifice the truth, attributing and hedging their claims on the one hand, while intensifying them on the other.

Different genre conventions apply in the press, and the more downmarket the publication is, the less likely the writer is to be worried about differences between *may be* and *is*. The tabloid press, in particular, does not operate within the epistemological paradigm of scientific research, but rather seeks to situate stories of this kind within the master-frame of science versus disease, or provide a straightforward answer to the question 'what does it mean for our readers?'.

These findings shed further light on what Martin and White (2005: 164–184) term 'evaluative key' in journalistic discourse. Key, in their system, encompasses the "sub-selections from the overall meaning-making potential" used in a particular type of text or register (2005: 164). They were able to show convincingly that 'hard news' articles are written in a different kind of 'voice' from editorials or commentary, and track the differences along the evaluative cline. In their analysis of these "re-settings of the language's global evaluative meaning making potential" across the range of 'attitude' (2005: 181), they were able to show that 'reporter voice' contained no inscribed judgement or authorial affect, and a low probability of inscribed appreciation, since the writer of 'hard news' generally "minimises interpersonal meanings which may act to reveal or foreground his/her subjective involvement in the meanings in the text" (White 2005: 107). Such judgement or affect as is present tends to be in statements attributed to persons involved in the events, which enables the writer to steer a middle course between appearing objective in order to assert his/her credibility as a news writer, and projecting strong interpersonal meanings in order to interest the reader (White 2005: 109). The evidence considered here sheds further light on what Wahl-Jorgensen has termed the 'neat trick' of "outsourcing of emotional labor to non-journalists" (2013: 130). In other voices, however, such as what Martin and White (2005) term 'commentator voice', the settings are different, so that, for example, it is quite usual for the author to proclaim his/her own judgements or affect.

5. Conclusion

In the present chapter, we have observed that such clinal distinctions are also present across the 'engagement-graduation' dimension. In this sample, the more downmarket the newspaper, the more likely it is for information to be presented as an assertion, or in a dialogically contractive manner. Since up-scaling resources are frequent in all these texts, we can observe that it is actually the type of engagement that marks the main difference between the press release and the popular press. High intensification and high dialogicity in the press release is subtly transformed into high intensification and low dialogicity in the downmarket media – which probably has serious consequences for the public understanding of scientific issues. Further research is needed to test out this observation, and to explore other ways in which 'reporter voice' varies across different types of publication.

In all this, we have seen that the engagement system provides tools to characterise media genres more precisely. It is particularly promising in this area, in that it reasserts the importance of the dialogic nature of text and negotiation of alignment between writer, the sources and the inscribed reader. However, use of this system is not exempt from difficulties. Two issues that arose in the present study are: the question of the status of attributed statements, particularly when these appear to come from authoritative sources; and the question of the interplay between engagement and graduation, in specific instances where the writer appears to apply resources of intensification, while simultaneously distancing him/herself from commitment by hedging or attribution.

First, the actual status of attribution raises a question that cannot easily be answered within the Appraisal system. The issue is this: is it admissible to regard statements such as “red grapes and blueberries boost immune system, scientists say” as a simple attribution? Or does the implication of expertise attaching to the word *scientists* turn them into endorsements, thereby weighting the dice and acting as a means of dialogic contraction instead of expansion? The patchwork texture of news writing has long fascinated linguists and discourse analysts. Within a Bakhtinian perspective, Ducrot (1984) drew attention to the way in which writers invoke other voices in order to shape their relationship with readers. Van Dijk (1988) devoted considerable attention to the relationship between information and commentary in supposedly objective news reporting. From an Appraisal perspective, Martin and White (2005: 115) suggest that whether or not writers align themselves with the voices cited can be best understood in terms of genre. In their words, “[s]ome texts operate under a regime by which it is assumed that it is possible for the speaker/writer to remain aloof from, and unimplicated in, any of the value positions which are contained in attributed material.” In their view, this regime operates in the so-called ‘hard news’ reporting found in quality newspapers, in which one generic convention supposes a certain kind of impartiality on the part of the writer, who can include direct quotations from his/her sources without being assumed to subscribe to the positions that they represent.

Nonetheless, while in ‘hard news’ such a convention may exist, scientific reporting might be understood to be located somewhere in the borderlands between ‘hard news’ and feature writing, where conventions are looser. Even in ‘hard news’, Martin and White (2005: 116) concede that when the sources are understood to have high status in the field, what they say has greater credibility. Here, the situation is more polarised: the textual evidence points to a considerable alignment of the writer with the agents cited. In the small sample of texts considered here, except in the case of the one quotation attributed to the head of the research team in person, the ‘scientists’ or ‘researchers’ are labelled generically as a collective, that is, an apparently homogeneous, consensual group (van Leeuwen 1996: 46). Moreover, this collective is discursively constructed as having authoritative status: the scientists' university affiliation is stressed, and their findings are mainly presented as conclusive rather than tentative. Just as in a certain type of advertising, the scientist in a lab coat is presented as an endorsement of the product's effectiveness, in media reports of this kind, what scientists or researchers have to say is likely to carry a particular weight (Calsamiglia/López Ferrero 2003: 155–156). Finally, most of the statements attributed to the scientific collective in the media texts analysed here are presented without quotation marks, as integrated or inserted citations brought into the main discourse of the text, voices that are clearly invoked or assumed by the writer.

Secondly, the way in which 'graduation' and 'engagement' are intertwined even in simple texts points to an interesting phenomenon, in which writers appear to point two ways when writing about certain types of issue. It would probably be going too far to say that writers of press releases intentionally blend intensification with hedging in the knowledge that the journalists who pick up their text will replicate the intensification and discard the hedging. However, they certainly operate within two parameters that are often difficult to reconcile: the need to be 'newsworthy', and the commitment to strict truth. Much scientific research proceeds extremely slowly, and results that are promising in a laboratory setting may take many years to bear fruit in clinical practice. Yet in the competition for funding and promotion, visibility is essential. Press releases are therefore in some sense a site of struggle (Fairclough 1989) where the intense intermingles with the tentative in almost equal degree. Close attention to resources of engagement and graduation at least helps to bring this struggle to light, even if it cannot fully explain it.

References

Calsamiglia, Helena / López Ferrero, Carmen 2003. Role and Position of Scientific Voices. Reported Speech in the Media. *Discourse Studies* 5/2, 147–173.

Dijk, Teun A. van 1988. *News as Discourse*. Hillsdale, NJ: Lawrence Erlbaum.

Ducrot, Oswald 1984. *El decir y lo dicho. Polifonía de la enunciación*. Barcelona: Paidós.

Fairclough, Norman 1989. *Language and Power*. London: Longman.

Fowler, Roger 1991. *Language in the News*. London: Routledge.

Hyland, Ken 2000. *Disciplinary Discourses. Social Interactions in Academic Writing*. London: Routledge.

Leeuwen, Theo van 1996. The Representation of Social Actors. In Caldas-Coulthard, Carmen R. / Coulthard, Malcolm (eds) *Texts and Practices: Readings in Critical Discourse Analysis*. London: Routledge, 32–70.

Martin, James R. / White, Peter R.R. 2005. *The Language of Evaluation: Appraisal in English*. London: Palgrave Macmillan.

Semino, Elena 2008. *Metaphor in Discourse*. Cambridge: Cambridge University Press.

Wahl-Jorgensen, Karin 2013. The Strategic Ritual of Emotionality: A Case Study of Pulitzer Prize-winning Articles. *Journalism* 14, 129–145.

White, Peter R.R. 2005. Death, Disruption and the Moral Order: the Narrative Impulse in Mass Media 'Hard News' Reporting. In Christie, Frances / Martin, James R. (eds) *Genres and Institutions: Social Processes in the Workplace and School*. London: Continuum, 101–133.

Texts

1. Guo, Chunxiao / Sinnott, Brian / Niu, Brenda / Lowry, Malcolm B. / Fantacone, Mary L. / Gombart, Adrian F. 2014. Synergistic induction of human cathelicidin antimicrobial peptide gene

expression by vitamin D and stilbenoids. *Molecultar Nutrition Food Research* 8/3, 528–536. <http://onlinelibrary.wiley.com/doi/10.1002/mnfr.201300266/abstract>.

2. Red grapes, blueberries may enhance immune function. *Oregon State University News and Research Communications.* 17/09/2013. <http://oregonstate.edu/ua/ncs/archives/2013/sep/red-grapes-blueberries-may-enhance-immune-function>.
3. Collins, Nick 2013. Red wine and blueberries could boost immune system. *Daily Telegraph*, 17/09/2013. <http://www.telegraph.co.uk/health/healthnews/10315217/Red-wine-and-blueberries-could-boost-immune-system.htmlv>.
4. Willey, Jo 2013. Revealed: the secret of living a berry healthy long life. Red wine and blueberries could protect against illness by boosting the immune system, researchers found. *Daily Express*, 18/09/2013. <http://www.express.co.uk/life-style/health/430247/Revealed-The-secret-of-living-a-berry-healthy-long-life>.
5. Red grapes and blueberries boost immune system, scientists say. *Mirror*. 17/09/ 2013. <http://www.mirror.co.uk/lifestyle/health/red-grapes-blueberries-boost-immune-2280755>.

María José Luzón

Recontextualizing Expert Discourse in Weblogs: Strategies to Communicate Health Research to Experts and the Interested Public[1]

1. Introduction

In the last few years science blogs have proliferated as a communication medium to share scientific research with experts and to inform the interested public of science-related news and discoveries. Medical weblogs, in particular, have become an increasingly popular way to disseminate health-related information to the end user (i.e. clinicians, patients). In addition to the high number of individual medical and health blogs, high profile journals, like the *British Medical Journal* (BMJ) or the *New England Journal of Medicine* (NEJM), also have their blogs and social media sites, intended to make research results more accessible to the interested public. Posts in medical blogs may contain information about diseases and treatments, information on current medical research, and discussion of recently published medical papers and of their relevance for clinical practice (Prasad/Kumar 2012). The objective is not only to share knowledge, but also to debunk myths and help readers take informed decisions. In their study of health research blogging, Shema et al. (2014) found that 90% of the posts in their corpus included a discussion and examination of issues dealt with in published articles, 30% included some criticism of issues discussed in the papers (e.g. criticism of claims, beliefs, methodology) and 27% recommended actions for the

1 This research has been carried out within the framework of the InterLAE research team (www.interlae.com), funded by the local educational authories (Diputación General de Aragón), and by the research project FFI2012-37346 (Spanish Ministry of Economy and Competitiveness).

readers. This reveals the blogger's desire to share knowledge with their audience, but also to influence them.

Medical blogs provide a public space with health-related information both for experts and non-specialist readers. Their audience is a diverse one, ranging from medical professionals to patients, with no clear boundary between specialist and non-specialist audience. Like any other type of blogs, medical blogs are not really intended for the world at large, but for those who share the blogger's interests and concerns (Myers 2010). Blogs enable the blogger not only to get to and connect with multiple publics with shared interests (Blanchard 2011), but also to cater for the information needs of these multiple audiences.

Science blogs rely on an approach to science communication based on dialogue (Miller 2001; Bucchi 2008). The underlying assumption in science blogs and therefore in medical blogs is that science communication is not a response to the public's deficit of scientific knowledge but communication of science based on a two-way exchange between scientists and the public audience (Miller 2001). As a matter of fact, most medical blogs have commenting capabilities, which enable the readers to contribute to the post discussion. The technological features of blogs facilitate this dialogue-based model of science communication and make them especially useful for public health science communication (Bjerglund/Söderguist 2012): new findings and ideas can be spread quickly to the relevant audiences, who can contribute to the discussion of the issue; blogs can connect different communities (e.g. researchers with health practitioners, interested public, students) and can be used to communicate public health research to these communities; information can be adjusted to the characteristics of these diverse audiences, i.e. information can be easily recontextualized to get to multiple audiences and to achieve new purposes.

The concepts of 'recontextualization' (Calsamiglia/Van Dijk 2004) and 'proximity' (Hyland 2010) are useful to explain the discourse processes in research blogs. Calsamiglia and Van Dijk (2004: 371) describe popularizations as being determined by the properties of the *communicative context* ("participants and *participant roles"*, as well as "their respective *purposes*, beliefs and *knowledge"*) and thus involving "not only a *reformulation*, but in particular also a *recontextualization* of scientific knowledge and discourse that is originally produced in specialized contexts". Similarly, research blogposts also involve a recontextualization of scientific knowledge and require the use of discourse strategies for that purpose. Hyland (2010: 117) uses the term 'proximity' to refer to a writer's strategic use of rhetorical features which involve "responding to the context of the text, particularly the readers who form part of that context". Proximity can be negotiated in several ways: by shaping material for the audience through different types of appeals, by adapting information to the assumed knowledge of potential readers, by expressing stance, and by using engagement markers to connect with the readers. Bloggers writing research blogposts recontextualize scientific discourse into another domain and use the affordances of the medium to adapt to the needs of a diverse audience. In order to meet the information needs of this diverse audience and make scientific knowledge accessible for the lay public, bloggers make use of various recontextualization or mediation strategies.

In this chapter I will focus on research-commenting posts, i.e. posts that comment and report on published research. Bloggers use them to share links to already published articles, but also to reflect on and evaluate the research or to share informal background information and personal commentary on the topic, in order to help public understanding of the issues involved in the research (Luzón 2013). The objective of the research presented here is to study the strategies used by bloggers to communicate and recontextualize the scientific discourse of academic journals in the realm of medical blogs. The chapter is intended to answer the following questions:

1. Which strategies do medical bloggers use to adjust information to the reader's knowledge, interest and expectations?
2. Which strategies do bloggers use to engage the reader?

2. Corpus and method

The data for this study consists of 75 blogposts which present and discuss new research in medicine. They were taken from <ResearchBlogging.org>, a website that aggregates blogposts about peer-reviewed research. I selected posts in the Medicine category at three different moments: October 17, 2013, November 25, 2013 and January 2, 2014. I selected the first 25 posts from these dates backwards, taking into account that only two posts by the same author could be selected at each moment. (See the appendix for a list of blogs from which posts have been taken.)

In order to determine the strategies used in the corpus and their frequency I used a coding scheme based on previous research on the rhetorical strategies in popularizing genres (e.g. Fahnestock 1998, 2004; Hyland 2010; Calsamiglia/Van Dijk 2004; Giannoni 2008). This coding scheme was developed for a study of the recontextualizing strategies in a corpus of blogposts taken from different academic disciplines (Luzón 2013). In this chapter I focus exclusively on medical blogs. The general public is increasingly turning to the Internet for health information and their opinion on health issues is particularly important, because it might affect decision-taking at higher levels. It is therefore assumed that medical blogs may use distinctive strategies to disseminate health-related information and engage the public.

In the following section the different recontextualization strategies used by medical bloggers are discussed and illustrated.

3. Results

3.1 Strategies to tailor information to the assumed knowledge of potential readers

When communicating science, writers adapt information to the knowledge and interests of potential readers. While writers of research papers write for peers and therefore use technical terminology or reference to disciplinary practices (Hyland 2010), writers of popularizations use rhetorical strategies to help the readers connect the new knowledge in the text to their existing knowledge, e.g. defining new concepts as they are introduced (Hyland 2010). Medical bloggers seek to frame content both for expert and non-specialist audiences. Table 1 shows the strategies used in the posts in the corpus to meet the information needs of the audience, with the number and the percentage of posts in which these strategies occur:

Strategies to tailor information	Overall number of posts	% out of number of posts
Links	66	88
Visuals conveying information (graphs, charts, medical pictures)	29	38.7
Explanation of terms and concept (Definition, elaboration of terms, explanation of concepts, paraphrases)	23	30.7
Comparisons and metaphors	3	4
Extended examples from daily life	3	4

Table 1. Strategies to adapt information to the audience's knowledge.

The most frequent strategy used in the corpus to tailor information to the readers is links (present in 88% of the posts). Bloggers take advantage of the hypertextual allowances of the medium to adapt the explanation and clarification of disciplinary concepts to the needs of the audience. Links create a hypertext co-constructed with the reader, who can decide whether to read the explanation/clarification in the link. Bloggers can thus provide for readers with different levels of expertise and enhance their texts both with clarifications for non-experts and specialized information for more knowledgeable readers.

The following example, with fragments from the posts 'Maternal diabetes and offspring autism risk' in the blog *Questioning Answers* helps to illustrate the types of links in medical blogs:

(1) The systematic review and meta-analysis reported by Xu and colleagues* (a)[2] caught my eye recently. Concluding that: "*maternal diabetes was significantly associated with a greater risk of ASD in the offspring*" my interest was truly piqued.

2 Underlining is used throughout the paper to mark hyperlinks. In example (1) each hyperlink has been assigned a letter to facilitate reference to these links in the text.

> Diabetes (b) in relation to autism has cropped up a few times on this blog. I've talked about the possibility of a more general connection (see here) (c) and also more specific as part of some of the CHARGE (d) results (see here) (e).
> Indeed those CHARGE results, based on the study by Paula Krakowiak and colleagues** (open-access) (f) I remember generated quite a bit of discussion (g) at the time of their publication given the suggested link with various facets making up metabolic syndrome (h) in mums.
> I'm not really surprised by the Xu results when you think that the association between gestational diabetes (i) and offspring autism risk has been talked about before based on some pretty strong association data. I note for example, that the study by Lyall and colleagues*** (open-access) (j) flagged up this association – "*gestational diabetes was associated with a significantly increased risk of ASD*" – based on quite a nice sample size. That and the paper by Hannah Gardener and colleagues**** (open-access) (k) who suggested that gestational diabetes was perhaps one of several factors which might elevate offspring risk as per the Krakowiak results.

Some of the links in the post provide information for more expert readers, e.g. links to research papers in specialized journals (links a, f, j, k), while others provide information for a more general audience, e.g. links to information on diabetes (b), metabolic syndrome (h) or gestational diabetes (i). Link (b) leads to the page 'What is diabetes' in the website *DIABETES UK*, the website of a diabetes charity addressed at a lay audience. Links (h) and (i) lead respectively to the entries 'metabolic syndrome' and 'gestational diabetes' in the page *NHS choices*. This is part of the section *Health A-Z*, an online medical encyclopaedia for lay people, where different conditions are explained in detail, providing information on symptoms, causes and possible actions. Interestingly, the blogger does not link to Wikipedia, a site to which science bloggers link frequently when they need to provide extended explanations for the lay public (Luzón 2013). The blogger here prefers to explain health conditions and treatments by linking to a highly reliable work of reference, *NSH choices*, which is presented in the following way in its 'about us' page:

> NHS Choices is the UK's biggest health website. It provides a comprehensive health information service to help put you in control of your healthcare. The website helps you make choices about your health, from decisions about your lifestyle, such as smoking, drinking and exercise, to finding and using NHS

services in England. [...] NHS Choices is certified by the Information Standard as a producer of reliable health and social care information (*NHS Choices*)

The blogger also uses several links, often to posts in his own blog, to provide background for the new post. In example (1) the blogger links to two of his previous posts (links c and d) ('Hey sugar: diabetes and autism', 'Maternal obesity and risk of autism') and to the website of a study on the environmental causes and risk factors for autism, the CHARGE (CHildhood Autism Risks from Genetics and the Environment) study. If readers want to know more about the topic (i.e. the relation between maternal diabetes and autism) and the blogger's view on it, they can read these texts.

In the following extract from the post 'Fear factor', the blogger assumes that many of the readers will be familiar with the 'Little Albert' experiment, so he does not consider it necessary to explain it in the post. However, he provides a link to the Wikipedia entry explaining the experiment so that readers not familiar with it can follow his text:

(2) It was shown in 'Little Albert' that phobias can be conditioned and by conditioning one could trigger the fear response to a stimuli that generally does not induce fear (for example, ringing a bell). While the 'Little Albert' experiment is considered as controversial and unethical, today. It does raise the questions *Why do we feel fear? What is it that triggers fear in us?* (*GTKSB*)

The links that bloggers incorporate have, therefore, different functions. First, they do not only provide information on concepts that may help understanding for some readers but also allow the blogger to contextualize the new post by providing background information. In addition, links are bibliographical references, which give direct access either to the commented papers or to their abstract in scientific databases. These links enable the specialist audience to read the original text and find information that only they may be interested in.

The next most frequent element used to tailor information to the audience was visuals conveying information, present in 38.7% of the posts in the corpus. In most cases the bloggers used the visuals that occurred in the commented paper, although the explanation was simplified and contextualized. In addition, bloggers often provided extra textual explanation to facilitate understanding of the visuals.

The third most frequent strategy to tailor information was explanation of terms and concepts (30.7% of the posts). Academic bloggers use different explanatory elements typical of popularizations (e.g. comparisons and metaphors, definitions or elaboration of terms, examples) to help non-specialist audiences integrate specialist knowledge (Luzón 2013). However, in the medical blogging corpus, comparisons (e.g. 3) and examples from daily life were rare. As for explanation of concepts, there were a few examples of definitions, explanation of technical terms or paraphrases (examples 4–5), but most frequently clarification of concepts in the corpus involved the description of diseases, conditions, proteins, bacteria, etc. in terms of their effects (examples 6–7), probably because this is what really concerns the reader. Example 7 shows that, although any reader will probably know what vitamin D is, what is important in this context is to know its effects and what happens when there is a lack of it.

(3) Inhibiting protein production has similar consequences as removing a selection of car engine parts. The car dies and so do bacteria treated with antibiotics. (*The Molecular Scribe*)

(4) Researchers call this difference weight suppression (WS, more specifically, the highest *adult* body weight and one's current weight). It can be thought of as the extent to which an individual has reduced their weight through dieting. (*Scienceofeds*)

(5) Runner's high, that feeling of euphoria that is supposed to come from long intense exercise. (*Biological Exceptions*)

(6) Multiple Sclerosis (MS) is a disease characterized by lesions in the nervous system induced by the loss of the protective sheaths that cover nerve fibers and assure the proper transmission of electric impulses. (*United academics*)

(7) Vitamin D is referred to as the 'sunshine vitamin'. It is a fat-soluble vitamin that acts as a steroid hormone. It is produced by the skin in response to ultraviolent light (sunlight). It also occurs naturally in a few foods such as egg yolks, fish oils, and cheese. Vitamin D is essential for strong bones because of its role in calcium metabolism, and it has immune-modulating functions. Vitamin D deficiency (VDD) can result in rickets, osteomalacia, skeletal muscle weakness, and a susceptibility to other conditions ranging from multiple sclerosis to tuberculosis and accelerated lung function decline. (*Science storiented*)

3.2 Strategies to engage the reader

Bloggers used a variety of devices to signal awareness of their audience, engage the readers and guide them to particular positioning (see Table 2). They engaged the readers by arousing their interest, by constructing common grounds, and using interaction to create intimacy and immediacy, and by evaluating scientific content with the purpose of influencing readers.

Strategies to engage the reader	Overall number of posts	% out of number of posts
Engaging title	75	100
Pictures	48	64
Questions	46	61.3
Markers of positive evaluation	42	56
Inclusive pronouns	35	46.66
Personal expression of feelings	27	36
References to reader	25	33.33
Features of conversational discourse	21	28
Personal expression of opinion	16	21.33
Self-disclosure	15	20
Markers of negative evaluation	15	20
References to popular lore, beliefs	12	16

Table 2. Strategies to engage the readers.

A strategy borrowed from popularization is that of changing the title of the original paper to frame the research in a way that may interest the reader. In most cases the bloggers provided an informative title, which presents the results of the research in a comprehensible manner (1, 2 in Table 3). Most frequently titles were used to engage the reader by showing that the results of scientific research may be relevant for their daily life. Sometimes bloggers used a shocking title, which was closer to the reality of the intended audience than the title of the original paper or piqued their audience's curiosity (see respectively 3–4, in the Table below).

Commented paper title	Post title
1) A regenerative approach to the treatment of multiple sclerosis (Deshmukh et al. 2013)[3]	Drugs for Parkinson may help attack multiple sclerosis (*United academics*)
2) Obesity-induced gut microbial metabolite promotes liver cancer through senescence secretome (Yoshimoto et al. 2013)[4]	Researchers discover link obesity and liver cancer: gut microbes facilitate obesity-induced liver cancer (*United academics*)
3) Prevalence rates of mental disorders in Chilean prisons (Mundt et al. 2013)[5]	Is America Less Mentally Healthy Than A Chilean Jail? (*Neuroskeptic*)
4) Surgical castration of the male common hippopotamus (Hippopotamus amphibious) (Walzer et al. 2014)[6]	Why it's nearly impossible to castrate a hippo (*fieldofscience*)

Table 3. Titles in research papers and in the blogposts discussing them.

Bloggers also used several strategies to construct a shared floor, including features typical of informal and private discourse. The most common feature of informal written discourse is visuals related to the title which do not convey information, whose only purpose is to attract, reinforce the message in the text, or shock the reader, e.g. pictures, drawings (present in 64% of the posts). For instance, the post titled 'It's an exercise resolution' includes a picture of a baby lifting heavy weights and the post 'Fear Factor' a picture of the work by Lichtestein *Screaming Lady*.

---

3 Deshmukh et al. 2013 V.A, V. Tardif, CA. Lyssiotis, CC. Green, B. Kerman, H.P. Kim, K. Padmanabhan, J.G. Swoboda, I. Ahmad, T. Kondo, et al. 2013. A regenerative approach to the treatment of multiple sclerosis. *Nature* 502/ 7471: 327–32.

4 Yoshimoto S., T.M.Loo, K. Atarashi, H. Kanda, S. Sato, S. Oyadomari, et al. 2013. Obesity-induced gut microbial metabolite promotes liver cancer through senescence secretome. *Nature* 499: 97–101.

5 Mundt A.P., R. Alvarado, R. Fritsch, C. Poblete, C. Villagra, S. Kastner, S. Priebe. 2013. Prevalence rates of mental disorders in Chilean prisons. *PloS One* 8: 1–8.

6 Walzer, C., T. Petit, G.L. Stalder, I. Horowitz, J. Saragusty, R. Hermes, 2014. Surgical castration of the male common hippopotamus (Hippopotamus amphibius). *Theriogenology* 81/3: 514–518.

Another related strategy intended to attract the audience is the reference to popular lore and beliefs, pop culture and common knowledge, present in 16% of the posts. For instance, the title of the post 'Fear factor', which discusses two papers reporting research on the causes of fear, makes reference to the American dare reality game show *Fear Factor* and the post itself includes a reference to Halloween celebrations ("Halloween is right around the corner, and everyone likes to get spooky! I do fear a lot, in the halloween sense"). In the post 'What's Vitamin D, Precious', there is explicit mention of *The Hobbit* ("The latest installment of The Hobbit trilogy has come to theaters. In honor of Bilbo's return to the screen…"), a picture of Gollum, and the title itself is a humorous reference to the well-known quote from the *Lord of the Rings: The Two Towers*: "What's 'taters', precious?"

Intimacy was also created through self-disclosure, i.e. details about the blogger's personal life (20% of the posts). Although self-disclosure is absent in most scientific discourse, it is frequent in weblogs, especially in personal blogs (Qian/Scott 2007). The details of the blogger's life that are disclosed are related to the content of the post and this contributes to showing the importance of research in 'our' lives (blogger's and readers' lives) and to bring medical research closer to our daily routines. For instance, example (8) is the beginning fragment of the post 'Christmas food for thought', a post which discusses the importance of gut microbes for our health. Examples (9a) and (9b) are respectively the first and the last fragments of the post 'Exercise in a pill… again!', where the blogger questions research that suggests that a drug can mediate the benefits of exercise in our health.

(8) The morning before Christmas eve, I'm sitting here in the dining room munching happily on the bits and pieces of what's left of our gingerbread house that was only erected to its full glory the night before. I have not consumed this amount of carbohydrates in over a year. Inside, a few species of my gut microbes are screaming bloody murder (*Neurorexia*)

(9) a. When life gets rough, I go out for a run. A sweet tune, a steady pace, a great view and all the anxiety and stress that plague me melt away.

b. Whether a single drug can mimic the mind-boggling spectrum of physiological and psychological effects of exercise though is another question. While scientists continue on their search, me? I'm going for a run. (*Neurorexia*)

Bloggers also engaged the readers through devices of dialogic involvement, such as questions, conversational elements or reader pronouns. Questions were the third most frequent strategy used by bloggers to engage the reader (61.33% of the posts). Questions were used for a range of different rhetorical functions in the posts in the corpus, the most important ones being: (i) to make the readers (often a clearly identified intended audience) reflect on the results of the commented paper for clinical or professional practice (10), (ii) to anticipate the topic, either of the whole paper or of the following fragment of text (11), (iii) to question what has been done by the authors of the paper on which the blogger is commenting (12):

(10) Questions for Discussion: As a healthcare professional, how often do you consider long-term consequences of treatment and interventions? As a clinician have you ever had an athlete with an augmentation device? [...] If you had to give advice for a patient going into surgery about the use of augmentation device what would you suggest? How did you come up with your suggestion? (*SMR*)

(11) An alternative strategy is to focus on *messengers* that link the body to the brain. In other words, how does exercise, which happens in the body, increase BDNF in the brain? (*Neurorexia*)

(12) The study recruited patients up to 2011, so I wonder how they got 5-year follow-up data from those admitted in 2010 and who, say, remitted in 2011? Are these researchers psychic? (*Scienceofeds*)

Informality and immediacy were also constructed by adopting discourse practices and linguistic features generally associated with conversational discourse, with 28% of the posts displaying one or more occurrences of these features. These included: parenthetical metalinguistic cues (e.g. "Hmm", "Hmr", "Wow"), oral discourse markers ("I know") and response forms ("yea"), syntactic structures typical of spoken grammar, e.g. omission of parts of the sentence ("Sounds pretty good, right?").

Another strategy to engage the readers is to draw them into the discourse with reader pronouns. Bloggers used both inclusive pronouns, i.e. *we, us* (46.66% of the posts) and second person pronouns (33.33% of the posts). These pronouns represent the readers as participants in the interaction and help the blogger guide the reader towards a particular interpretation. In the corpus of medical blogs the main function of reader pronouns is to present the results of the research reported on as relevant for the reader. Reader pronouns tend to appear at the beginning of the posts, in the introductory paragraphs, to show that the topic of the post may be relevant for the readers' lives and encourage them to go on reading (13–15), or at the end of the posts (16–17), usually to call practitioners to action: the blogger uses expressions of inclusiveness and solidarity to influence the reader. The blog from which examples 16 and 17 have been taken is a group blog, whose purpose, stated in its homepage, is "to bridge the gap between research and clinical practice related to sports medicine" (*SMR*).

(13) Antibiotic therapy is also troubled by the problematic core concept that it lacks specificity, and wipes out good and bad bugs alike. This is particularly worrying as *we* continue to discover just how much the trillions of good bugs that live in *our* gut contribute to *our*[7] health and wellbeing. (*Scilogs*)

(14) There are two major questions to be answered as to a 'getting fit' resolution. The first is obvious – why would more exercise be good for *me*? *We* all know about how expending more energy than *you* take in will help *you* control your weight. So that's an easy one. Exercise also helps *your* health by building muscle, improving flexibility, increasing bone density, and improving both cardiac and pulmonary function. (*Biological Exceptions*)

(15) Inhibitory processes form a crucial part of *our* lives – we use them to delay gratification, bite our tongue in social situations and update our beliefs when confronted with new evidence. (*Neurofractal*)

(16) As a clinician there are many situations in which coaches and athletes desire short-term outcomes. [...] This study should cause *us* to step back and re-assess the use of augmentation devices by considering if the possible short-term benefits are sufficient to justify their use. (*SMR*)

7 Italics have been added in examples 13–30 to highlight some words.

(17) Questions for Discussion: As a healthcare professional, how often have *you* seen athletes physically suffer from dehydration that may be attributed to alcohol consumption? (*SMR*)

The last type of strategy used by medical bloggers to engage the readers is related to the expression of evaluation or stance. The posts in the corpus displayed a high frequency of evaluative devices, both expressing affective attitude (e.g. "This study is an *important* advancement in the research for MS treatment") and epistemic attitude (i.e. commitment to the truth of a proposition) (e.g. "I'm not sure").

56.54% of the posts included positive evaluation of previous research, especially in terms of interest, importance or relevance of the results. In example (18) evaluation is used to structure the post. The post begins by introducing the paper by Campisi et al. and explaining the objective. It then focuses on the originality of the paper, emphasizing that the authors had adopted a 'different' approach (18a). The results are then presented as "interesting" (18b). The post concludes by referring to the high impact of the paper (the number of citations being a measurement of academic quality) and by stressing its significance in the field (18c). Positive evaluation was frequent at the beginning of the post, to attract the readers' interest (18a/b), but also at the end of the post, as a way of conclusion (18c, 19 and 20).

(18) 'The contagion of age'

a. […] until Campisi and her co-workers published their PLOS Biology article in 2008, what goes on when cells senesce had mostly been investigated at the level of genes and their transcripts. Campisi and colleagues tried something *different* [*Brief explanation of the method/ approach*. Not included]
b. What they found was rather *interesting*. [*Report of the results*. Not included]
c. Having had almost 31,000 views and 389 citations, this study defining the SASP is *clearly a significant* one in the field (*PLOS biologue*)

(19) The Taylor paper is an *interesting* one and no doubt will generate some discussion about the numbers of cases of autism. (*Questioning Answers*)

(20) In each case, *important lessons were learned* that should help inform and refine the design of future animal studies. (*PLOS biologue*)

Unlike in research papers, there was also a relatively high percentage of posts displaying expressions of explicit negative evaluation of previous research (20% of the posts). Examples (21–24) show how bloggers used negative evaluation to criticize the research methodology or reject the results or claims presented in the paper. These criticisms are related to the values of the scientific community and to the criteria by which members of this community are judged, e.g. competence in research and argument. As can be seen, bloggers often raise criticism regarding methodological issues, as a way to challenge the reliability of the claims, and in some posts it is suggested that the peer-review process did not work properly and that these papers should not have been published as they are (examples 23–24).

(21) I'm not a statistician. Not even close. But it seems *disingenuous* to calculate remission rates this way. (*Scienceofeds*)

(22) And here is where a very intriguing study hits a road block with me. Although the claim that these 11 participants are synesthetes has the weight of multiple statistical analyses behind them [...] the connection to the fridge magnets *is not statistical at all*. Instead, all we get is a picture, showing the colors identified for each letter of the alphabet by each synesthete. (*Contemplating Cognition*)

(23) I assume vertebrate genome alignments are the source, though the authors don't explicitly state where they got the phyloP values *(come on, peer reviewers!)*. (*Massgenomics*)

(24) *this lack of clarity is unacceptable for a peer-reviewed paper.* (*Scienceofeds*)

In the posts analyzed there were also several examples of harsh and explicit criticism, and even insults, to debunk what bloggers considered misconceptions about a scientific issue (25). The blogger in example 25 is fully aware of the power of social media to spread views on public health and he acts as a 'civic scientist' (Kyvic 2005)[8] advocating against a theory ("AIDS is not caused by HIV") that he calls "pseudoscientific bullshit". He uses emotional appeals to try to persuade the readers that this theory is false and suggests that intelligent people are not deceived

8 Kyvik (2005: 289) defined a civic scientist as "a scientist who communicates with general audiences and brings knowledge and expertise into the public arena to increase awareness about science and/or facilitate discussion and decision making on issues of importance to society".

by pseudoscientists who defend it. Although direct criticism of peer-reviewed articles may occur in some medical genres, like journal editorials or book reviews (Salager-Meyer 2001; Salager-Meyer et al. 2007), insults and ad-hominem attacks are not allowed in traditional genres of medical discourse. The use of insults to express socioemotional meaning seems to be a feature adopted from other types of CMC, such as online fora, where flaming is not unusual (Angouri/Tseliga 2010).

(25) […] the idea that AIDS is not caused by HIV. The main defender of this *irrational* theory is [XX], a professor of Molecular and Cellular Biology in the University of California, Berkeley. Since 1987 (i.e., almost 27 years ago!) he defends such an *absurd* idea that is *rejected by the main research groups working on AIDS* worldwide. […] Anyway, [XX] and his followers' ideas are so *absurdly ridiculous* that the scientific community in general tends to simply ignore him; The problem happens when someone with such a view decides to express it in media for the non-scientific community. […][XX] and his friends are only *pseudoscientific rioters* trying to spread conspiratory ideas. Be smart and don't get trapped in this *pseudoscientific bullshit* (*Earthlingnature*)

The high incidence of both positive and negative explicit evaluation in these posts suggests their relation to academic genres where evaluation of research plays a prominent role, e.g. review articles and editorials (Salager-Meyer 2001) or peer reviews (Hewings 2004), and indicates that some of these posts are intended as post-publication peer reviews. This is a new genre that harnesses the affordances of the medium for new social practices. In their study of peer-reviewed journal article references, Cole and Cole (1971, cited in Shema et al. 2014) found a low rate of critical references and they argued that researchers only criticize works that they consider significant enough to be taken seriously, ignoring those papers that they consider to be of low quality. This is clearly not what happens in medical research-commenting blogs, where all the papers can be the target of criticism, but it is the case of those that bloggers consider especially influential and therefore harmful because they contribute to spreading misconceptions about science (and may misinform the lay public) and those that, in the bloggers' view, should not have passed the peer review process.

Another striking difference between conventional genres of academic discourse and medical research blogposts is the high frequency of personal evaluation. A high percentage of posts in the corpus

(21.33%) displayed personal expressions of epistemological stance, i.e. expressions of stance which include a first person pronoun ("I think", "I'm not surprised that"), revealing the contingency and informality of this type of discourse. Another evaluative element typical of personal discourse that was frequent in the posts analyzed (36.4% of the posts) was the expression of the blogger's feelings or emotional reactions:

(26) *I'm not really surprised* by the Xu results when you think that the association between gestational diabetes and offspring autism risk has been talked about before based on some pretty strong association data. (*Questioning Answers*)

(27) As a biologist, the undead zombie *troubles me* for several reasons. (*Biological exceptions*)

(28) *It is sad to* see how easily people are convinced by what the unskilled media communicates (*Earthlingnature*)

(29) This part of the paper really *infuriated me.* (*Scienceofeds*)

(30) *I was particularly worried* about the importance of stochasticity after seeing the relapse threshold of just 200 stem cells in Horn et al. (2013) (*Egtheory*)

4. Conclusions

The purpose of this study was to analyze how the scientific research reported in academic journals is recontextualized in medical blogs. The chapter has shown that medical research-commenting posts are intended to provide personalized information for readers (i.e. information simultaneously adapted to the needs and interests of diverse audiences), but also to arouse the readers' interest in health research, bring it closer to the readers' daily life and help them make informed decisions.

The adaptation of the information to the background knowledge and interests of a diverse audience is mainly done by linking to websites and online texts which provide reliable health-related information at different levels of expertise, thus harnessing the hypertextual nature of online texts. Strategies typically found in popularizations to make content more understandable by the lay audience (e.g. comparisons, definitions) were not frequent. This contrasts with the relatively high incidence of explanations of medical concepts (e.g. conditions, proteins) in terms of their effects, which reveals the bloggers' desire to spread useful information for readers and to make them aware of the importance of these concepts for people's daily lives. Bloggers are fully aware that promoting the public understanding of science, by informing/persuading the general public of the relevance of medical research, is critical, because this understanding can influence government decisions regarding science policy and funding.

The analysis has also revealed the large variety of strategies to engage the readers used by medical bloggers, and the high number of occurrences of such strategies. Many of these strategies are also intended to help readers perceive the relevance of scientific research for their daily life and to persuade health professionals that the results of the research should be taken into account in their medical practice. Some of the strategies intended to engage the audience are typical of a contingent repertoire (Gilbert/Mulkay 1984) and personal discourse: bloggers attempt to construct intimacy and solidarity and thus align the readers' interests and view with their own.

To conclude, the use of these recontextualizing strategies shows that blogs have become a new medium to communicate health-related science, with the advantages both of public and personal spaces. Bloggers can discuss and evaluate research in a public forum, which enables them to get to different audiences, adopting a personal position, which fosters solidarity and involvement, and facilitates the connection with the general public.

References

Angouri, Jo / Tseliga, Theodora 2010. 'You Have No Idea What You are Talking About!' From E-disagreement to E-impoliteness in Two

Online Fora. *Journal of Politeness Research. Language, Behaviour, Culture* 6/1, 57–82.

Bjerglund, Nina / Söderguist, Thomas 2012. *Social Media and Public Health Research.* <http://bjerglund.files.wordpress.com/2012/11/final-social-media-and-public-health-research1.pdf>.

Blanchard, Antoine 2011. Science Blogs in Research and Popularization of Science: Why, How and for Whom? In Cockell, Moira / Billotte, Jérôme / Darbellay, Frédéric / Waldvogel, Francis (eds) *Common Knowledge: The Challenge of Transdisciplinarity,* Lausanne: EPFL Press, 219–232.

Bucchi, Massimiliano 2008. Of Deficits, Deviations and Dialogues: Theories of Public Communication of Science. In Bucchi, Massimiliano / Trench, Brian (eds) *Handbook of Public Communication of Science and Technology*, London: Routledge, 57–76.

Calsamiglia, Helena / Van Dijk, Teun 2004. Popularization Discourse and Knowledge about the Genome. *Discourse & Society* 15/4, 369–389.

Cole, Jonathan / Cole, Stephen 1971. Measuring the Quality of Sociological Research. Problems in the Use of the Science Citation Index. *American Sociologist* 6/1, 23–29.

Fahnestock, Jeanne 1998. Accommodating Science: The Rhetorical Life of Scientific Facts. *Written Communication* 15, 330–350.

Fahnestock, Jeanne 2004. Preserving the Figure: Consistency in the Presentation of Scientific Arguments. *Written Communication* 21, 6–31.

Giannoni, Davide 2008. Popularizing Features in English Journal Editorials. *English for Specific Purposes* 27/2, 212–232.

Gilbert, G. Nigel / Mulkay, Michael 1984. *Opening Pandora's Box: a Sociological Analysis of Scientists' Discourse.* Cambridge: Cambridge University Press.

Hewings, Martin 2004. An 'Important Contribution' or 'Tiresome Reading'? A Study of Evaluation in Peer Reviews of Journal Article Submissions. *Journal of Applied Linguistics* 1, 247–274.

Hyland, Ken 2010. Constructing Proximity: Relating to Readers in Popular and Professional Science. *Journal of English for Academic Purposes* 9/2, 116–127.

Kyvik, Svein 2005. Popular Science Publishing and Contributions to Public Discourse among University Faculty. *Science Communication* 26, 288–311.

Luzón, María-José 2013. Public Communication of Science in Blogs: Recontextualizing Scientific Discourse for a Diversified Audience. *Written Communication* 30/4, 428–457.

Miller, Steve 2001. Public Understanding of Science at the Crossroads. *Public Understanding of Science* 10/1, 115–120.

Myers, Greg 2010. *The Discourse of Blogs and Wikis*. London: Continuum.

Prasad, Murali / Kumar, Vijaya 2012. Specialty Medical Blogs: A Tool to Disseminate Health Information. *National Journal of Research in Community Medicine* 1/4, 178–241

Qian, Hua / Scott, Craig 2007. Anonymity and Self-disclosure on Weblogs. *Journal of Computer Mediated Communication* 12/4, 1428–1451.

Salager-Meyer, Françoise 2001. From Self-highlightedness to Self-effacement: A Genre Based Study of the Socio-pragmatic Function of Criticism in Medical Discourse. *LSP and Professional Communication* 1/2, 63–84.

Salager-Meyer, Françoise / Alcaraz, María Ángeles / Pabón, Maryelis 2007. Collegiality, Critique and the Construction of Scientific Argumentation in Medical Book Reviews: A Diachronic Approach. *Journal of Pragmatics* 39/10, 1758–1774.

Shema, Hadas / Bar-Ilan, Judit / Thelwall, Mike 2014. How is Research Blogged? A Content Analysis Approach. *Journal of the Association for Information Science and Technology*. <10.1002/asi.23239>.

Appendix

List of blogs from which posts to make up the corpus have been taken

- As many exceptions as rules <http://biologicalexceptions.blogspot.com.es/> (Biological Exceptions)
- Blastocystis parasite blog <http://www.blastocystis.net/>
- Brainposts <http://brainposts.blogspot.com.es/>
- Companion Animal Psychology <http://www.companionanimalpsychology.com/>
- Contemplating Cognition <http://contemplatingcognition.wordpress.com/>
- Cracking the enigma <http://crackingtheenigma.blogspot.com.es/>
- Earthlingnature <https://earthlingnature.wordpress.com/>
- Garden of the mind <http://gardenofthemind.com/>
- Getting to know structural bioinformatics <http://structuralbioinformatician.wordpress.com/> (GTKSB)
- Inkfish <http://inkfish.fieldofscience.com/>
- Kevin O'Brien's Orthodontic Blog <http://kevinobrienorthoblog.com/>
- Massgenomics <http://massgenomics.org/page/5>
- Medical reference Net <http://www.medical-reference.net/>
- Mmmbitesizescience <http://mmmbitesizescience.com/>
- Neurocritic <http://neurocritic.blogspot.com.es/>
- Neurofractal <http://neurofractal.tumblr.com/>
- Neurorexia <http://www.neurorexia.com/>
- Neuroskeptic <http://blogs.discovermagazine.com/neuroskeptic/>
- PLOS Biologue <http://blogs.plos.org/biologue/>
- Questioning Answers <http://questioning-answers.blogspot.com>
- Science of Eating Disorders <http://www.scienceofeds.org/> (Scienceofeds)
- Science storiented <http://storiented.blogspot.com.es/>
- Scilogs <http://www.scilogs.com/>
- Sports Medicine Research <http://www.sportsmedres.org/> (SMR)
- Steam cells freak <http://www.stemcellsfreak.com/>
- The molecular scribe <http://www.molecularscribe.com/>
- The unsilenced science <http://theunsilencedscience.blogspot.com.es/>
- Theory, Evolution, and Games Group <http://egtheory.wordpress.com/>
- United academics <http://www.united-academics.org/>

Davide Mazzi

Semantic Sequences and the Pragmatics of Medical Research Article Writing

1. Introduction

In today's medical profession, there is increasing recognition that doctors should develop clinical as well as research-oriented skills. In this respect, the medical discourse community demands that they become ever more active members of the discipline in both doing and writing about the research they undertake (Swales 2004). One implication of such a complex training process is that doctors are expected to familiarise themselves with the communicative requirements of medical research texts, and more precisely with their key pragmatic aspects.

This may request that doctors acquire sound knowledge of the relationship between the discourse structures of the discipline and its underlying epistemology (Dahl 2004; Engberg 2010). This is an overall challenging task in terms of language-teaching methodology and syllabus design, whereby the need for a grammar addressing fluency as well as context-based accuracy goes hand in hand with the expectation that "descriptions of language will be based on quantities of authentic data rather than on a course writer's intuitions and/or language prejudices" (Hunston/Francis 1998: 45).

It is within such an educational setting that specialised corpora (Hunston 2002; McEnery/Hardie 2011; Gabrielatos et al. 2012) deserve to be acknowledged as a source of significant insights to socialise medical students along with practitioners into the distinctive communicative practices of scientific communities. This aspect should become central when it comes to the prolific output of corpus investigation to show the recurrence of co-occurring items in text. In that regard, the adoption of corpus-based approaches to the study of naturally-occurring language has shed light on remarkable discourse regularities, among which the tendency of words to go together and make meaning by virtue of their combination has been a favourite subject of investigation over the last two decades.

Co-occurring items have been variously termed. For instance, Sinclair (1996) talks about 'units of meaning' as longer sequences to be described in terms of collocation, colligation and semantic preference. These respectively denote firstly the regular co-occurrence of words; secondly, the co-occurrence of grammatical choices; and thirdly, "the restriction of regular co-occurrence to items which share a semantic feature" (Sinclair 2004: 142) as in the case, for instance, of an adjective co-occurring with nouns from the lexical field of sports.

Likewise, in their project aimed at a corpus-driven pedagogic grammar, Hunston and Francis (1998) look at the close association between 'verb patterns' and meaning in the 250-million-word Bank of English; Biber et al. (1999: 990) conduct a cross-register investigation of 'lexical bundles', i.e. "sequences of word forms that commonly go together in natural discourse" regardless of their idiomaticity; and Wray (2002) discusses 'formulaic expressions or sequences' as linguistic units composed of multiple words, which she analyses in the light of different frames of interpretation, e.g. individual motivations for achieving novelty and pragmatic notions of shared knowledge between speaker/writer and listener/reader. Co-occurring patterns have been variously ascribed to such widespread phenomena as Sinclair's (2004) idiom principle, Hoey's (2005) lexical priming and Goldberg's (2009) construction grammar, and they represent the primary focus of the present chapter as well.

In this vein, the aim of this study is to focus on yet another suitable candidate for the description of regularity in text, i.e. 'semantic sequences'. These are defined by Hunston (2008: 271) as "recurring sequences of words or phrases […] more usefully characterized as sequences of meaning elements rather than as formal sequences", and they are analysed here as a clue to the main aspects related to the presentation and discussion of research findings in specialised journals. In particular, semantic sequences were studied on the basis of a corpus of authentic research articles, the genre with the lion's share in specialised medico-scientific knowledge dissemination. In Section 2, the materials on which the research is based are discussed and analytical criteria are clarified, whereas Section 3 is devoted to the presentation of findings to be discussed in Section 4.

2. Materials and methods

The study was undertaken on a small synchronic corpus of 280 authentic medico-scientific research articles (RAs) taken from fourteen specialised journals.[1] The first strand of corpus texts (140) dates back to the period June/September 2007, and it was later supplemented with a second, more recent strand including just as many texts covering the same time span (June-September) from the year 2012. Altogether, the corpus consists of 984,304 running words.

From a methodological perspective, the study began with the computer-assisted (Scott 2009) corpus-based retrieval of the most frequent semantic sequences at two main levels. First of all, sequences were identified by starting with 'closed-class' grammar words: these "would seem to be of no interest to the discourse analyst at all" yet may be taken as a sound basis to identify patterns that define "the conventional meanings and values expressed in corpus texts" (Groom 2010: 61). Secondly, sequences were detected by starting with a grammar pattern acknowledged by the literature (Halliday/Matthiessen 2004; Hunston 2008) to be both outstandingly frequent and significant in scientific writing. This is

1 The specialised journals were selected on the basis of chiefly exogenous criteria, i.e. the feedback provided by the staff of the Ph.D. School in Clinical and Experimental Medicine of the University of Modena and Reggio Emilia (Italy). In particular, the following publications were included: *British Journal of Dermatology* (BJD), *Journal of the American Academy of Dermatology* (JAAD), *Blood Cells, Molecules and Diseases* (BCMD), *Proceedings of the National Academy of Sciences of the United States* (PNAS), *Cancer Research* (CR), *British Journal of Haematology* (BJD), *Artificial Organs* (AO), *Proteome Science* (PS), *Clinical Chemistry* (CC), *Journal of Pharmaceutical and Biomedical Analysis* (JPBA), *Science* (SC) and *Current Opinions in Genetics and Development* (COGD).

the 'N *that*' pattern, where a noun "indicates the epistemic status of the proposition" expressed in the upcoming *that*-clause (Hunston 2008: 278).

The second stage of the investigation lay in the concordance-based (Stubbs 2001) quantitative and qualitative study of both the most frequent 3/6-grams including the selected grammar words, and the most common 'N *that*' patterns highlighted in the corpus. As a result, the analysis focused on items such as *of patients with*, *in response to* and *depending on the* on the one hand, and *the possibility that*, *the hypothesis that* as well as *the finding that* on the other.

As such, the above elements were taken as a basis for the isolation of semantic sequences in context. More specifically, the collocational, colligational and semantic-preference patterns displayed by the items were a clue to the semantic sequences and the main discourse functions these were observed to perform across research-article sections ('Introduction', 'Methodology', 'Results' and 'Discussion'), from a convincing presentation of research findings to expressions of alignment of current research with a body of mainstream literature.

3. Results

The study of semantic sequences in context tends to reveal interesting patterns related to their distribution and functions across research article sections. For this reason and for the sake of clarity, the use of the most frequent sequences is illustrated with a view to the RA section they were observed to typically occur in, with §3.1 devoted to the 'Introduction', §3.2 to 'Methods', §3.3 and §3.4 dealing with 'Results' and 'Discussion' respectively.

3.1 Semantic sequences in RA Introductions

The 'Introduction' is by far one of the most extensively studied sections of RAs. This is largely due to its considerable rhetorical complexity

(Swales/Feak 2012), which all too often has a two-fold cause. First of all, a remarkable variety in the steps through which its structure may be formed, with a range of different options allowing writers to situate their contribution within the broader research field either with a sense of continuity, or with a more challenging attitude pointing to the limitations of prior research. Secondly, the wealth of information for potential inclusion, from a broad review of items of previous research to more or less substantial anticipations of the contents of the rest of the paper.

In this context, the occurrence of semantic sequences in this RA section appears to be primarily linked to two inter-related phenomena. On the one hand, their use is correlated to the writer's attempt to make topic generalisations: this facet is distinctive of the first part of several scientific introductions, where authors survey their well-established research tradition through wide knowledge-claims about the state of the art of clinical practice, the implementation of diagnostic tools or laboratory techniques, to name but a few. From a discursive point of view, this function is best served by the three-word prepositional cluster *for patients with*, embedded within semantic sequences of the kind ['Current knowledge on available therapeutic options' + *for patients with* + 'Disease'] highlighted in (1) below:[2]

(1) **Currently**, chemotherapy, radiation, and surgery **are the only choices** for patients with **basal breast cancers**, but all show poor outcomes[(6)]. The need for a specific targeted therapy for basal breast cancer remains urgent. (CR_16)

On the other hand, the same cluster may signal that writers are uncovering fresh and genuine evidence that will be further explored in the rest of their paper. In this case, they provide more than a simple overview of present-day knowledge; rather, in anticipating the core elements of their original contribution, they begin by shedding light on new and attractive therapeutic options clinicians are likely to benefit from in the near future. This is forcefully expressed by means of the

2 In all numbered examples, underlining and bold typeface are mine. More specifically, the former is utilised to identify the node of the semantic sequence, whereas bold typeface marks the other elements that typically characterise the meaning pattern defined by the sequence. In addition, the source of each example is reported in brackets with both journal initials and an anonymised file number (e.g. CR_1 for the first corpus text from *Cancer Research*).

sequence ['New treatment strategy' + *for patients with* + 'Disease'] instantiated in (2):

(2) For patients who fail initial therapy and are either refractory or relapsed, there is no standard therapy. **Novel agents** such as thalidomide, bortezomib, and lenalidomide **offer new treatment options** for patients with **AL amyloidosis.** (BL_14)

Taken together, the two sequences examined so far amount to 26.9% of the 63 occurrences of the expression *for patients with*, i.e. the fifth most common 3/6-word cluster retrieved for *with* at a corpus level.

3.2 Semantic sequences in 'Methods'

In his seminal work on research genres, Swales (2004) notes the somewhat decreasing rhetorical effort channelled into 'Methods' owing to the overall standardised nature of experimental procedures. This means that in a large number of published papers, researchers tend to replicate well-established methods that do not need full elucidation at the outset. Nonetheless, the fact remains that the methodological section is still required to play a key-role in the reconstruction of the relevant research setting. With the aim of providing accurate information about the criteria behind patient recruitment or data collection, the type of procedure applied – e.g. statistical or other – and the devices/facilities that make for the necessary research apparatus, scientific contributors often avail themselves of two prominent semantic sequences encompassing the top cluster of both *for* and *on*.

The first one is ['Methods/Tools' + was + *used for the* + 'Research goal'], which concerns 55.7% of the 61 entries of *used for the* and is designed to reconcile the adoption of a certain method with the key research goal this was elected to pursue (cf. (3) below). The second sequence suggests a close parallel with the first: accordingly, ['Procedure' + *on the basis of* + 'Underlying criteria'] emphasises the writer's care in relating an experimental procedure with the criterion or purpose underlying its choice. Of note, the sequence applies to 22.4% of the corpus tokens of *on the basis of*. Moreover, the first element in the pattern ('Procedure') is invariably expressed through verbs sharing a recognisable semantic preference of 'procedural requirement' – e.g. *recruit*, *assess*, *sort*, *exclude* or *select* – and employed in the passive voice, as can be seen in example (4):

(3) Two different sampling **devices** were used for the **dissolution experiment**. (JPBA_6)

(4) This PET imaging agent **was developed** on the basis of **a 14-mer peptide** identified by phage display technology.[15] (CR_19)

3.3 Semantic sequences in 'Results'

'Results' are by definition a most eagerly awaited section of RAs. Its interest predictably lies in the presentation of the findings of the study, which by all accounts deserves to be seen as a truly creative endeavour on the writer's part. In spite of the distinctive traits 'Results' have been observed to exhibit on a cross-disciplinary basis (Thompson 1993; Brett 1994; Williams 1999), there is convincing evidence that the section may yet display a number of repetitive phraseological patterns. In the case of medico-scientific articles, semantic sequences serve three major functions: pointing out, firstly, the salient feature(s) of the observed phenomenon; secondly, the description of cause-effect relationships in the data; and finally, an assessment of what brings about noticeable changes in the items under investigation.

To begin with, the effort to draw the readers' attention to any feature writers consider as conspicuous about the clinical data they scrutinised, is well orchestrated through two semantic sequences. Perhaps not surprisingly, they both begin with verbs sharing a clear semantic preference of 'sight' (e.g. *see*, *detect*, *observe*, *identify* and *highlight*). Still, a peculiarity of the first sequence is that it displays a marked preference for the passive voice of such verbs, whereas the second one suggests a stronger inclination towards the active form.

The first sequence, i.e. ['Key-element' + Verb of sight $_{\text{(passive)}}$ + 'Location' + *of patients with* + 'Disease'] concerns 5% of the 184 occurrences of the node phrase *of patients with*, and it points out what was detected as significant in the blood, plasma, serum or skin of patients affected by a certain illness (cf. example 5 below). Likewise, the second is [Verb of sight + *as a potential* + 'Determinant' + *for*/*of* + 'Disease']: it reveals the element isolated as the potential trigger (e.g. *biomarker for* or *risk factor of*) of a critical condition, and it applies to 29.4% of the corpus tokens of *as a potential*, as documented in (6):

(5) Because low-to-moderate avidity EphA2-specific **CD8+ T cells have been detected in the peripheral blood** of patients with **renal cell carcinoma or prostate carcinoma** [19, 20], levels of circulating CD8+ T cells could also be amplified by vaccination for improved immune targeting of EphA2+ tumor cells in vivo. (CR_14)

(6) In this work, five novel proteins associated with alcohol induced hepatic fibrosis were detected. **We have** specifically **identified annexin A3 and annexin A6** as a potential **biomarker for** predicting **alcohol-induced liver cirrhosis**. (PS_13)

Establishing cause-effect relationships in the data is the second fundamental aspect emphasised by semantic sequences in 'Results'. In this respect, the two sequences concerned involve the paradigmatically interchangeable presence of the node prepositional phrases *in the pathogenesis of* and *in the regulation of*, and their role is to show what elements are implicated in a certain biological or pathophysiological process (e.g. *cell adhesion* and *inflammatory states* in 7 and 8, respectively). To mention but two of the combinations embedding the above phrases, ['Element' + be involved + *in the regulation of* + 'Process'] occurs in 39.5% of the hits for *in the regulation of*, whereas ['Element' + play + a critical/central/important role + *in the pathogenesis of* + 'Process'] is attested in 30.5% of *in the pathogenesis of*, as illustrated in (7) and (8) below:

(7) In the current study, three cytoskeletal proteins, vimentin (intermediate filaments), tubulin (microtubules) and actin (microfilaments) were identified with enhanced S-nitrosylation under rosuvastatin treatment. In addition, TPM, which regulates actin movement, was also found to be S-nitrosylated. **These proteins are involved** in the regulation of **cell shape, cell adhesion and migration**. (PS_20)

(8) As a prototypic damage-associated molecular pattern (DAMP) molecule, **HMGB1 plays a central role** in the pathogenesis of **many inflammatory states** released following tissue damage or injury, and is found in the serum-including cancer [38, 42] as well as other settings. (CR_11)

The last function carried out by semantic sequences in the findings section of scientific articles essentially looks like a minor variant of that documented in (7) and (8) above. It is represented by the writers' retrieval of first-hand empirical information about what changes vis-à-vis a certain type of input or determinant. In 17.5% of the entries of *in response to*, for instance, the phrase is part of the sequence ['Element' + Verb of 'change' + *in response to* + 'Input']. At the same time, 23.3% of *depending on the* can be observed to be part of the sequence ['Element' + Verb of 'change' + *depending on the* + 'Determinant']: here, a factor (e.g. *molar mass*, *molecular weight* or *the mode of injury*) is shown to explain the variation of some entity under the researchers' looking-glass, as it were. What gives both sequences their characteristic flavour is the colligation between the node and verbs sharing a typical semantic preference of 'change' – e.g. *change*, *alter*, *differentiate*, *vary*, *differ*, *degrade* – as can be appreciated in (9) and (10):

(9) **Several genes** involved in proliferation, metabolism or structure **were** also **altered** in response to **FLT3 signalling** including BCL7A, CLIC1, MRPL12, ATAD2, VIM and UBE2J1, as were genes involved in receptor-mediated signalling (IL1RAP, CDC42EP3, PLAUR, CD180 and GHRH). (BJH_3)

(10) Fig. 4 demonstrates that **the major products** formed **vary** depending on the **sample solvent**. (JPBA_19)

3.4 Semantic sequences in 'Discussion'

The 'Discussion' section is a key-moment in the process of specialised knowledge dissemination: at this stage, the specifics of experimental findings to which readers are often re-oriented in the opening segment of the section are expected to be contextualised within the broad disciplinary framework outlined in the literature review. In this vein, discussions should be a convenient place to establish the news value of research findings presented earlier on, and it is interesting that the writer's interpretation of data and consolidation of the research space occupied in the 'Introduction', very often leads to the expression of authorial stance. This can be defined as a dimension of discourse including features which refer to the ways writers present themselves and convey their opinions and commitments (Hyland 2005). As such, stance denotes the strategies through which "writers intrude to stamp their personal authority onto their arguments or step back and disguise their involvement" (McGrath/Kuteeva 2012: 163).

Following Biber et al. (1999) and Conrad/Biber (2000), it can be argued that the most frequently occurring semantic sequences in discussions are highly instrumental in expressing two kinds of stance. The first one is attitudinal stance, conveying attitudes, feelings and value judgments about the entities reported in the text. The sequences that suit this purpose are characterised by the collocation of *in patients with* and *the finding that* with evaluative markers through which writers express a markedly positive stance on the overall significance of the findings recorded in 'Results'. In [Evaluative marker + *in patients with* + 'Disease'], which concerns 7.4% of *in patients with*, evaluation may take the form of stance adverbials (cf. 11 below), nouns (e.g. *efficacy*, *interest*) or adjectives that show the benefits of a procedure, tool, therapy or predictor investigated in the current study (*effective*, *useful*). By contrast, [*the finding that* + 'Element' + Evaluative marker], applying to 14.7% of *the finding that*, overwhelmingly involves the choice of evaluative adjectives (e.g. *encouraging*, *novel*) to promote the putative validity and genuineness of research findings, as shown in example (12):

(11) **Interestingly**, no DSRAD mutation has been found in patients with **DUH**.[29] (JAAD_6)

(12) The finding that **CCR5 antagonists block FBS-induced invasion** is **novel** and suggested that CCR5 activation contribute to the production of metastasis in vivo where different chemotactic and growth signals are present. (CR_16)

The second kind of stance is epistemic, related to the expression of degrees of certainty attached to the truth-value of the attendant proposition. On the one hand, 25.5% of the corpus hits of *the possibility that* are embedded in the sequence ['Re-statement of results' + Hedge + *the possibility that* + 'Implication']: in this co-text, the N *that* pattern co-occurs with hedges – e.g. *we cannot rule out*, *these data do not exclude* – the aim of which is to more tentatively draw the implications foreshadowed by the findings briefly summarised earlier on (cf. 13). At the top end of the epistemic scale, on the other hand, 24.4% of the occurrence of *the observation that* is part of the sequence ['Re-statement of findings' + Booster + *the observation that* + 'Back-up finding']. Here, the three-gram invariably collocates with boosters (e.g. *is consistent with*, *fits with*, *is upheld by*) that strengthen authorial claims about the convincing nature of findings or even more so, their mutual consistency. These aspects are emphasised in passages (13) and (14), respectively.

(13) **Our results**, which **suggest that rhBMP-7 protects the heart by inhibiting TGF-1-induced EndMT**, are consistent with a study showing that, in a mouse model of ischemic injury, rhBMP-7 injected into the heart stabilizes the micro-vasculature.[33] **We cannot exclude** the possibility that rhBMP-7, in addition to inhibiting EndMT, might also elicit anti-inflammatory effects, promote myo-genesis or prevent apoptosis of endothelial cells.[34] (NM_6)

(14) **Figure 1A also shows that** although p53 is important in determining the out-come of AAV infection, **the downstream transcriptional target** of p53, p21, **is similarly important. This is highlighted by** the observation that **HCT116 p21-/- cells**, despite expressing functional p53 protein, **also undergo apoptosis** following AAV infection. (CR_8)

What passages such as (14) emphasise is that the idea of consistency in findings is highly-prized by the parent scientific community of professional writers. Corpus evidence suggests that this is more than a mere first impression, as is documented by two semantic sequences evenly distributed across 'Results' and 'Discussion', i.e. ['Finding' + Verb of 'continuity' + *our hypothesis that*] and ['Finding' + Verb of 'continuity' + *the notion that*]. These demonstrate that the solidity of findings in today's big science is frequently attributed to their consistency with either the initial hypothesis formulated in the 'Introduction', or helpful suggestions from authoritative sources in the literature.

Consistency between results and the initial working hypothesis is a regularity of *our hypothesis that*, where 58.2% of the occurrences of the pattern are inscribed in the sequence ['Finding' + Verb of 'conti-nuity' + *our hypothesis that*]. Moreover, consistency between findings and suggestions from the relevant literature is the norm in 68.7% of the entries of *the notion that*, where the pattern is incorporated in the sequence ['Finding' + Verb of 'continuity' + *the notion that*]. The mean-ings conveyed by the two patterns are effectively communicated by the colligation between the N *that* patterns and verbs sharing a definite semantic preference of 'continuity', such as *confirm*, *support*, and *be consistent/in keeping/in line with* exemplified in (15) and (16) below:

(15) **These results were consistent with** our hypothesis that extracellular Prxs induce the IL-23–IL-17 inflammatory pathway through TLR2 and TLR4 and promote post-ischemic inflammation and infarct volume growth. (NM_14)

(16) On the other hand, similar treatment to the normal-glucose cultivated keratinocytes did not significantly alter the pSTAT-1 expression (see Fig. S3) and increased the hBD2 levels by 4·6 ± 14·7%, which is not statistically signifycant. **These results validated and strengthened** the notion that AGE formation in the high-glucose cultivated keratinocytes contributed to hBD2 reduction in our experimental conditions. (BJD_20)

4. Conclusions

The study of co-occurring items has become a prominent feature in present-day corpus and discourse studies. Whether we take Erman/Warren's (2000) claim that at least 55% of the words in English texts are part of pre-fabricated multi-word units, or Biber et al.'s (1999) finding that 21% of words in academic prose occur in a recurrent lexical bundle, there is more than a reason to believe that co-occurrence patterns warrant proper consideration in descriptive accounts of both general and specialised language.

With reference to medico-scientific knowledge dissemination, this chapter has shed light on the wide array of meanings semantic sequences can be observed to codify across RA sections, from writers' generalisations about the state of the art of clinical practice, the implementation of diagnostic tools or laboratory techniques in introductions (cf. §3.1), to the expression of authorial stance in consolidating research findings in discussions (see §3.4). In spite of the specificity of each method used to identify semantic sequences – i.e. by starting with a grammar word or the N *that* pattern – there is remarkable continuity between the one and the other, insofar as they provide a useful link between lexis and grammar. Accordingly, evidence showed that not only do closed-class words and N *that* maintain a regularity in terms of their attested corpus use, but more interestingly, words sharing homogeneous patterns typically fall into groups based on mutually agreed, institutionalised and purposeful aspects of meaning inherent in the genre investigated here.

In this respect, data indicate a wide range of well-established, pre-constructed forms in use within the medical research community, when the draft of scholarly papers comes to the rhetorical turning points implied by a convincing presentation of research findings – whether it is accuracy in investigating cause-effect mechanisms, or consistency with the literature. As Hyland (1998) puts it, whereas individual factors may inform writers' choices in the step-by-step creation of an RA, key-meanings ultimately arise from the interaction between writers themselves and readers in specific social circumstances. As a result, writing as a medical researcher implies being capable of talking to the expert members of the relevant discourse community in ways they find most effective, which may eventually take the form of the reiterated semantic sequences examined here.

The qualitative and quantitative findings in Section 3 suggest that the capability of corpus-based teaching of highlighting semantic sequences may provide a large amount of information about disciplinary ideologies. If, as a matter of fact, the study of individual word forms in context is well suited to the description of the subject matter of a discipline, the phraseologies at the heart of semantic sequences are indicative of its epistemology, because they are less linked to the subject matter than they are to well-established meanings and functions (Hunston 2008).

On these grounds, a sequence-based approach to word behaviour is likely to prove an essential tool for language instructors in devising awareness-raising activities based on authentic written text rather than intuition, especially at the top end of specialised-knowledge dissemination represented by high-profile RAs to be submitted to scholarly journals. With a view to practitioners' needs, sequences should indeed be seen as a firm basis for vocabulary building, so that the availability of lists of widespread sequences stands out as a resource for teachers to avert the chaos of individual word use through "an order based on meaning" (Hunston/Francis 1998: 70). Hence, the opportunity arises of including sequences such as those accounted for in the present study in a reference book providing learners with a more apt description of the language they will be expected to master, by contributing to their overall accuracy and fluency.

References

Biber, Douglas / Johansson, Stig / Leech, Geoffrey / Conrad, Susan / Finegan, Edward 1999. *Longman Grammar of Spoken and Written English*. London: Longman.

Brett, Paul 1994. A Genre Analysis of the Results Section of Sociology Articles. *English for Specific Purposes* 13, 47–60.

Conrad, Susan / Biber, Douglas 2000. Adverbial Marking of Stance in Speech and Writing. In Hunston, Susan / Thompson, Geoff (eds) *Evaluation in Text. Authorial Stance and the Construction of Discourse*. Oxford: Oxford University Press, 56–73.

Dahl, Trine 2004. Textual Metadiscourse in Research Articles: a Marker of National Culture or of Academic Culture?. *Journal of Pragmatics* 36/10, 1807–1825.

Engberg, Jan 2010. Knowledge Construction and Legal Discourse: The Interdependence of Perspective and Visibility of Characteristics. *Journal of Pragmatics* 42/1, 48–63.

Erman, Britt / Warren, Beatrice 2000. The Idiom Principle and the Open Choice Principle. *Text* 20/1, 29–62.

Gabrielatos, Costas / McEnery, Tony / Diggle, Peter J. / Baker, Paul 2012. The Peaks and Troughs of Corpus-based Contextual Analysis. *International Journal of Corpus Linguistics* 17/2, 151–175.

Goldberg, Adele 2009. The Nature of Generalization in Language. *Cognitive Linguistics* 20/1, 93–127.

Groom, Nicholas 2010. Closed-class Keywords and Corpus-driven Discourse Analysis. In Bondi, Marina / Scott, Mike (eds) *Keyness in Text*. Amsterdam: Benjamins, 59–78.

Halliday, Michael A.K. / Matthiessen, Christian 2004. *An Introduction to Functional Grammar*. London: Arnold.

Hoey, Michael 2005. *Lexical Priming: A New Theory of Words and Language*. London: Routledge.

Hunston, Susan 2002. *Corpora in Applied Linguistics*. Cambridge: Cambridge University Press.

Hunston, Susan 2008. Starting with the Small Words. Patterns, Lexis and Semantic Sequences. *International Journal of Corpus Linguistics* 13/3, 271–295.

Hunston, Susan / Francis, Gill 1998. Verbs Observed: A Corpus-driven Pedagogic Grammar. *Applied Linguistics* 19/1, 45–72.

Hyland, Ken 1998. Boosting, Hedging and the Negotiation of Academic Knowledge. *Text* 18/3, 349–382.

Hyland, Ken 2005. Stance and Engagement: A Model of Interaction in Academic Discourse. *Discourse Studies* 7/2, 173–192.

McEnery, Tony / Hardie, Andrew 2011. *Corpus Linguistics*. Cambridge: Cambridge University Press.

McGrath, Lisa / Kuteeva, Maria 2012. Stance and Engagement in Pure Mathematics Research Articles: Linking Discourse Features to Disciplinary Practices. *English for Specific Purposes* 31, 161–173.

Scott, Mike 2009. *WordSmith Tools 5.0*. Liverpool: Lexical Analysis Software.

Sinclair, John 1996. The Search for Units of Meaning. *Textus* 9/1, 75–106.

Sinclair, John 2004. *Trust the Text. Language, Corpus and Discourse*. London: Routledge.

Stubbs, Michael 2001. *Words and Phrases: Corpus Studies on Lexical Semantics*. Oxford: Blackwell.

Swales, John 2004. *Research Genres. Explorations and Applications*. Cambridge: Cambridge University Press.

Swales, John / Feak Christine 2012. *Academic Writing for Graduate Students. Essential Tasks and Skills*. Ann Arbor: The University of Michigan Press.

Thompson, Dorothea K. 1993. Arguing for Experimental 'Facts in Science: A Study of Research Article Results Sections in Biochemistry. *Written Communication* 10, 106–128.

Williams, Ian A. 1999. Results Sections of Medical Research Articles: Analysis of Rhetorical Categories for Pedagogical Purposes. *English for Specific Purposes* 18/4, 347–366.
Wray, Alison 2002. *Formulaic Language and the Lexicon*. Cambridge: Cambridge University Press.

Stefania M. Maci

'Health slips as the financial crisis grips': Tensions and Variations in Medical Discourse

1. Introduction

In 1992 the *Journal of American Medical Association* (*JAMA*), published an article (Evidence Based Medicine Working Group 1992) dealing with the rise of a new medical practice – evidence-based medicine – which integrates individual clinical expertise with the best available external clinical evidence deriving from systematic research (Sackett *et al.* 1996). This article was in some respects foretelling, since such a new paradigm in medical practice was claimed to be a consequence of the fact that medicine would "continue to face an exploding volume of literature, rapid introduction of new technologies, deepening concerns about burgeoning medical costs, and increasing attention to the quality and outcomes of medical care" (Evidence Based Medicine Working Group 1992: 2424). New skills would be required, such as efficient literature searching and the application of formal rules of evidence in evaluating the clinical literature. Indeed, such systematic analysis of medical protocols gave rise to studies and their relevant publications – all of them being evidence-based rather than narrative-based medical investigations, disease- and doctor-oriented examinations relying on randomized clinical trials and scientific research (Bensing 2000). At the same time, concerns about medical costs increased and greater attention was paid to medical research quality resulting in outstanding publication. The *JAMA* predictions regarding the increase in medical literature were indeed confirmed in 2005 when the editor of the *British Journal of Plastic Surgery* claimed that "these are times of rapid development all around, as e-publishing takes off and the medical publishing market globalises" (Kay 2005: 1041). The accent on change and globalization was a fundamental issue. As was later disclosed in the editorial, the developments dealt with in the document seemed to prompt action: a new editorial policy required journal changes in order to cope with global medical competition – and the starting point was the dismissing of the parochial image conveyed by the adjective *British* in the journal title *British Journal of Plastic Surgery*: switching to the acronym title *BJPS* was in fact meant to emphasize the inclusive cultural and societal quality of the journal.

It seems, therefore, that one of the main concerns of the scientific community – both in academic and clinical practices – has been to cope with changes in research, scientific literature and media publication, changes that seem to be more urgent in our globalised era. Although at first the concept of globalisation was regarded quite positively, in the long term it has acquired negative connotations when related to the financial world, and globalisation has begun to be regarded as a synonym for global crisis.

On 1st April 2009 the World Health Organization (WHO) issued a public statement which, while confirming pessimistic predictions about the global financial crisis, disclosed a growing concern for health care in terms of economic investments and developments (Chan 2009). Such a feeling seems to be confirmed by the editorial published on April 18th, 2009 in *The Lancet* (Horton 2009). Here the recent G20 summit in London was seen as a failure because of the disappointing address regarding global health issues. The WHO's accent was on the necessity for the G20 *communiqués* to understand that the 'global society' they were speaking of also included the international health community "which must seize the moment by noisily raising the possibility of providing a global social security net, *financed internationally and progressively*, and build on national social protection mechanisms" (Horton 2009: 1311, my emphasis).

Nowadays – like almost two decades ago – medicine and business seem to be strongly interrelated. Overall, business interests have gained such an important place in medicine that members of the medical community have progressively adopted a business mentality while coping with the economic crisis (without losing the fundamental values of professional and academic medicine) because clinical research mainly depends on funds. Indeed, medical care seems to have acquired a more corporate identity.

In this development from medical virtue to medical business, scientific investigation has been affected so much that scientists now more than ever before have to cope with publication pressure requiring high standards of quality research to be carried out within financial constraints. Despite the crisis and the absence of private and public funds, the yardstick for measuring the quality of research still depends on the number of contributions reporting research results.

Scientific knowledge and medical discourse are formally constructed in research articles (RAs).[1] This is, indeed, confirmed by the proliferation of new specialised medical journals (in 2015, PubMed, the U.S. National Library of Medicine,[2] listed approximately 26,000 medical publications), which seems to substantiate the fact that, despite the crisis, findings of contemporary scientific research need to be circulated as quickly as possible because of increasing specialization and

---

1 Medical discourse has been the object of in-depth research, from both a synchronic (Gotti/Salager-Meyer 2006) and a diachronic viewpoint (Taavitsainen/Pahta 2004; Tardy 2004; Gotti 2008; Maci 2012a, 2012b, 2014a). In particular, RAs have been studied from various perspectives. Among the phletora of scientific research on the topic, the most recent investigation has been focussed particularly on issues of cultural and authorial identity in medical academic prose (Breivega/Dahl/Fløttum 2002; Hyland 2002a; Fløttum 2005, 2006; Maci 2010, 2014b) and on generic analysis (Maci 2009, 2011, 2012c, 2012d, 2012e) examining medical RA *Introductions* (Swales 1990; Samraj 2002), *Method* and *Discussion* sections (see, for instance, Nwogu 1997; Martinez 2003; Maci 2012d, 2012e). Scholarly attention has also been given to meta-discursive features of medical writing (Dahl 2003, 2004), hedging devices used in medical academic discourse (Hyland 2006; Salager-Meyer 2006). The problem of the representation of truth in medical science has also been taken into consideration (Koutsantoni 2004). Similarly, issues of argumentation and persuasiveness have been keypoints in this domain (Ferguson 2001; Hyland 2002b). Finally, further linguistic analysis has been carried out by members of the medical community. Noteworthy are the ANSI/NISO *Guidelines for Abstracts* (1997), the *International Committee of Medical Journal Editors* (2008) and the various 'technical' guidelines for written medical texts (Skelton/Edwards 2000).

2 The US National Library of Medicine (NLM) has been the world's largest biomedical library since 1835 and produces print documents and makes electronic resources searched by millions of people all over the world available. Data available at <www.nlm.nhi.gov> [17/03/2015].

fast-paced progress. This, in turn, forces authors to establish a new priority in their research: their aim is to publish their findings before others do.

RAs, as an expression of formality in scientific discourse, seem to be continually reshaped in the course of social practices. According to Fairclough (2001), social practices can be defined as stabilized forms of social activities (such as teaching, family meals, news reporting, etc.) in which diverse social moments[3] interact (Fairclough 2007). These moments are not discrete: each of them internalizes in itself other moments without being reducible to them. When the relation between them varies, variation occurs, indicated as *change*, in the internal equilibrium characterizing the social practice. In the formal realization of the RA, there is indeed a change as scientific discourse goes through various stages: from facts to generalisations, from generalisations to theories and from theories to formal knowledge accepted by peers (Iedema 1999). The internal equilibrium represented by the interrelation between the elements characterizing the (medical) social practice of detecting facts is therefore re-arranged and re-contextualised as a formal organizational meaning which takes the aspect of the RA. When examined at a global level, such re-contextualisation of formality seems dependent upon transnational societal changes which include discourse and its role within these processes of change. As Hyland (2000: 85) remarks, "One consequence of this is that genres have quickly emerged and changed in response to the social and intellectual activity they are part of".

It is the aim of this chapter to investigate processes of change in medical discourse provoked by globalisation, the global crisis and the pressures based on rapid and competitive publishing. It also aims to explore the extent to which medical discourse globally creates and appropriates corporate thinking. In order to carry out this research, a Critical Discourse Analysis (CDA) approach will be adopted, drawing on Fairclough (2001, 2007).

3 Fairclough (2007) identifies the following moments which are dialectically (i.e., dialogically) related in a social process: discourse, power, beliefs, values, desires, social relations, institutions and ritual, other practices.

2. CDA and medical discourse

Any change is perceived by people as a form of 'crisis'. Indeed, as aptly defined by the OED, a 'crisis' is "a turning-point; also, a state of affairs in which a decisive change for better or worse is imminent; now applied especially to times of difficulty, insecurity, and suspense in politics or commerce". When the change is economic, political or social, it may affect people's lives, identities, and culture on the basis of the different (re)distribution of pre-existing power relations within social practices,[4] which may result in different power relations, and hence in discrete political and economic decisions and strategic choices. As a consequence, a shuffling and reallocation of power distribution within society occurs. The strategies exploited to change social practices are expressed through discourse, and "connect the present with the past with predictive or perspective imaginaries for the future" (Fairclough 2007: 12).

When social practices, strategies and discourses change, they are recontextualised, since they move from one context to another. Furthermore, such recontextualization requires a colonization of the new context and the appropriation of all 'new' social practices, discourse included, from 'old' practices (Fairclough 2007). This may give rise to unpredictable results (Fairclough 2001) because in this process not only does discourse interpret and represent social change but also the way in which discourse itself has been appropriated and recontextualised in the new domains.

An example can be given by the process of globalization. Globalization can be interpreted as a worldwide process characterised by a network of social practices calling for harmonization and social relations (Salkov-Iversen/Hansen/Bislen 2000), facilitating the coordination of national and local systems in order to think and act transnationally. Nevertheless, such core concept has not been considered because

4 Social practices are determined by the different networked connections existing between the elements constituting the practice itself, namely activities, subjects (and their social relations), instruments, time and place, form of consciousness, values and discourse (Fairclough 2001).

the theoretical model of management thinking at a local level has prevailed. This is particularly true when a welfare crisis occurs: as Salkov-Iversen/Hansen/Bislen (2000) claim, managerial thinking in public institutions, or New Public Management (NPM), emerges whenever a crisis emerges.[5]

The conceptualization of NPM in medical discourse is evident in the International Campaign to Revitalise Academic Medicine (ICRAM) manifesto.[6] ICRAM was a *global* initiative launched in 2003 by the *British Medical Journal*, *The Lancet*, and 40 other partners, and focussing on redefining the core values of academic medicine as well as aiming at creating better career paths and improving relationships with 'customers' (i.e. clients, policy makers, practitioners, etc.). As indicated by Salkov-Iversen/Hansen/Bislen (2000), the narrative employed by NPM is generally developed in three stages:

(i) a set of representations of rapid change;
(ii) a set of representations of the relationship between global and local realities; and
(iii) a set of representations of the internal organizational changes needed to achieve the desired standard of performance.

The same three-level structure can be identified on the ICRAM homepage, where we can read that these are "time[s] of increasing health burden, poverty, globalisation, and innovation" ((i) – rapid changes), in which "academic medicine is [perceived as being] in crisis around the world" ((ii) – rapid changes *and* relationship between global and local realities) and because of this ICRAM is "recommending strategies for building capacity in academic medicine" ((iii) –representtations of the internal organizational changes needed to achieve the desired standard of performance) in order to be actively responsive to the crisis rather than passively experiencing the crisis. Interestingly, despite the fact that

5 NPM is created as *political rationalities* (programs, plans, working papers and other documents, that constitute discourses, i.e. genres, texts and styles), and *technologies of government* (tools and methods) the local institution employs to actuate the political rationalities. In its realization, NPM follows three principles: i) custom-orientation; ii) service-orientation; iii) performance standards (i.e., responsiveness and efficiency) (Salkov-Iversen/Hansen/Bislen 2000).

6 Available at <http://www.bmj.com/content/329/7469/787/> [17/03/2015].

ICRAM's desire is to revitalize academic medicine, managerial thinking is consistently substantiated by the presence of 'customers' who, in the ICRAM members' opinion, are the recipients of the academic medicine services, that is "patients, policy makers, practitioners, and others", as found on ICRAM homepage, including, among others "stakeholder advisory groups representing the interests of academics, business groups, government representatives and policy makers, patients, professional associations, journal editors, and students and trainees", thus putting an emphasis on economics, as far as the relationships between the ICRAM academia members and society is concerned.

As Bhatia (2004: 87) claims, the "colonization of one genre by the other by invading its integrity" results when rhetorical and discoursal generic conventions deriving from a particular genre in the realization of another are used. Such colonization is evident in the ICRAM discourse, which confirms the presence of NPM and, as argued by Fairclough (2007), these global dynamics mediated by the local configurations of resources and ideas are context-dependent and give rise to a complex blending of texts in which social variations and tensions coexist.

3. Change and change again: the research letter

In such a critical setting, and in response to the new economic conditions where the academia has adopted a NPM approach, specialised genres are developing and hybridising at an unprecedented rate. Indeed, while the IMRD[7] model offered by the hard sciences is imitated by the

7 The structure of medical RAs is so strictly codified that transcends national cultures (Dahl 2004). Such structure (the latest version of which is downloadable from <http://www.icmje.org/>), was published in 1991 by the International Committee of Medical Journal Editors (ICMJE) in the *British Journal of Medicine*; its constraints were set out in the *Uniform requirements for the manuscripts submitted to biomedical journals* in 1978 and are usually known as the *Vancouver Style.* The recommendations indicated in the *Vancouver Style* cover an ample range of topics, including RA genre organization, according to which

soft sciences, in the medical field it has apparently acquired new forms of expression. This seems to be supported by the fact that, as claimed by previous research (Maci 2008, 2009, 2012c), editors of the most important international medical journals have decided to introduce a new genre: the research letter (RL).[8] RLs, also called *fast track papers* or *communications*, are designed for the medical academic community and are usually primary research papers of exceptional clinical importance and urgency, thus warranting rapid dissemination. They are extremely short and have a text usually ranging from 600 to 1,600 words, including references, tables and figures.[9]

An initial investigation was carried out on the type of medical journals from which the RL corpus could be collected. The selection of medical journals was based on their reputation, (web) accessibility and representativeness, as well as on their Impact Factor (I.F.). To avoid differences in the RAs due to editorial constraints and which might affect the results of our research, only two journals were selected among those which conform to the standard requirements formulated by ICMJE: *JAMA* and *The Lancet*. Fifty RLs collected in the CADIS corpus, the University of Bergamo corpus of academic discourse,[10] were

---

RAs are structured following the Introduction-Method-Results-Discussion (IMRD) pattern.

8 Hyland (2000) identifies such a genre for physics, chemistry, and microbiology only. Yet the scope and purpose of the letters Hyland found are different from those of medical RLs, since Hyland's letters highlight the brief report of new results and ideas to a wider community than specialists and are a means of promoting young scientists. On the contrary, as our corpus suggests, medical RLs specifically target medical specialists; furthermore, RL authors range from young scientists to renowned specialists.

9 For an in-depth analysis of medical RL moves and steps, see Maci (2008, 2009, 2012c).

10 As part of the national research project funded by the Italian Ministry of University (project number 2005109911), CADIS (the University of Bergamo Corpus of Academic Discourse) was collected with the purpose of carrying out an in-depth analysis of variation in intercultural communication and of identifying textual variants arising from the use of English as a first language, second language, or lingua franca of the scientific community. Further information is available at <http://dinamico.unibg.it/cerlis/page.aspx?p=138>, 17/3/15.

downloaded or scanned and digitalized in Word format to produce a small corpus of 75,241 words (see Table 1).[11]

Journal	Publication year	Item #	Word #	Total words	I.F.
Lancet	2005	25 RLs	27,639	75,241	28.638
JAMA	2005	25 RLs	47,602		25.547

Table 1. Medical RL corpus.

RLs do not seem to differ from RAs in that they are precisely organized according to the IMRD pattern. Apparently RLs seem to confirm the integrity of the genre they belong to. Indeed, at a superficial level, words occurring in the RL corpus appear to belong to the medical semantic field, as the tag cloud in Figure 1 suggests.

As shown in Maci (2009, 2012c), argumentation in RLs is apparently lacking due to the fact that these texts are extremely short. Indeed, as argued by Maci (2008, 2009, 2012c), RLs are characterised by different rhetorical strategies from RAs. In order to persuade their readers, while presenting their theory or experiment, RL authors tend to use scientific discourse in a direct way, so as not to be subjected to counterclaims, featured by an ample use of first person pronouns, the present tense (especially in the *Discussion* section), and comparatively few lexical hedges. This does not prevent the writer from employing hedging devices whenever s/he is on the verge of being so over-confident as to seem presumptuous in the concluding remarks. As usual, caution is used, not only to diminish negative face threat, but also to prevent possible attacks from future investigation denying cognitive consensus.

11 In our study percentages have been normalized per 10,000 words in order to make results comparable across the corpus. For the purpose of this research, the RL titles, tables, figures, footnotes and references – though interesting because of their value as 'visual' evidence of the RL methodological procedures – were not taken into consideration.

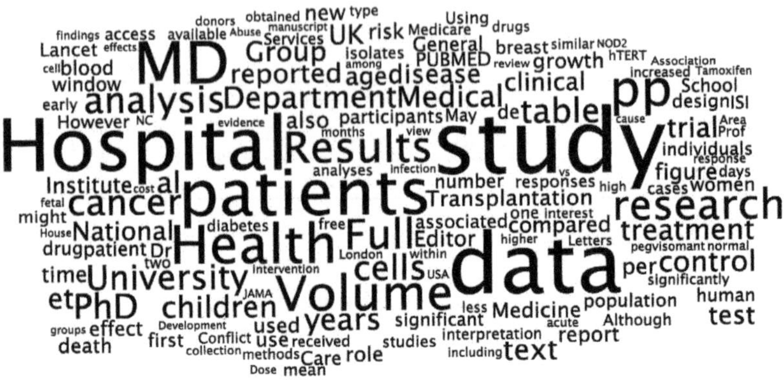

Figure 1. RL tag cloud.

From a lexico-grammatical point of view, there is, however, the perception that RLs contain elements that have been colonised by NPM. Simply by superficially looking at the tag cloud represented above, we can see that there are such lexical items as *services*, *costs*, *free* and *medicare*, which, despite being depicted in minor fonts, are indeed relevant precisely because they do not belong to the scientific register of medical discourse. Tag clouds are usually computed by creating a sort of keyword list within the corpus, which *per se* does not carry great weight: in a medical corpus, we would not expect anything different from medical register. The reason why *services*, *costs* and *medicare* do occur in our corpus lies in the fact that these are indeed words which are essential within the corpus itself. In order to see whether the significance of the words could be confirmed in linguistic terms, a keyword list with Wordsmith Tools (Scott 2004) was created through a comparison between the RL wordlist and the BNC wordlist. The RL keyword list has underpinned the occurrence of lexical elements belonging to the managerial domain (excerpted in Table 2 below), which were in part found in the tag cloud:

N Key word	Freq.	%	RC.	Freq.	RC. %	Keyness P
1 MEDICARE	56	0,07	65		623,06	0,0000000000
2 FUNDING	47	0,05	4.302		151,40	0,0000000000

N Key word	Freq.	%	RC.	Freq.	RC. %	Keyness P
3 DISCLOSURES	18	0,02	204		129,34	0,0000000000
4 FUNDED	25	0,03	1.550		98,60	0,0000000000
5 UNINSURED	9	0,01	41		79,89	0,0000000000
6 FREE	66	0,08	20.566	0,02	76,53	0,0000000000
7 SPONSOR	16	0,02	686		74,26	0,0000000000

Table 2. Excerpt from the RL Keyword List.

Not only are the words found in the tag cloud relevant within the medical corpus; they have been detected as keywords in it: they are also statistically *significant*. They express concern about financial constraints, medical business and ethical practice. As we can see in Table 2 above, the first keyword is *Medicare*. Medicare[12] is the US Federal health insurance program for elderly people and the young who suffer from disabilities or terminal stage diseases. The authors' main worry is apparently linked to official administrative acceptance of any medical service cost in the clinical practices described in the RL. The most common collocates characterizing the word *medicare* are *plan*, *discount*, *services*, *beneficiaries* and *free*. Patients are therefore *benefitciaries* who, following a *medicare plan*, can receive *discounted* or *free services* conditional upon the *medicare* program:

(1) We examined trends in annual house call volume and expenditures, as well as the types of clinicians making house calls to free-for-service *Medicare* beneficiaries. [J25]

Funding and *funded* occur 79 times altogether (TTR[13] 10.5) and are mainly linked to financial *disclosures* (18 hits / TTR 2.39) by means of which researchers claim that no conflicts occur in their investigation and that the role their *sponsor* had in their study has not biased scientific objectivity on financial grounds, as in examples (2) and (3):

(2) Access to Data: Dr Adachi-Mejia had full access to all of the data in the study and takes responsibility for the integrity of the data and the accuracy of the data

12 See the link at <http://www.medicare.gov/> [17/03/2015].
13 Type/Token Ratio.

analysis. Financial Disclosures: None reported. *Funding*/Support: This study was *funded* by National Cancer Institute grants CA-94272 and CA77026. Role of the *Sponsor*: The study's *sponsor* had no role in the design and conduct of the study, in the collection, analysis, and interpretation of the data, or in the preparation, review, or approval of the manuscript. [J10]

(3) The *sponsors* of this study had no role in the study design, data collection, data interpretation, data analysis, or writing of the report. [L4]

The attention to financial aspects related to the (U.S.) medical system and the vain attempt to adapt it to medical ethics is evident in the occurrence of the adjective *uninsured*:

(4) Every respondent reported inability to obtain at least 1 mental health service for *uninsured* patients. [J4]

66 hits (TTR 8.8) of the item *free* occur at the top of the keyword list. Yet a manual extraction of the results evidences that the adjective *free* has no connection with the financial world, as in general it refers to the possibility the medical community has to download the reference or the text the RL author is citing (44 hits out of 66 occurrences, corresponding to TTR 5.84):

(5) 1. Papadakis MA. The step 2 clinical-skills examination. N Engl J Med. 2004;350:1703–1705. *FREE* FULL TEXT

2. Barzansky B, Etzel SI. Education programs in US medical schools, 2002–2003. JAMA. 2003;290:1190–1196. *FREE* FULL TEXT. [L6]

In some ways, however, this is indirectly connected to the financial constraints imposed over scientific research: high quality investigation is subservient to financial limitations. Qualitative research can, nevertheless, be carried out thanks to the free link to scientific academic literature – this complying with the paradigm of evidence-based medicine according to which practicing clinicians assess the clinical relevance of the best studies carried out on the basis of strict criteria for the quality and validity of research.

One of the words appearing in the tag cloud and strongly linked to the NPM paradigm is *cost*. In NPM, the combined impact of budget cuts needed to restore fiscal balance and the growing application of information technology is expected to lead to reduction in public health service. Although medical research is carried out beyond the immediacy of politics and public services, the application of any research to clinical practice has a concrete realization conditional upon *costs*. There are 88 occurrences (TTR 11.69) of the stem *cost** (the asterisk standing for any possible suffix), an extract of which can be seen in Figure 2:

N	Concordance	Set	Tag	Word #	t. #
1	Petty EA, Szydlowski JS. The use and cost of health services prior to death: a			65.984 085	
2	errors click to sort ty of the diagnosis or cost data has not been established.			65.650 068	
3	When using the last-diagnosis and cost methods, there is the potential for			65.635 068	
4	directly into account. However, the cost method is sensitive to differences in			65.610 067	
5	care utilization closest to death. The cost method could result in more reliable			65.589 066	
6	than 50%. The last-diagnosis and cost methods had relatively high			65.393 061	
7	within these categories. For the cost method, we identified the category			65.246 056	
8	major diagnosis, and the health care cost during the final year of life. We			65.203 053	
9	files, we extracted utilization and cost data for 12 808 VA users who died			65.150 052	
10	for the most resource use near death (cost method) 4-5 We assessed the			65.102 051	
11	problematic data quality,1 prohibitive cost of obtaining National Death Index			65.025 049	
12	have a significant impact on the overall cost of the Medicare prescription drug			63.670 956	
13	regimens at a substantially decreased cost. This suggests that adopting a			63.393 946	
14	and Modernization Act would cost substantially less if the federal			62.933 933	
15	Phelps CE. Economic foundations of cost-effectiveness analysis. J Health			43.242 818	
16	(2003) Webtable 4 - Sensitivity of cost per life year saved to variation in			43.074 805	
17	in US dollars (2003) Webtable 3 - Total cost of training and equipment provision			43.052 805	
18	Web Extra Material Webfigure - Cost structure of trial Webtable 1 –			43.025 805	

Figure 2. *Cost* concordance list.

The set of lexical items, other than function words and auxiliary verbs, forming the collocational framework with *cost** are *effectiveness*, *average*, *prescription*, *annual*, *health*, *data*, *total*, *assistance*, *technical* and *start,* as revealed by Table 3 below. Apart from the adjectives *annual*, *total*, *technical* and the noun *effectiveness*, which is the head of the noun group having *cost* as the premodifier, all the collocates are nouns in an adjectival position. This is in line with medical discourse, which is generally characterised by an information-packaging framework with high lexical density.

N	Word	With	Relation	Total
1	EFFECTIVENESS	cost*	10,201	9
2	AVERAGE	cost*	9,254	6

N	Word	With	Relation	Total
3	PRESCRIPTION	cost*	9,254	6
4	ANNUAL	cost*	9,616	6
5	HEALTH	cost*	5,794	6
6	DATA	cost*	5,244	6
7	TOTAL	cost*	8,161	5
8	ASSISTANCE	cost*	9,254	5
9	TECHNICAL	cost*	9,701	5
10	START	cost*	10,161	5

Table 3. Collocates for *cost**.

The meaningful aspect of *cost* is that this item occurs in patterns revealing the *cost analysis process* of medical procedures from which the average cost and revenues for the case under investigation result, as the quotations below reveal:

(6) For islet transplants to becomc a widespread clinical reality, diabetes reversal needs to be achieved with one donor only, *to reduce risks and costs* and to increase the availability of transplantation. […] Our successful transplantation might have implications for the ongoing transition of the procedure, from clinical investigation to routine clinical care. [L10]

(7) In our sample regimens, the new Medicare prescription discount cards offered a *modest saving* when compared with the Internet mail order pharmacy site. Alternatively, the Denver VAMC could purchase and fill both regimens at a substantially *decreased cost*. This suggests that adopting a strategy of negotiating drug prices could significantly *lower costs* in the future Medicare prescription plan. [J16]

What seems to result from this cost analysis process is that the medical community acquires a critical role in the discussion regarding forms of investment or change of the 'top-down' type. In this discussion researchers offer 'bottom up' reforms because of their being expert members of the medical social practice subject to global development. Thus, they confirm their active position within society.

Cost analysis processes cannot be conducted without the presence of a manager. The concordance list of the lexical stem *manage** indicates its high frequency, as it occurs 46 times within the corpus corresponding to TTR 6.11 (see Figure 3).

N	Concordance	Set	Tag	Word #	t. #	os.
1	team —Haleema Shakur (trial manager from 2002). Ian Roberts (clinical			21.643	923	6%
2	(trial administrator). Lin Barnetson (data manager from 2004). Janice Fernandes			21.661	923	0%
3	(Chair). Charles Warlow (1999–2001). Management group —Phil Edwards.			21.608	922	7%
4	secretary from 2003). Nin Ritchie (trial manager to 2002). Reshma Mashru (data			19.025	848	7%
5	to 2002). Reshma Mashru (data manager to 2004). Catherine Godward			19.031	848	2%
6	secretary from 2003). Nin Ritchie (trial manager to 2002). Reshma Mashru (data			21.711	923	8%
7	patients, physicians, nurses, and data managers who participated in the			36.317	543	0%
8	support for central coordination, data management, and statistics provided by			36.355	544	9%
9	at 14-weeks' gestation. The donor was managed by a medical team			31.720	356	5%
10	to 2002). Reshma Mashru (data manager to 2004). Catherine Godward			21.717	923	3%
11	an appropriate programme of medical management. Follow-up questionnaires			26.714	145	0%
12	(trial administrator). Lin Barnetson (data manager from 2004). Janice Fernandes			18.977	848	0%
13	with AstraZeneca for operational management and to support some of the			1.631	63	2%
14	the trial investigators, nurses, data managers, pharmacists, and other			1.712	69	1%
15	analysis. G Y Locker participated in the management of the trial. J S Tobias			1.470	52	3%
16	A Buzdar participated in the trial management and data interpretation. J			1.382	46	3%
17	in design issues, the overall operational management of the trial, and the			1.452	51	0%
18	the local sites, the monitors and data management staff of AstraZeneca, and			1.726	69	5%
19	(Chair). Charles Warlow (1999–01). Management group —Phil Edwards.			18.924	847	7%

Figure 3. *Manage** concordance list.

The term *manage** is central to medical discourse based on the NMP paradigm where quality management is the necessary background for service quality improvement. The core concept of management is that it offers the solution for an improvement in the performance of critical medical and business applications. Although OED defines *management* in medical terms as "the care of a patient or treatment of a disease or condition" and "the coordinated course of action determined for this purpose", in RLs the stem *manage** occurs in contexts where the reference is to business reasoning:

(8) The main outcome measures were annual number of house calls, house calls per 1000 enrollees, allowed charges for house calls, house calls by clinician type, number of house call visits and their charges as a percentage of outpatient evaluation and *management* services, and changes in these data over time [J24]

(9) Dr [...] holds a contract with AstraZeneca for operational *management* and to support some of the monitoring of the trial. [L12]

*Manage** refers to the collection, administration and control of the medical data resulting from the investigation. The managerial activity described in each study is necessary in order to deploy, monitor, analyze and optimize results so as to recognize information for correct decision-making within medical research. It highlights priorities, adapts services to needs and changing situations, makes the most of limited resources, and improves the standard and quality of services. Management principles and methods applied in medicine offer, therefore, a positive and eulogistic image of the medical community in a period of financial limitations where expert medical members, while persevering in economic constraints, never lose sight of basic medical principles.

4. Conclusions

Globalisation and the welfare crisis have caused not only financial limitation, but also changes in governance. Such changes are mirrored in discoursal changes, which become operational and require new forms of communicative interaction (Fairclough 2005). When this occurs, interdiscursivity takes place. Indeed, we have seen that under the influence of globalisation, the application of NPM in medical governance and practices has determined the rise of interdiscursivity.

As defined by Bhatia (2007: 393), interdiscursivity is established when hybrid genre frameworks are created by adopting conventions associated with other genres and professional practices, "often resulting in mixing, embedding and bending of generic norms in professional contexts".

In this case, the first step towards interdiscursivity is realised by the ICRAM manifesto, where the NPM's thought is evident: the whole medical academia, in the form of *participating democracy* (Fairclough 2005, 2007), actively and strategically takes part in the social change proposing plans to cope with the crisis by adopting a NPM mentality, where the participants are seen as 'customers'.

Such a corporative view is perceivable in the RLs. Although at the most superficial level (the layout) RLs maintain the IMRD integrity, at a lexico-grammar level they evidence items that are more typical of NPM discourse. Indeed, the type of keywords found in the corpus (*funding*, *cost**, *manage**) underlines a financial emphasis in medical discourse which has probably been absent so far. Yet most lexical items pertaining to the corporate representation of the medical world occur in a RL section defined either as *Financial disclosure* (in U.S. RLs) or *Conflict of interest statement* (in British RLs). As indicated by both editorial boards of *The Lancet*[14] and *JAMA*,[15] a conflict of interest exists when authors and/or their institutions have financial or personal relationships or affiliation with other people or organisations that could influence their actions; for this reason, all authors are required to disclose all potential conflicts of interest, including specific financial interests and relationships and affiliations relevant to the subject of their manuscript. Such an aspect is so relevant within medical genres that it has become a generic constraint. In some ways, we may see that the *conflict of interest statement* is one of the possible actions that NPM has taken in order to grant the best possible performance standards in medical practices and discourses.

References

ANSI/NISO 1997. *American Standard Guidelines for Abstracts*. Bethesola, Maryland: Niso Press.

Bhatia, Vijay 2004. *Worlds of Written Discourse*. London: Continuum.

Bhatia, Vijay 2007. Interdiscursivity in Critical Genre Analysis. *Proceedings of the 4th International Symposium on Genre Studies*. Available at <http://www3.unisul.br/paginas/ensino/pos/linguagem/cd/English/36i.pdf> [16/03/2015].

14 At <http://www.thelancet.com/writing-for-the-lancet> [17/03/2015].

15 <http://jama.ama-assn.org/misc/ifora.dtl#ConflictsofInterestandFinancialDisclosures> [17/03/2015].

Bensing, Jozien 2000. Bridging the Gap. The Separate Worlds of Evidence-Based Medicine and Patient-Centered Medicine. *Patient Education and Counseling* 39, 17–25.

Breivega, Kjersti R. / Dahl, Trine / Fløttum, Kjersti 2002. Traces of the Self in Research Articles. A Comparative Pilot Study of English, French and Norwegian Research Articles in Medicine, Economics and Linguistics. *International Journal of Applied Linguistics* 12/2, 218–239.

Chan, Margaret 2009. *Impact of Financial Crisis on Health: A Truly Global Solution is Needed*. World Health Organization. Available at <http://www.who.int/mediacentre/news/statements/2009/finan cial _crisis_20090401/en/index.html> [13/03/2015].

Dahl, Trine 2003. Accommodating the Reader: Metatext in Research Articles. *New Direction in LSP. Proceedings of the 14th Symposium on LSP 18–22 August 2003, Surrey.* Available at <www.sur rey.ac.uk/lcts/cts/events/LSP2003-preceedings.pdf>. [14/03/15].

Dahl, Trine 2004. Textual Metadiscourse in Research Articles: a Matter of National Culture or of Academic Discipline? *Journal of Pragmatics* 36, 1807–1825.

Evidence Based Medicine Working Group 1992. Evidence-Based Medicine. A New Approach to Teaching the Practice of Medicine. *JAMA* 268/17, 2420–2425.

Fairclough, Norman 2001. The Dialectics of Discourse. *Textus* 19/2, 231–242.

Fairclough, Norman 2005. *Governance, Partnership and Participation: Cooperation and Conflict.* Unpublished paper given at the conference of the International Association for Dialogue Analysis, Bucharest. Available at <http://www.ling.lancs.ac.uk/profiles/263> [17/03/2015].

Fairclough, Norman 2007. Introduction. In Cortese, Giuseppina / Fairclough, Norman / Ardizzone, Patrizia (eds) *Discourse and Contemporary Social Change*. Bern: Peter Lang, 9–14.

Ferguson, Gibson 2001. If you Pop Over There: A Corpus-Based Study of Conditional in Medical Discourse. *English for Specific Purposes* 20, 61–82.

Fløttum, Kjersti 2005. The Self and the Others: Polyphonic Visibility in Research Articles. *International Journal of Applied Linguistics* 15/1, 30–44.

Fløttum, Kjersti 2006. Medical Research Articles in Comparative Perspective of Discipline and Language. In Gotti/Salager-Meyer (eds), 251–270.

Gotti, Maurizio 2008. Developments in Medical Discourse in Early Modern English. In Douthwaite, John / Pezzini, Domenico (eds) *Words in Action*. Genova: ECIG, 92–105.

Gotti, Maurizio / Salager-Meyer, Françoise (eds) 2006. *Advances in Medical Discourse Analysis: Oral and Written Contexts*. Bern: Peter Lang.

Iedema, Rick 1999. Formalizing Organizational Meaning. *Discourse Society* 10, 49–65.

Horton, Richard 2009. Health Slips as the Financial Crisis Grips. *The Lancet* 373, 1311.

Hyland, Ken 2000. *Disciplinary Discourses: Social Interactions in Academic Writing*. Harlow: Longman.

Hyland, Ken 2002a. Authority and Invisibility: Authorial Identity in Academic Writing. *Journal of Pragmatics* 34, 1019–1112.

Hyland, Ken 2002b. Directive: Argument and Engagement in Academic Writing. *Applied Linguistics* 23/2, 215–239.

Hyland, Ken 2006. Medical Discourse: Hedges. In Brown, Keith (ed.) *Encyclopedia of Language and Linguistics*, Elsevier. Available at <http://www.sciencedirect.com.ezproxy.unibg.it:2048/science/referenceworks/0080448542> [16/03/15].

ICRAM program. Available at <http://www.bmj.com/academicmedicine/> [16/03/2015].

International Committee of Medical Journal Editors 2008. *Uniform Requirements for Manuscripts Submitted to Biomedical Journals: Writing and Editing for Biomedical Publication*. Available at <http://www.icmje.org/> [16/03/2015].

Kay, Simon 2005. Change and Change Again. *British Journal of Plastic Surgery* 58, 1041–1042.

Koutsantoni, Dimitri 2004. Attitude, Certainty and Allusion to Common Knowledge in Scientific Research Articles. *Journal of English for Academic Purposes* 3, 163–182.

Maci, Stefania M. 2008. The Research Letter: An Emerging Medical Genre. In Di Martino, Gabriella / Polese, Vanda / Solly, Martin (eds) *Identity and Culture in English Domain-specific Discourse*. Napoli: Edizioni Scientifiche Italiane, 367–390.
Maci, Stefania M. 2009. The Migration of Scientific Knowledge into Alternative Forms of Research Articles: The Case of Medical Research Letters. In Torretta, Domenico / Dossena, Marina / Sportelli, Annamaria (eds) *Forms of Migration. Migration of Forms*. Bari: Progedit, 479–495.
Maci, Stefania M. 2010. The Argumentative Structure in American and Italian Medical Research Articles. In Garzone, Giuliana / Archibald, John (eds) *Discourse and Identity in Specialized Communication*. Bern: Peter Lang, 343–363.
Maci, Stefania M. 2011. Genre Variation in Medical Discourse: The Case of Medical Posters. In Sarangi, Srikant / Polese, Vanda / Caliendo, Giuditta (eds) *Genre(s) on the Move. Hybridization and Discourse Change in Specialized Communication*. Napoli: Edizioni Scientifiche Italiane, 169–190.
Maci, Stefania M. 2012a. Poster Makers Should Think as Much about Show Business as Science. The Case of Medical Posters in a Diachronic Perspective. In Garzone, Giuliana / Catenaccio Paola / Degano, Chiara (eds) *Genre Change in the Contemporary World*. Bern: Peter Lang, 77–98.
Maci, Stefania M. 2012b. Abstracts of Poster Presentations: A Diachronic Analysis (1980–2010). *Papers from the Lancaster University Postgraduate Conference in Linguistics and Language Teaching (LAEL PG)* 6, 93–113.
Maci, Stefania M. 2012c. Fast-Track Publications: The Genre of Medical Research letters. In Gotti, Maurizio (ed.) *Academic Identity Traits*. Bern: Peter Lang, 243–262.
Maci, Stefania M. 2012d. The Genre of Medical Conference Posters. In Gotti, Maurizio (ed.) *Academic Identity Traits*. Bern: Peter Lang, 283–301.
Maci, Stefania M. 2012e. Medical Discourse from a Quantitative Perspective. The Case of Poster Abstracts. In Dalziel, Fiona / Gesuato, Sara / Musacchio, Maria T. (eds) *A lifetime of English Studies*. Padova: Il Poligrafo, 217–229.

Maci, Stefania M. 2014a. The Popularisation of Scientific Discourse for the Academia from a Diachronic Perspective: The Case of Nobel Lectures. In Chiavetta Eleonora / Sciarrino Silvia (eds) *Perspectives on the Popularisation of Natural Sciences in a Diachronic Overview*. Newcastle on Tyne: Cambridge Scholars Publishing, 97–118.

Maci, Stefania M. 2014b. Investigating Variation in Medical Poster Abstracts. In Evangelisti Allori, Paola / Bateman, John / Bhatia, Vijay K. (eds) *Evolution in Genre. Emergence, Variation, Multimodality*. Bern: Peter Lang, 67–94

Martinez, Iliana A. 2003. Aspects and Theme in the Method and Discussion Sections of Biology Journals Articles in English. *Journal of English for Academic Purposes* 2, 103–123.

MEDICARE. Available at <http://www.medicare.gov/> [17/03/2015].

Nwogu Ngozi, Kevin 1997. The Medical Research Paper: Structure and Functions. *English for Specific Purposes* 16/2, 119–138.

Sackett, David L. / Rosenberg, William M. C. / Gray, J A Muir / Haynes, R. Brian / Richardson, W Scott 1996. Evidence Based Medicine. What it is and What it isn't. *BMJ* 312,71–72.

Salager-Mayer, Françoise 2006. *I Think that Perhaps you Should: A Study of Hedges in Written Scientific Discourse*. Available at <www.exchanges.state.gov/education/engteaching/pubs/BR/functionalsec3_8.htm> [12/03/2015].

Salkov-Iversen, Dorte / Hansen, Hans K. / Bislen Sven 2000. Governmentality, Globalization and Local Practice: Transformation of a Hegemonic Discourse. *Alternatives* 25, 183–222.

Samraj, Betty 2002. Introductions in Research Articles: Variations across Disciplines. *English for Specific Purposes* 21, 1–17.

Scott, Micheal 2004. WordSmith Tools version 4, Oxford: Oxford University Press.

Skelton, John, R. / Edwards, Sarah J. 2000. The Function of the Discussion Section in Academic Medical Writing. *British Medical Journal* 320, 1269–1270.

Swales, John M. 1990. *Genre Analysis. English in Academic and Research Settings*. Cambridge: Cambridge University Press.

Taavitsainen, Irma / Pahta, Päivi 2004. *Medical and Scientific Writing in Late Medieval English*, Cambridge, Cambridge University Press.
Tardy, Christine 2004. The Role of English in Scientific Communication: *Lingua Franca* or *Tyrannosaurus Rex*? *Journal of English for Academic Purposes* 3, 247–269.

Anna Stermieri

Knowledge Dissemination in Genetics Blogs

1. Introduction

Linguistic phenomena related to processes of knowledge dissemination (KD) and popularization have been increasingly attracting the interest of researchers in recent years. While at the beginning researchers focussed their attention on discourse pertaining to the hard sciences (Calsamiglia/Van Dijk 2004; Ciapuscio 2003; Moirand 2003), more recent studies have widened the span of the research to include also topics more closely related to humanities, such as legal discourse (Anesa 2012; Preite 2012) and applied linguistics (Giannoni 2012). Therefore, an interesting and detailed mapping of the different ways in which strategies of specialized knowledge simplification act as a communicative interface in the relationship between experts in a specific field or discipline and laypeople has thus begun to be drafted.

Interestingly, the concept of science popularization began to be associated with the idea of 'bringing science to the people' (O'Connor 2009: 333) as early as the 19th century, in a context in which the leading modes of science communication were largely elitarian and addressed specific discourse communities – e.g. lectures, personal correspondence, scientific treatises, transactions of learned societies (Topham 2013) – thus bringing about a wealth of genres aimed at the dissemination of knowledge, such as reviews, abstracts, synopses, etc.

In today's connected world, Internet has become the main channel for knowledge dissemination, and in particular it has become one of the main, if not the first, source of information, especially for non-experts looking for a comprehensible explanation of specialized notions. The extent of the information available, the fact that it is free and easily accessible and the fact that it is possible to find an answer to one's questions though remaining anonymous are possibly some of the reasons behind this phenomenon. In particular, it has been pointed out how patients are increasingly browsing the web for medical advice and information (Eysenbach/Diepgen 1999; Tustin 2010), and how this opens up issues related to information reliability (cf. Eysenbach *et al.* 1998 on medical information, but also Facchinetti 2012 on reliability of unmediated news content).

Conversely, Web 2.0 content producing dynamics (Sokól 2012: 266–268), allowing users to freely contribute to the information available on line, has increased the number of experts (or semi-experts) willing to share their ideas and knowledge with a wider audience. From a practical point of view, free blogging software and hosting platforms, seem to have been central to this process, having provided users with accessible and easy to use suites of tools which allow the updating of the pages, the automatic construction of an archive of the published posts and a customizable layout (Baron 2008; Garzone 2012; Halavais 2002; Herring *et al.* 2005; Krishnamurty 2002; Myers 2010; Nardi *et al.* 2004, Puschmann 2013; Riboni 2014).

Blogs have thus become "a way for individuals of any technical caliber to create an attractive, easy-to-read website that can be readily followed by an audience" (Jones *et al.* 2010: 101). These platforms are one of the instances of the processes of democratization that have been going on in the web at a fast pace in the last twenty years (Baron 2002; Myers 2010). The undeniable success of scholarly blogging (Bonetta 2007; Puschmann/Marht 2012) has attracted the interest of linguists towards the phenomenon, and in particular has led to a wealth of studies concerning the communicative strategies of KD used by scholars in popularizing science in a web-based blog environment (Blanchard 2011; Colson 2011; Gregg 2009; Kouper 2010; Luzón 2013).

In a similar way, in this chapter I will discuss KD strategies associated with medical discourse in the context of academic blogs written by scientists working in the field of genetics. Genetics appears as an interesting field for popularization, as it seems to occupy a linking position between medicine and scientific research.

The analysis is based on a small corpus of blog posts written by geneticists working as academics. Drawing on a combination of qualitative and quantitative methodologies, deriving from both discourse analysis and corpus linguistics, the study aims at unveiling the linguistic features realising KD in this particular context and the implications, in terms of the interaction among experts and non-experts, generated by the use of this particular medium.

2. Materials and methods

2.1 Corpus description

A small corpus has been collected for the purpose of the study, while an already existing reference corpus of blog posts has been used in order to generate a keyword list of lexical items revealing specific traits of the academic blog in the field of genetics. Both corpora have been manually tagged, in order to separate post text from comment text, by means of two simple tags, marking the beginning and the end of each section.[1] The *GeneBlog Corpus* includes the contents of four blogs by geneticists working in academia, for a total of 277 texts and 298,688 words. The following criteria led the selection of the blogs: the rank of each blog according to Technorati, and the references made to each blog in other blogrolls. Two of the blogs are independently published on regular blogging platforms[2] whereas two belong to a dedicated academic platform: *scienceblogs.com*.[3] All the texts in the *GeneBlog Corpus* were posted online between 2008 and 2013. Table 1 provides a detailed description of the contents of the *GeneBlog*.

1 The tags used in both corpora were <POST> and </POST> ; <COMM> and </ COMM>.

2 <http://www.genetic-inference.co.uk/blog> retrieved on 15/09/14; <http://new songenetics.blogspot.com retreived on 15/09/14>.

3 <http://scienceblogs.com/geneticfuture> retrieved on 15/09/14; <http://genoto pia.scienceblog.com> retrieved on 15/09/14.

Blog	*#posts*	*<post> tokens*	*<comment> tokens*	*Total tokens*
Genetic inference	80	60,943	20,435	81,378
Genetic future	90	52,040	86,372	138,412
Genotopia	83	58,971	14,315	73,286
News on genetics	24	5,434	180	5,612
Totals	277	177,388	301,122	298,688

Table 1. The GeneBlog corpus in figures.

The reference corpus, called the *BLOGcorpus* (Seidenari 2012) includes texts posted on-line between September 2008 and September 2009, on a wide variety of different topics, i.e. business; entertainment; science and technology; lifestyle; politics; sports. The *BLOGcorpus*, which amounts to about 1,600,000 words in total, includes about 300,000 words in the post section, and 1,300,000 words in the comments section.

2.2 *Keywords selection and preliminary analysis*

The two corpora have been analysed, and compared, by means of the software for lexical analysis WordSmith Tools 5.0 (Scott 2008). Since this study focussed only on the posts section of the *GeneBlog Corpus*, a keyword list was produced comparing the post section of the *GeneBlog Corpus* against the post section of the *BLOGcorpus*. The aim of this step was to identify lexical items pertaining to blogging in the field of genetics. Then I focussed my attention on the first one hundred items in the keyword list, which I have assigned to different semantic categories devised for the purpose of this study.

The classification has emerged as a result of the study of the concordance profile of each keyword. The categories identified are six. The first five are strictly semantic: *Medicine; Academic research; People/ companies; Grammar words; Blog*. The last one includes items that could not be classified after a thorough observation of their concordances (*n.c.*). In this phase, two items have been selected i.e. *disease* and *risk*, and their concordances analysed to investigate how research-related topics and concepts are represented in blog posts.

3. Keywords analysis

3.1 Sematic categories: an overview

Of the six semantic categories outlined in the previous section, two appear to be particularly prominent. The category including the majority of items is the first one, Medicine (41 keywords), followed by Academic research (30 keywords). The prominence of both these semantic categories seems to reveal a twofold orientation of this discipline, that seems to be lexically constructed as bridging a gap between medicine and research. It seems in fact that in their posts, geneticists are both engaged in describing and explaining symptoms (1), and in doing research and interpreting data (2):

(1) **Crohn's disease** is a type of Inflammatory Bowel **Disease**; it is a rare autoimmune disorder in which the immune system overreacts to microbes in the intestine wall, attacking tissue and causing inflamed, sore patches to appear throughout the gut.

(2) Interestingly, they even have a somewhat opposite <u>interpretation of the primary research data presented in our paper:</u> our original purpose is to **demonstrate** how rare variants may contribute to human diseases.

The third most frequent category, People\companies, highlights the actors involved in the geneticists' professional environment, mapping the internal divisions of the discourse community gravitating around these blogs. In the list we see two proper names, which as Sokól (2012) has noted, are a fairly typical element in academic blogs, where it is possible to make reference to colleagues citing their work or point of view with a certain degree of familiarity and intimacy. However, even if we found examples in the corpus of this kind of 'familiar attribution', in this specific case, they are simply the names of two of the bloggers recurring in their post headers or footers (3):

(3) <POST>
My genetic future
Posted by Daniel MacArthur on February 16, 2010
My wife and I have embarked on our first collaborative genetic experiment.
</POST>

The world of academia is further represented by the surnames of scientists which have contributed to the field, as in (4) and (5):

(4) Arthur quotes Joel Parker berating as 'embarrassing' biologists who claim that it was **Darwin**, and not Lamarck, who came up with the idea of an evolutionary tree.

(5) Eugenics has been defined in many ways over the last 130 years, viz.: "The study of the agencies under social control, that improve or impair the racial qualities of future generations either physically or mentally". (**Galton**, 1883)

Various forms of attribution are shown in (4) and (5): in (4), the quote is introduced by a strongly evaluative verb (*berating*) which would be less acceptable in a traditional academic environment, while in (5) the quote follows the rules of academic citation, reporting the author surname and the year of publication.

The fourth group of participants includes the private companies working in genetics (i.e. *23andMe*, in example 8), in contrast with the academic environment in which the bloggers work, while the fifth group includes the laypeople involved in the field, i.e. the *patients* (6), the *population* (7) and the *customers* (8), again drawing a line between the world of academia and the world of privately funded research.

(6) Whatever the benefits that accrue to **patients** from genomic technology, they cannot possibly live up to the hype.

(7) For me, these are compelling evidence that **population** stratification does not explain the signal, though I think that functional studies are certainly necessary to identify causal variants and to study their roles.

(8) **23andMe customers** have responded, and there is a petition calling for continued access to genetic information.

While the items included in the Blog category are quite self-explanatory and depend on the communicative environment under investigation, Grammar words are interesting under a variety of aspects. Items in this category are adjectives, adverbials, connectors and prepositions. Interestingly, among the first one hundred keywords we have items like *however* and *such*, which can be used in problematizing and exemplifying concepts and in expressing contrast, in the first case, and for creating links of similarity, in the second.

Three interesting items are *complex*, *common* and *rare*, which are often collocates of *disease*, to identify three different types of diseases which are an object of study for the geneticist:

(9) A more serious motivation comes from those suffering from a **rare genetic disease** for which the underlying mutation is currently unknown.

(10) That's the (biologically entirely plausible) hypothesis that most **complex disease** geneticists are working under right now.

(11) In April, I cited an excellent article by McClellan and King, who argued that "many rare alleles account for **common diseases**".

The analysis of the keyword included in each category and of the way in which each keyword would interact with other keywords (e.g. *disease*, in examples 9 to 11 above) led me to the selection of two items to investigate: *disease* and *risk*.

3.2 Popularizing strategies: disease

Our analysis begins with the study of the concordance profile of the word *disease*. There are 390 occurrences of the item in the </post> *GeneBlog* sub-corpus, and it is the highest ranking keyword to have been selected, as it ranks third in the keyword list produced comparing the *GeneBlog* to the *BLOGcorpus*. From the observation of the concordances of the item listed below, it is evident that it is often used as part of an expression naming a specific type of disease, either as part of a proper name (e.g. *Crohn's disease*) or as part of a name identifying a certain class of diseases which have a set of characteristics in common (e.g. *hereditary disease, complex disease*).

prevention of **hereditary disease** would lead to th
a serious **monogenic heart disease** without even kno
ering from a **rare genetic disease** with an unknown
will be useful in **complex disease** will depend stro
d at a very large **Crohn's disease** whole-genome seq

iabetes or **coronary heart disease**. While the prima
ome-wide studies of **human disease**, which is worth
rld with a **severe genetic disease**, when this situa
ics of **inflammatory bowel disease**. We genotyped ov
ants that underlie **common disease**. We will need to

Table 3 presents the collocates that form proper names of diseases central to the debate in genetic research.

Proper names	*Total Occurrences*	*Popularizing Occurrences*
Crohn's Disease	15	4
Inflammatory Bowel Disease	8	2
Parkinson's Disease	4	0
Sickle Cell Disease	3	1
Celiac Disease	2	1
Huntington Disease	1	0
Reagan's disease	1	1
Sydney disease	1	0
Total	35	9

Table 3. Collocates identifying a specific disease.

Table 4, on the other hand, lists the collocates that identify a class of diseases rather than a particular one.

General names	*Total Occurrences*	*Popularizing Occurrences*
Genetic disease	22	0
Complex disease	15	1
Heart disease	15	4
Common disease	10	0
Human disease	10	0
Infectious disease	7	2
Molecular disease	4	0
Auto-immune disease	1	1
Cardiovascular disease	1	0

General names	*Total Occurrences*	*Popularizing Occurrences*
Hereditary disease	1	0
Metabolic disease	1	1
Polygenic disease	1	0
Rare disease	1	0
Total	89	9

Table 4. Collocates identifying a class of diseases.

Items in Table 3 mainly refer to the name of the scientists who have discovered each particular disease. In Table 4 on the other hand, the collocates of *disease* are mainly adjectives, pointing at what is affected by the disease or to the effects it has on the body, or to its distinctive traits, thus describing classes of diseases that can include more than one. Interestingly, while *genetic* and *molecular* are very clearly identifiable scientific terms, *complex* and *common* seem more vague and possibly carrying an evaluative meaning. Observing the items in context though, it is possible to note that they are actually very context-specific and that they are used to distinguish diseases on the basis of the variants that cause their insurgence (as shown in 12 and 13).

(12) That's the (biologically entirely plausible) hypothesis that most **complex disease** geneticists are working under right now.

(13) We have discovered dozens of SNPs associated with **common disease**.

While the items in Table 3 seem to be less frequently used in the corpus than the items in Table 4 (35 total occurrences for the former, 89 total occurrences for the latter), it is important to note how there seems to be a tendency for proper names of diseases to be used more frequently as part of phraseological structures typical of popularization (26% of cases, i.e. 9 out of 35 total occurrences), whereas general names seem to occur less frequently in such phraseological structures (10% of cases, i.e. 9 out of 89 total occurrences).

In order to interpret these results, it might be useful to look at some examples: in (14) the blogger provides an explanation for what

Crohn's disease is and for what its main symptoms and effects on the body are:

(14) **Crohn's disease** is a type of Inflammatory Bowel **Disease**; it is a rare autoimmune disorder in which the immune system overreacts to microbes in the intestine wall, attacking tissue and causing inflamed, sore patches to appear throughout the gut.

This explanation is not aimed at experts in the field, as is revealed by the presence of terms such as *sore patches* or *the gut*, which do not appear to be scientific or medical. Moreover, reformulation strategies, as for example predicative structures in which a specialized term is explained in terms of "*x* is *y*", can be seen as a way to 'unpack' the information for the reader. Such structures expand the context and provide a set of information the expert recognizes as part of the meaning of the specialized term, while the non-expert needs it to be clarified explicitly. Table 4 provides a pattern of how such structures work, on the basis of example (14) above:

Specialized concept	*Reformulation 1*	*Reformulation 2*
Crohn's disease **is**	a type of Inflammatory Bowel Disease;	
It [Crohn's disease] **is**	a rare autoimmune disorder	**in which** the immune system overreacts to microbes in the intestine wall, attacking tissue and causing inflamed, sore patches to appear throughout the gut

Table 5. Reformulation of the name *Crohn's disease.*

As shown in Table 5, by expanding the amount of information concerning the specialized core concept, a recontextualization of the concept is provided by the expert, so as to reduce the gap existing between the specialized content and the ability of comprehension of a layperson.

3.3 *Communicating* risk: *a scientist's perspective on a medical condition*

The inherently harmful nature of diseases makes it central to our analysis to understand the discursive practices used by geneticists in their blogs in order to introduce, discuss and represent risk, and therefore to communicate risk to their readership. In particular, this may shed light on the preferred strategies used in disseminating knowledge about risk among a mixed audience looking for health information, while at the same time unveiling common academic and professional practices, values and attitudes towards this specific issue in the field of genetics. Due to the relevance of the issue, the following section will only aim at providing a preliminary investigation of how risk is approached in scholarly blogs dealing with genetics, since it is evident that it is a complex notion which deserves a much more extensive investigation (cf. Zinn 2010 on risk as discourse, and Marko 2010 on risk in popular health discourse).

3.3.1 Typologies of risk

The two main collocates of risk are *disease* (51) and *genetic* (44) – cf. examples 15 and 16 – accounting respectively for 23% and 20% of its overall occurrences (220). These two collocations introduce us to the areas of interest of the geneticist, suggesting again a double nature of their professional role, as both researchers and medical experts.

(15) It's worth noting that discrepancies between the predictions made by the companies don't necessarily mean that they are doing something wrong – predicting **disease risk** from genetic variants is still a new and uncertain field, and there is still plenty of room for valid disagreement on the best approach to use.

(16) We know that the assumptions you make can drastically change (for instance, whether you think **genetic risk** prediction will be useful in complex disease will depend strongly on what model of **genetic risk** you use).

There is no clear-cut difference between the two typologies of risks, i.e. a genetic risk can also be a disease risk, and both collocate with a similar set of items (e.g. *prediction*, *predicting* in examples 15 and 16). They can also be used in combination, as in (17):

(17) Learning of your genetic risk is unlikely to be harmful. Long profoundly exaggerates the risks of learning of one's own **genetic disease risk**:

Nonetheless, it is evident that the semantics of the two terms highlight different aspects of risk: on the one hand, *disease risk* concentrates the focus on the possibility of contracting a disease, but not on the factors leading to its insurgence; on the other hand, *genetic risk* highlights the fact that the set of factors leading to the insurgence of a disease are unavoidable, as they are part of the genetic history of the patient.

Interestingly, observing the collocates of *risk* which co-occur either with *genetic* or with *disease* (cf. concordances below), it seems possible to find further evidence of this distinction: for example, *factors* (9 occurrences) only collocates with *risk* (4 occurrences) or with *genetic risk* (5 occurrences), but never with *disease risk.* On the other hand, *associations* (1 occurrence,) and *associated* (8 occurrences) only co-occur either with *risk*+the name of a disease, or with *disease risk.*

N	*Concordance risk+ factors*
1	**of risk factors. Basically,** genetic risk factors **are**
2	**eptional relative to other types of** risk factors.
3	**ates. 5) Excluding the HLA,** genetic risk factors **for**
4	**etic risk. This states that** genetic risk factors **act**
5	**ame amount regardless of what other** risk factors **are**

N	*Concordance: associated +risk*
1	**very weakly** associated **with** disease risk**, but the au**
2	**which are** associated **with increased** risk of breast and ovarian cancers

N	*Concordance: associations+ risk*
1	**ore well-powered to pick up** disease risk associations **given their more**

It seems then that while *genetic risk* is determined by a set of characteristics which are independent from the actions and habits of the patients as they are inscribed in their DNA, *disease risk* is assessed as a consequence of the observation of a state of things, which are not direct causes of the disease, but which are associated with its insurgence.

In both cases, risk is communicated as a notion which can be investigated, but most importantly, as an entity that can be measured, since it emerges as a consequence of a set of causes, either external or internal to the patient.

3.3.2 Assessing risk

We mentioned *factors* in the previous section as an interesting collocate of *risk* pointing to its nature as a potential consequence of a set of causes either internal or external to the patient. The second most frequent collocate of *risk* (the first being *of* with 27 occurrences) is *variants* (23 occurrences).

(18) Goldstein's argument is straightforward: although GWAS have been "strikingly successful" in identifying sites of common genetic variation associated with complex diseases, the **variants** they have found – both individually and altogether – explain a small fraction of the overall genetic contribution to common disease risk. These common **variants** typically only increase risk by 10 to 70% – so for a disease that affects 2% of the population, carrying one of these variants means your disease risk increases to 2.2 to 3.4%. For even heavily studied diseases the variants found to date typically explain less than 20% of the heritable variance in disease risk.

Again, in (18) the notion of risk is constructed as a quantifiable entity. Risk depends on a set of causes that cannot be entirely determined in advance, in that they assume different combinations from patient to patient, but that can be identified and measured to a certain degree of extent and precision. Reducing risk to its basic components (variants, or factors) allows for its manipulation and allows the researcher to describe risk, representing it in figures and percentages. In this scientific perspective where risk is described by means of data, figures and percentages, it is no more an obscure, looming possibility: it can be quantified, represented, observed and manipulated, at least in part.

Further evidence is provided by the fact that the third and the fourth most frequent collocates of *risk* (on the right side of the node) are *prediction* (12 occurrences) and *predictions* (12 occurrences):

(19) Two of these are very important: there needs to be a strong research focus on examining whether receiving genetic risk information actually changes behavioural outcomes, and on performing large prospective studies (that is, studies in

which large numbers of people are genotyped and then followed to see if they develop common diseases) to validate **risk prediction** algorithms.

(20) Personal genomics customers should of course treat their current risk predictions with caution – for most diseases, current **risk predictions** are barely better than noise – and bear in mind that their profiles will alter over the next few years as increases in scientific understanding of the genetic basis of disease improves, and as their **predictions** become steadily more accurate.

Risk, we stated above, is constructed in discourse as a quantifiable entity, depending on a set of recognizable factors or variants, which can be measured. While scientists are aware of the limits of their investigation (cf. "for most diseases, current risk predictions are barely better than noise", in example (20)), they are also aware of the potential of their work, as it allows to provide prediction which "become steadily more accurate" (cf. example (20)). Therefore, on the basis of this observation, a hypothesis can be made and risk can be predicted. Risk is thus rationalized by means of a scientific process, and reduced to a comprehensible notion that can be understood and investigated. Most importantly, on the other hand, the limits of the research are never kept secret. The process of risk assessment emerges from the blog posts as being the result of:

- a phase of *observation*, during which the correlation between the presence of certain risk factors and the insurgence of specific diseases is revealed;
- a phase during which *hypotheses* are made: a prediction of the chances of insurgence of a certain disease is determined on the basis of the observed factors influencing risk.
- A phase of *investigation* during which risk is calculated and measured to the best of the scientist's possibilities.

For example, let us observe the way *disease risk* (40 occurrences, Table 6) is conceptualized, in order to see how the above described process is reflected in discourse:

Observation	associated with (3) associations (1) linking … to… (1)	relationship between … and … (1) see changes to (1)
Hypothesis	to predict (4) prediction (2) predictions (3)	predictive power (1) predictor (1)
Investigation	explain (3) increase (2) learning (2) testing (2) effects on (2) affect (1) be source of (1) contribution to (1)	evaluate (1) figure out what has an impact on (1) get information (1) model (1) think about the things that effect (1) uncover (1) work on (1)

Table 6. Collocates of *disease risk*

The first category of items signals the identification of relation between a cause of risk and a specific disease:

(21) Extreme paternalism would suggest that gatekeepers control access to ancestry information or to studies **linking** normal traits to **disease risk**, but this level of paternalism could hinder education and active participation in one's own health.

The second category includes items related to the prediction of the disease risk:

(22) From the outset the aim of genome-wide association studies has been two-fold: (1) identifying markers that can be used to predict individual **disease risk;** and (2) highlighting the molecular pathways underlying disease, providing potential targets for therapy.

Disease risk is thus the object of a hypothesis-making process that projects it in the future, while the present is devoted to the third phase of the process, i.e. investigation, represented by the items in the third category. Investigation is constructed in text by means of items that mirror the professional activity of the researcher, i.e. *test*, *evaluate* and *model*, but also by means of a set of expressions describing the behavior of the data, as in (23):

(23) now reporting on less common genetic **variants** with much ***larger effects*** **on disease risk**

It is possible to note how such items are usually part of a phraseological structure including: one item pointing at the risk factor (e.g. *variant*) and another pointing at the type of effect produced by the risk factor on disease risk (e.g. *larger effects*). This highlights relevant items which are worth investigating within the geneticists' research field. The semantic categories listed above in Table 6 highlight and narrow the scope of the geneticists' research interests, revealing their disciplinary and professional approach to risk and disease.

3.4 Epistemic values and educational intentions in genetics blogs

We noted earlier, when mapping the corpus keywords, that one of the semantic categories included the names of private companies working in the field of genetics. In their blogs, geneticists working in academia appear to express a negative opinion towards the services offered to the public by such companies (24):

(24) The potential customer is left with a clear if implicit message that there is a gene for speed and that for $299 you can find out if you have it. The discussion of variation and the importance of training and other factors is lost. Where it gets lost, not surprisingly, is in the sales pitch, which brings up my second **risk:** commercialization. 23AndMe is not a charity. Although I have no reason to doubt the humanitarian impulses of anyone at the company, it's no secret that their first allegiance is to their shareholders. Their primary task is making money. This of course does not immediately invalidate it as a socially beneficial enterprise, but it does and should make us alert to potential conflicts between profit and benevolence. As an advocate for patients, one feels responsible for raising questions and maintaining transparency so that the medical benefits Angrist rightly emphasizes don't get lost in the commercialism Brandom exposes.

In (24) the blogger establishes a clear-cut distinction between himself ("an advocate for patients") and the companies marketing at-home DNA tests that can be freely purchased by the customers. Moreover, this distinction brings about a second dichotomy: patients – i.e. the academic perspective on those interested in mapping their DNA – and customers – i.e. the private company perspective on the same people, in that such companies are "not a charity" and "Their primary task is making money".

The distinction bloggers establish between themselves and the private companies finds further confirmation in the ways bloggers construct risk in their posts. In their opinion, private companies minimize risk and provide limited information to their patients ("The potential customer is left with a clear if implicit message that there is a gene for speed and that for $299 you can find out if you have it. The discussion of variation and the importance of training and other factors is lost").

Geneticists, on the contrary, construct risk in discourse as a quantifiable entity emerging from a combination of factors that can be observed, investigated and that can be the basis of a prediction concerning the percentage of risk each patient is subject to, depending on either internal or external causes. If we consider again examples (18), (19) and (20) another aspect of the notion of risk emerges: risk is quantifiable but there are limits to this quantification process, which a scientist cannot ignore. In (18), for example, it is stated that "although GWAS have been 'strikingly successful' in identifying sites of common genetic variation associated with complex diseases, the **variants** they have found – both individually and altogether – explain a small fraction of the overall genetic contribution to common disease risk." In (20), the blogger points out that "for most diseases, current **risk predictions** are barely better than noise". Evaluative items expressing epistemic modality emerge in these examples as an important feature of geneticists' writing, balancing the factuality provided by data with a cautious perspective on the conclusions that such data may lead to.

While hedging strategies aimed at mitigating, balancing or downtoning claims of certainty are a typical feature of academic writing, in this particular context they seem to have a specific purpose: by clearly reporting results and data in full, without making explicit claims of certainty, and by means of epistemic discursive strategies belonging to their professional field, i.e. academic writing, geneticists construct themselves as reliable and trustworthy sources of information in the eyes of their lay readership, as opposed to private companies which are discursively constructed as providing misleading information and as being only profit oriented.

4. Discussion and conclusion

Science blogs blur the boundaries of science communication: the scientific discussion is no more confined to conference environments or academic journals, but rather it becomes accessible to wider audiences through the Web. Interestingly, this happens because the experts themselves make their scientific debate available to others, by posting their ideas and contributions on a blog. The Web allows for a wider readership to access their writing, in comparison to academic journals or academic publications. Moreover, lay people are increasingly turning to the Web in order to collect medical information (Tustin 2010). The presence of a non-expert component of the readership does not emerge clearly from the analysis of the geneticists' blog comments carried out in this chapter, as it seems that lay audiences reading scientific blogs are less likely to comment and actively participate in the online discussion, which on the contrary features the active contributions of other experts, possibly because they feel either excluded or not able to contribute in a pertinent way to the debate (Stermieri 2013), but the use of popularizing strategies on the part of the bloggers shows their awareness of the heterogeneous nature of their audience.

Investigating the keywords of the corpus has allowed for a first rough mapping of the areas of interest of geneticists who blog, pointing out not only their hybrid position as both academic researchers and medical experts, but also pointing at the complex network of actors populating the field of genetics research. As far as popularizing strategies are concerned, we noted how there seems to be a preference for the use of KD strategies to re-contextualize terms such as the names of specific diseases, while more general names often remain unexplained, even if they might be obscure to the lay audience. A possible interpretation for this phenomenon lies in the above mentioned hybrid nature of the geneticists as academics with both a medical and technical background, which becomes particularly evident in the case of those who decide to disseminate their knowledge by means of a blog. Geneticists who blog, in fact, enter in contact with a wide and mixed audience including both experts (e.g. colleagues) and non-experts. The latter category seems to be more interested in the medical aspects of the geneticists' work, rather than in the academic and laboratory-related ones, and thus geneticists appear to respond to this demand by means of a diversified approach to specialized notions and language. Interestingly, items for which recontextualization is offered are names of diseases which are known to the audience at large. Such items, e.g. *Crohn's disease*, seem to pertain more to the 'medical' sphere, as opposed to names such as *genetic disease* or *complex disease*, which seem to be more academic and research-bound, and less familiar to non-experts or lay people. Geneticists appear to feel free to use their everyday, working lexis knowing that a portion of their readership will understand it and at the same time consider them reliable as members of the same academic and discourse community, recognizing the lexical and discursive conventions characterizing their professional and academic communicative environment. At the same time, they seem to perceive a need to explain and disseminate knowledge when it comes to more widely used terms identifying hereditary diseases, which attract the attention of the lay portion of their readership. Another possible explanation is that bloggers might be more familiar with technical terms pertaining to their discipline, thus not feeling a pressing need to 'popularize' concepts they have interiorized as part of their professional and academic practice.

We introduced the idea that genetics might occupy a bridging position between medicine and academic research: this seems to find a confirmation in the way the notion of *disease* and *risk* are constructed in the posts: *disease* is conceptualized mainly in terms of its risk of occurring. Risk is evaluated and calculated following a scientific method of analysis (observation – hypothesis – investigation). Most importantly, no attempt is ever made at suggesting cures: diseases are recognized, and the risk of their insurgence calculated and measured on the basis of a set of factors or variants that may influence it, but no mention is ever made to treatment, which is clearly a task beyond the medical expertise of a geneticist.

Another interesting point that has emerged from the analysis is that a negative semantic prosody seems to be preferred when discussing the predictability of a risk, thus paving the way to an academic discursive strategy aimed at hedging claims of certainty. In so doing, bloggers are able to construct their identity as trustworthy sources of information, balancing facts (i.e. data and figures) with a cautious approach and the awareness of the actual limits of research. They construct this identity as opposed to private genetic companies, which are strongly criticised in their blogs. In so doing, bloggers draw upon the opportunities offered by the blog expanding the range of issues they discuss beyond the traditional boundaries of academic publishing. They exploit the freedom provided by their own web space to warn lay audiences of the possible dangers of relying on genetics companies, thus opening up spaces for both knowledge dissemination and lay-audiences education.

References

Anesa, Patrizia 2012. *Jury Trials and the Popularization of Legal Language: A Discourse Analytical Approach.* Bern: Peter Lang.

Baron, Naomi 2002. Who Sets E-Mail Style? Prescriptivism, Coping Strategies, and Democratizing Communication Access. *The Information Society* 18, 403–413.

Baron, Naomi 2008. *Always On: Language in an Online and Mobile World*. Oxford: Oxford University Press.

Blanchard, Antoine 2011. Science Blogs in Research and Popularization of Science: Why, How and for Whom? In Cockell, Moira / Billotte, Jérôme / Darbellay, Frédéric / Waldvogel, Francis (eds) *Common Knowledge: The Challenge of Transdisciplinarity*. Lausanne: EPFL Press, 219–232.

Bonetta, Laura 2007. Scientists Enter the Blogosphere. *Cell* 129/3, 443–445.

Calsamiglia, Helena / Van Dijk, Theun. A. 2004 Popularization Discourse and Knowledge about the Genome. *Discourse & Society* 15/4, 369–389.

Ciapuscio, Guiomar E. 2003. Formulation and Reformulation Procedures in Verbal Interaction between Experts and (Semi)laymen. *Discourse Studies* 5/4, 207–233.

Colson, Vinciane 2011. Science Blogs as Competing Channels for the Dissemination of Science News. *Journalism* 12/ 7, 889–902.

Eysenbach, Gunter / Diepgen, Thomas 1999. Patients Looking for Information on the Internet and Seeking Teleadvice: Motivation, Expectations, and Misconceptions as Expressed in E-mails Sent to Physicians. *Archives of Dermatology* 135/2, 151–156.

Eysenbach, Gunter / Diepgen, Thomas L. 1998. Towards Quality Management of Medical Information on the Internet: Evaluation, Labelling, and Filtering of Information. *Bmj* 317/7171, 1496–1502.

Facchinetti, Roberta 2012. News Writing from the 1960s to the Present Day. In Facchinetti, Roberta / Brownlees, Nicholas / Bös, Birte / Fries, Udo (eds) *News as Changing Texts. Corpora, Methodologies and Analysis*. Newcastle on Tyne: Cambridge Scholars Publishing, 145–196.

Garzone, Giuliana 2012. Where do Web Genres Come From? The Case of Blogs. In Campagna, Sandra / Garzone, Giuliana / Ilie, Cornelia / Rowley-Jolivet Elizabeth (eds) *Evolving Genres in Web-mediated Communication*. Bern: Peter Lang, 217–242.

Giannoni, Davide S. 2012. Evaluation and Popularisation in Journal Editorials: Medicine vs Applied Linguistics. In Gotti, Maurizio (ed.) *Academic Identity Traits: A Corpus-Based Investigation*. Bern: Peter Lang, 173–186.

Gregg, Melissa 2009. Banal Bohemia. Blogging from the Ivory Tower Hot-desk. *Convergence: The International Journal of Research into New Media Technologies* 15/4, 470–483.

Halavais, Alexander 2002. Blogs and the 'Social Weather'. Paper presented at *Internet Research 3.0*. Maastricht, The Netherlands.

Herring, Susan C. / Scheidt, Lois A. / Wright, Elijah / Bonus, Sabrina 2005. Weblogs as a Bridging Genre. *Information, Technology & People* 18, 142–171.

Jones, Brant / Spigel, Ben / Malecki, Edward J. 2010. Blog Links as Pipelines to Buzz Elsewhere: the Case of New York Theater Blogs. *Environment and Planning B: Planning and Design*. 37, 99–111.

Kouper, Inna 2010. Science Blogs and Public Engagement with Science: Practices, Challenges, and Opportunities. *Journal of Science Communication* 9/1, 1–10.

Krishnamurthy, Sandeep 2002. The Multidimensionality of Blog Conversations: The Virtual Enactment of September 11. Paper presented at *Internet Research 3.0*. Maastricht, The Netherlands.

Luzón, Maria José 2013. Public Communication of Science in Blogs: Recontextualizing Scientific Discourse for a Diversified Audience. *Written Communication* 20/10, 1–30.

Marko, Georg 2010. Heart Disease and Cancer, Diet and Exercise, Vitamins and Minerals: The Construction of Lifestyle Risks in Popular Health Discourse *CADAAD Journal* 4/2, 147–170.

Moirand, Sylvie 2003. Communication and Cognitive Dimensions of Discourse on Science in the French Mass Media. *Discourse Studies* 5/2, 175–206.

Myers, Greg 2010. *The Discourse of Blogs and Wikis*. London: Continuum.

Nardi, Bonnie A./ Schiano Diane J. / Gumbrecht, Michelle. 2004. Blogging as Social Activity, or, would you Let 900 Million People Read your Diary? In *Proceedings of the ACM Conference on Computer Supported Cooperative Work* (CSCW '04). New York: ACM Press, 222–231.

O'Connor, Ralph 2009. Reflections on Popular Science in Britain. Genres, Categories and Historians. *Isis* 100/2, 333–345.

Preite, Chiara 2012. Le fiches del Ministère de la Justice et des Libertés de la Republique Française come genere divulgativo: un esempio di trasmissione del sapere giuridico. In Diani, Giuliana / Preite, Chiara (eds) *La trasmissione del sapere nelle diverse comunità accademiche: una prospettiva plurilingue*. Roma: Officina edizioni, 167–179.

Puschmann, Cornelius 2013. Blogging. In Herring, Susan C. / Stein, Dieter / Virtanen, Tuija (eds) *Pragmatics of Computer-Mediated Communication.* Berlin: De Gruyter Mouton, 83–108.

Puschmann, Cornelius / Mahrt, Merja 2012. Scholarly Blogging: A New Form of Publishing or Science Journalism 2.0? In Tokar, Alexander / Beurskens, Michael / Keuneke, Susanne / Mahrt, Merja / Peters, Isabella / Puschmann /, Cornelius / van Treeck, Timo / Weller, Katrin (eds) *Science and the Internet*. Düsseldorf: Düsseldorf University Press, 171–181.

Riboni, Giorgia 2014. *Nuovi media e discorso politico. I blog nelle elezioni presidenziali americane*. Saarbrücken: Edizioni Accademiche Italiane.

Scott, Michael. 2008, *WordSmith Tools version 5*, Liverpool: Lexical Analysis Software.

Seidenari, Corrado 2012. *Evaluative Phraseologies in English and Italian Blog Discourse: A Corpus-based Study*. PhD Thesis, University of Modena and Reggio Emilia (unpublished).

Sokól, Malgorzata 2012. Metadiscourse and the Construction of the Author's Voices in the Blogoshphere: Academic Weblogs as a Form of Self-promotion. In Campagna, Sandra / Garzone, Giuliana / Ilie, Cornelia / Rowley-Jolivet Elizabeth (eds) *Evolving Genres in Web-mediated Communication*. Bern: Peter Lang, 265–287.

Stermieri, Anna 2013. 'Wow… you're on scienceblogs – congrats!' Blogs and Knowledge Dissemination: the Case of Genetics. Paper presented at: *CLAVIER13 conference: Discourse in and through the Media. Recontextualizing and reconceptualizing expert discourse*. Modena, 6–8 November 2013.

Topham, Jonathan R. 2013. Anthologizing the Book of Nature: The Circulation of Knowledge and the Origins of the Scientific Journal in Late Georgian Britain. In Lightman, Bernard / McOuat, Gordon / Stewart, Larry (eds) *The Circulation of Knowledge Between Britain, India and China: The Early-Modern World to the Twentieth Century*. Leiden: Brill, 119–152.

Tustin, Nupur 2010. The Role of Patient Satisfaction in Online Health Information Seeking. *Journal of Health Communication: International Perspectives* 15/1, 3–17.

Zinn, Jens O. 2012 Risk as Discourse: Interdisciplinary Perspectives. *CADAAD Journal* 4/2, 106–124.

Notes on Contributors

Miriam Bait is Assistant Professor in English Language and Translation at the Faculty of Political and Social Sciences, University of Milan, Italy, where she teaches language and communication-related courses. Her research interests include English for Specific Purposes, intercultural business communication, language in the media, and Special Educational Needs in EFL Teaching. Her current work focuses on textual and discursive variations in corporate and institutional communication in English, English as a lingua franca, Neurolinguistics and Learning aids for special needs. She has participated in nationally funded research projects based in Italy and has been on the organizing committee of numerous academic conferences. She conducts seminars and workshops for Italian companies and multinationals, training managers in intercultural business communication, public speaking, meetings and negotiations, and strategic communication.

Carol Berkenkotter is Professor of Rhetoric and Communication in the Department of Writing Studies, University of Minnesota. Her interests are in the rhetoric of medicine and psychiatry. Over the last decade she has used the techniques of discourse and genre analysis to study the evolution of the case history narrative resulting in the book, *Patient Tales: Case Histories and the Uses of Narrative in Psychiatry*. She is currently working with Cristina Hanganu-Bresch on a book-length manuscript, tentatively titled, *Madness and Identity: Diagnosing, Constructing, and Interpreting the Psychiatric Patient, 1850–1920.*

Ruth Breeze (MA, PhD) has researched and published widely in the area of media language, legal language and professional communication. She is a member of the GradUN research group within the Instituto Cultura y Sociedad at the University of Navarra, Spain. Her recent publications include the monograph *Corporate Discourse* (Bloomsbury Academic, 2013) and *Interpersonality in Legal Genres* (edited with Maurizio Gotti and Carmen Sancho Guinda, Peter Lang, 2014).

Rebecca R. Burson is a psychiatrist currently working with the United States Air Force on an inpatient ward in San Antonio, TX. She is adjunct faculty with the University of Texas Health Science Center where she works daily teaching resident physicians. She also is the Principal Investigator of a research grant investigating sleep, biomarkers and psychiatric outcomes. She is keenly interested in the interaction between trauma, mental health and physical health.

Paola Catenaccio is Associate Professor of English Linguistics and Translation at the University of Milan. Her research interests lie primarily in the field of discourse analysis, which she applies to a variety of domains (legal discourse, business communication, the discourse of news production, the discourse of science and popularization) in combination with other methodological perspectives, adopting a multi-method approach to linguistic research, especially in an intercultural perspective. Her most recent contributions focus on linguistic aspects of corporate communication, especially corporate social responsibility. She has authored numerous articles, which have appeared in international journals and edited collections. Some of her latest publications are: *Understanding CSR Discourse: Insights from Linguistics and Discourse Analysis* (2012); 'Social and environmental reports. A diachronic perspective on an emerging genre' (2011); 'Green advertising and corporate CSR communication: hybrid discourses, mutant genres' (2011); *Corporate Press Releases: An Overview* (2008); 'De-humanising the alien: The construction of migrants' rights in EU legislation' (2007); 'Press releases as a hybrid genre: Addressing the informative/promotional conundrum' (2008). She is also co-editor of *Identities Across Media and Modes: Discursive Perspectives* (2009) (with G. Garzone) and *Genre Change in the Contemporary World* (2012, with G. Garzone and C. Degano).

Kira Dreher is a PhD student in Rhetoric & Scientific & Technical Communication in the Department of Writing Studies at the University of Minnesota, Twin Cities. She is interested in the rhetoric of plain language in technical communication and its implications for genre studies. Her dissertation investigates the rhetorical assumptions of plain language in the Minneapolis City Charter and its use as an authorizing document in government action. She is a co-author of 'Arab Women in

Arab News: Old Stereotypes and New Media' (2012, with Al-Malki, Kaufer, and Ishizaki).

Celina Frade has a PhD in Linguistics and is Professor of English for Specific Purposes (ESP) at the Multidisciplinary Institute of the Rural Federal University of Rio de Janeiro, Brazil. Her main research interests include discourse analysis, genre analysis, translation and semiotics with particular focus on legal discourse. Recent works have also included sociological and anthropological approaches to affirmative action legislation. She also delivers ESP courses for Brazilian undergraduates and professionals in the areas of Tourism and Law.

Maurizio Gotti is Professor of English Language and Translation, Head of the Department of Foreign Languages, Literatures and Communication, and Director of the Research Centre for LSP Research (CERLIS) at the University of Bergamo. His main research areas are the features and origins of specialized discourse (*Robert Boyle and the Language of Science,* 1996; *Specialized Discourse: Linguistic Features and Changing Conventions*, 2003; *Investigating Specialized Discourse*, ^{3}2011). He is also interested in English syntax and English lexicology and lexicography, with particular regard to specialized terminology and canting. He is a member of the Editorial Board of national and international journals, and edits the *Linguistic Insights* series for Peter Lang.

Syelle Graves is a faculty member at LaGuardia College in New York City, where she teaches communication studies courses. She is also a PhD candidate in linguistics at the Graduate Center of the City University of New York.

Cristina Hanganu-Bresch is an Assistant professor of Writing and Rhetoric at University of the Sciences, Philadelphia, where she teaches composition and scientific writing. She is interested in rhetoric of medicine and psychiatric discourse. Among her recent publications are 'Occult Genres and the Certification of Madness in a 19th Century Victorian Asylum' (*Written Communication* 2010, with Carol Berkenkotter), 'Narrative Survival: Personal and Institutional Accounts of Asylum Confinement' (*Literature and Medicine* 2012, with Carol Berkenkotter), and 'Treat Her with Prozac: Four Decades of Direct-to-Physician Antidepressant Advertising' (in *Drugs & Media: New Perspectives on Communication, Consumption and Consciousness* 2012).

MARÍA JOSÉ LUZÓN is Senior Lecturer at the University of Zaragoza, Spain. She has a PhD in English Philology and has published papers on academic and professional discourse and on language teaching and learning in the field of English for Specific Purposes. Her current research interests include online academic genres, especially academic blogs, and English as a Lingua Franca in written academic discourse and online genres. She has recently published papers on the discourse of academic blogs in the journals *Written Communication, Discourse, Context and Media, Text&Talk* and *Applied Linguistics.*

STEFANIA M. MACI is Associate Professor of English Language and Translation at the University of Bergamo, where she teaches English linguistic courses at graduate and undergraduate level. Her research is focused on the study of the English language in academic and professional contexts, with particular regard to the analysis of medical, legal and tourism discourse. Her most recent publications include: the volume *Tourism Discourse: Professional, Promotional, Digital Voices* (2013); and the papers 'What Does he Think This is? The Court of Human Rights or the United Nations?' (2014). '(Plain) Language in the Written Memories of Arbitral Proceedings: A Cross-Cultural Case Study' (2014); 'Investigating Variation in Medical Poster Abstracts' (2014); 'Institutional Popularization of Medical Knowledge: the Case of Pandemic Influenza A (H1N1)' (2014); 'Popularizing Scientific Discourse for an Academic Audience: the Case of Nobel Lectures' (2013).

ROSITA MAGLIE is a researcher and lecturer in English Language and Translation at the University of Bari. Her main research interests are in Specialized Discourse, Corpus-based Translation Studies, and Applied Linguistics. Her PhD dissertation, along with other publications, focuses on the use of domain-specific parallel and comparable *corpora* specially collected in order to investigate English and Italian medical discourse (2004, 2005, 2007, 2009, 2011). Another area of interest includes cross-cultural communication in fashion advertising, a topic on which she has published different papers (2010, 2011, 2012). Her publications include two volumes: *Understanding the Language of Medicine* (Aracne 2009), and *English4Fashion* (Wip Edizioni 2010). An additional area of study she is interested in, examines approaches to teaching English to young learners by engaging with cross-cultural differences and gender variance. Two of her recent articles are on this research topic (2012, 2014).

DAVIDE MAZZI is research fellow in English Language and Translation at the University of Modena and Reggio Emilia (Italy). His research activity has essentially focused on the following areas: discourse analysis, corpus linguistics and argumentation studies. In particular, his research interests and related publications have concentrated on legal, academic, and news discourse. His recent publications include: *The 'Other's' Gaze. The Discursive Construction of Journalists' Professional Identity across Italy and the US*, Boca Raton, Brown Walker Press, 2012; and 'Our reading would lead to…': Corpus Perspectives on Pragmatic Argumentation in US Supreme Court Judgments (*Journal of Argumentation in Context*), 2014.

GREG MYERS is Professor of Rhetoric and Communication in the Department of Linguistics and English Language, Lancaster University, UK. He has written on academic discourse, advertising, and research methods; his most recent book is *The Discourse of Blogs and Wikis* (Continuum, 2010). He was Editor (2012–2014) of the Elsevier journal *Discourse Context & Media*.

ANNA FRANCA PLASTINA is Assistant Professor at the University of Calabria, Italy, where she teaches ESP at undergraduate/postgraduate levels. She holds habilitation qualifications as Associate Professor of English Language and Translation, and of Glottology and Linguistics. Her most recent publications include: 'Diagnostic News Delivery: A Microanalysis of the Use of Shields' (co-author) in Zuczkowski et al. (eds), John Benjamins, 2014; 'A European Approach to Language Teaching: Developing Competency in the Usage of Web 2.0 Tools' in Pérez Cañado / Ráez Padilla (eds), Peter Lang, 2014; 'Multimodality in English for Specific Purposes: Reconceptualizing Meaning-making Practices' *Revista de Lenguas para Fines Específicos,* 2013.

Michele Sala, PhD (University of Bergamo), MA (Youngstown State University, Ohio), is a researcher in English Language and Translation at the University of Bergamo, where he teaches English linguistic courses at graduate and undergraduate level. He is a member of CERLIS (Centro di Ricerca sui Linguaggi Specialistici) and a member of the scientific and editorial board of the *CERLIS Series* (international peer-reviewed volumes on specialized languages). His research activity and major publications deal with language for specific purposes and, more specifically, the application of genre and discourse analytical methods to a corpus-based study of legal-academic discourse and to the analysis of the linguistic, textual and pragmatic aspects of legal translation. He has also published in the field of academic discourse (*Persuasion and Politeness in Academic Discourse*, 2008, *Genre Variation in Academic Communication. Emerging Disciplinary Trends*, 2012 [co-edited with S. Maci]; *Corpora in specialized communication*, 2013 [co-edited with C. Desoutter and D. Heller]) and in the domain of pragmatics and cognitive linguistics (*Differently Amusing*, 2012).

Srikant Sarangi is currently Professor in Humanities and Medicine and Director of the Danish Institute of Humanities and Medicine (DIHM) at Aalborg University, Denmark. He is Honorary Professor at Cardiff University and Fellow of the Academy of Social Sciences, UK. His research interests are in institutional/professional discourse studies (e.g., healthcare, social work, bureaucracy, education) and applied linguistics. He is author and editor of twelve books, guest-editor of five journal special issues and has published nearly two hundred journal articles and book chapters. He is editor of *Text & Talk*; *Communication & Medicine* and co-editor of *Journal of Applied Linguistics and Professional Practice.*

Anna Stermieri holds a PhD in Human Sciences from the University of Modena and Reggio Emilia (Italy). She currently holds a research grant at the University of Modena and Reggio Emilia. Her research interests focus on genre analysis and discourse studies. Her publications explore the features of theatre criticism from a genre-based and ESP point of view, also in a diachronic perspective. Her current research interests are directed towards the discourse of blogs and the investigation of the strategies of popularization and knowledge dissemination in academic blogs and in educational videos.

ANNA TERESZKIEWICZ is a lecturer at the Institute of English Studies at the Jagiellonian University in Krakow, Poland. Her current research mainly focuses on various aspects concerning computer-mediated communication and online genres. Some of her latest publications are: 'Do Poles flame? Aggressiveness on Polish discussion groups and social networking sites' (2012), 'Headlines in British and German Online Newspapers' (2012), 'Rhetorical Strategies on User-Contributory Sites' (2013), 'Tweeting The News: A Contrastive Study of English and German Newspaper Tweets' (2013).

GIROLAMO TESSUTO is Associate Professor of English, Linguistics and Translation at the University of Naples 2, Italy. He also teaches at the Law Department of University of Federico II and the Medicine Department of University of Naples 2. His research interests are in applied linguistics, genre analysis of academic, institutional and professional discourses in legal contexts. Several of his publications have appeared as research papers, book chapters and co-edited volumes. His most recent publications include 'Generic structure and rhetorical moves in English-language empirical law research articles: sites of interdisciplinary and interdiscursive cross-over' (*Journal of English for Specific Purposes*) and *Investigating English Legal Genres in Academic and Professional Settings* (Cambridge Scholars). He is Chief Editor of the *Legal Discourse and Communication* series (formerly *Explorations in Language and Law*), and Editorial Board member of international linguistic journals.

JUDITH TURNBULL is an English language assistant at the Faculty of Economics, 'Sapienza' University of Rome. Her research interests include discourse analysis applied to the fields of economics and law and cross-cultural business communication, with a particular focus on websites. Her recent publications include: 'Expert to layman communication: legal information and advice on the Internet' (2014); *A Linguistic Analysis of English Online. Knowledge Dissemination and the Empowerment of Citizens* (2013); 'Tracking the evolution of Genres: The Case of Corporate Websites' (2013); 'The Blogs of the European Commission: Public-private Space in a Professional Institutional Context' (2013).

Linguistic Insights

Studies in Language and Communication

This series aims to promote specialist language studies in the fields of linguistic theory and applied linguistics, by publishing volumes that focus on specific aspects of language use in one or several languages and provide valuable insights into language and communication research. A cross-disciplinary approach is favoured and most European languages are accepted.

The series includes two types of books:

- **Monographs** – featuring in-depth studies on special aspects of language theory, language analysis or language teaching.
- **Collected papers** – assembling papers from workshops, conferences or symposia.

Each volume of the series is subjected to a double peer-reviewing process.

Vol. 1 Maurizio Gotti & Marina Dossena (eds)
Modality in Specialized Texts. Selected Papers of the 1st CERLIS Conference.
421 pages. 2001. ISBN 3-906767-10-8 · US-ISBN 0-8204-5340-4

Vol. 2 Giuseppina Cortese & Philip Riley (eds)
Domain-specific English. Textual Practices across Communities and Classrooms.
420 pages. 2002. ISBN 3-906768-98-8 · US-ISBN 0-8204-5884-8

Vol. 3 Maurizio Gotti, Dorothee Heller & Marina Dossena (eds)
Conflict and Negotiation in Specialized Texts. Selected Papers of the 2nd CERLIS Conference.
470 pages. 2002. ISBN 3-906769-12-7 · US-ISBN 0-8204-5887-2

Vol. 4 Maurizio Gotti, Marina Dossena, Richard Dury, Roberta Facchinetti & Maria Lima
Variation in Central Modals. A Repertoire of Forms and Types of Usage in Middle English and Early Modern English.
364 pages. 2002. ISBN 3-906769-84-4 · US-ISBN 0-8204-5898-8

Editorial address:

Prof. Maurizio Gotti Università di Bergamo, Dipartimento di Lingue, Letterature Straniere e Comunicazione, Piazza Rosate 2, 24129 Bergamo, Italy
Fax: +39 035 2052789, E-Mail: m.gotti@unibg.it

Vol. 5 Stefania Nuccorini (ed.)
Phrases and Phraseology. Data and Descriptions.
187 pages. 2002. ISBN 3-906770-08-7 · US-ISBN 0-8204-5933-X

Vol. 6 Vijay Bhatia, Christopher N. Candlin & Maurizio Gotti (eds)
Legal Discourse in Multilingual and Multicultural Contexts.
Arbitration Texts in Europe.
385 pages. 2003. ISBN 3-906770-85-0 · US-ISBN 0-8204-6254-3

Vol. 7 Marina Dossena & Charles Jones (eds)
Insights into Late Modern English. 2nd edition.
378 pages. 2003, 2007.
ISBN 978-3-03911-257-9 · US-ISBN 978-0-8204-8927-8

Vol. 8 Maurizio Gotti
Specialized Discourse. Linguistic Features and Changing Conventions.
351 pages. 2003, 2005.
ISBN 3-03910-606-6 · US-ISBN 0-8204-7000-7

Vol. 9 Alan Partington, John Morley & Louann Haarman (eds)
Corpora and Discourse.
420 pages. 2004. ISBN 3-03910-026-2 · US-ISBN 0-8204-6262-4

Vol. 10 Martina Möllering
The Acquisition of German Modal Particles. A Corpus-Based Approach.
290 pages. 2004. ISBN 3-03910-043-2 · US-ISBN 0-8204-6273-X

Vol. 11 David Hart (ed.)
English Modality in Context. Diachronic Perspectives.
261 pages. 2003. ISBN 3-03910-046-7 · US-ISBN 0-8204-6852-5

Vol. 12 Wendy Swanson
Modes of Co-reference as an Indicator of Genre.
430 pages. 2003. ISBN 3-03910-052-1 · US-ISBN 0-8204-6855-X

Vol. 13 Gina Poncini
Discursive Strategies in Multicultural Business Meetings.
2nd edition. 338 pages. 2004, 2007.
ISBN 978-3-03911-296-8 · US-ISBN 978-0-8204-8937-7

Vol. 14 Christopher N. Candlin & Maurizio Gotti (eds)
Intercultural Aspects of Specialized Communication.
2nd edition. 369 pages. 2004, 2007.
ISBN 978-3-03911-258-6 · US-ISBN 978-0-8204-8926-1

Vol. 15 Gabriella Del Lungo Camiciotti & Elena Tognini Bonelli (eds)
Academic Discourse. New Insights into Evaluation.
234 pages. 2004. ISBN 3-03910-353-9 · US-ISBN 0-8204-7016-3

Vol. 16 Marina Dossena & Roger Lass (eds)
Methods and Data in English Historical Dialectology.
405 pages. 2004. ISBN 3-03910-362-8 · US-ISBN 0-8204-7018-X

Vol. 17 Judy Noguchi
The Science Review Article. An Opportune Genre in
the Construction of Science.
274 pages. 2006. ISBN 3-03910-426-8 · US-ISBN 0-8204-7034-1

Vol. 18 Giuseppina Cortese & Anna Duszak (eds)
Identity, Community, Discourse. English in Intercultural Settings.
495 pages. 2005. ISBN 3-03910-632-5 · US-ISBN 0-8204-7163-1

Vol. 19 Anna Trosborg & Poul Erik Flyvholm Jørgensen (eds)
Business Discourse. Texts and Contexts.
250 pages. 2005. ISBN 3-03910-606-6 · US-ISBN 0-8204-7000-7

Vol. 20 Christopher Williams
Tradition and Change in Legal English. Verbal Constructions in Prescriptive Texts.
2nd revised edition. 216 pages. 2005, 2007. ISBN 978-3-03911-444-3.

Vol. 21 Katarzyna Dziubalska-Kolaczyk & Joanna Przedlacka (eds)
English Pronunciation Models: A Changing Scene.
2nd edition. 476 pages. 2005, 2008. ISBN 978-3-03911-682-9.

Vol. 22 Christián Abello-Contesse, Rubén Chacón-Beltrán, M. Dolores López-Jiménez & M. Mar Torreblanca-López (eds)
Age in L2 Acquisition and Teaching.
214 pages. 2006. ISBN 3-03910-668-6 · US-ISBN 0-8204-7174-7

Vol. 23 Vijay K. Bhatia, Maurizio Gotti, Jan Engberg & Dorothee Heller (eds)
Vagueness in Normative Texts.
474 pages. 2005. ISBN 3-03910-653-8 · US-ISBN 0-8204-7169-0

Vol. 24 Paul Gillaerts & Maurizio Gotti (eds)
Genre Variation in Business Letters. 2nd printing.
407 pages. 2008. ISBN 978-3-03911-681-2.

Vol. 25 Ana María Hornero, María José Luzón & Silvia Murillo (eds)
Corpus Linguistics. Applications for the Study of English.
2nd printing. 526 pages. 2006, 2008. ISBN 978-3-03911-726-0

Vol. 26 J. Lachlan Mackenzie & María de los Ángeles Gómez-González (eds)
Studies in Functional Discourse Grammar.
259 pages. 2005. ISBN 3-03910-696-1 · US-ISBN 0-8204-7558-0

Vol. 27 Debbie G. E. Ho
Classroom Talk. Exploring the Sociocultural Structure of Formal ESL Learning.
2nd edition. 254 pages. 2006, 2007. ISBN 978-3-03911-434-4

Vol. 28 Javier Pérez-Guerra, Dolores González-Álvarez, Jorge L. Bueno-Alonso & Esperanza Rama-Martínez (eds)
'Of Varying Language and Opposing Creed'. New Insights into Late Modern English.
455 pages. 2007. ISBN 978-3-03910-788-9

Vol. 29 Francesca Bargiela-Chiappini & Maurizio Gotti (eds)
Asian Business Discourse(s).
350 pages. 2005. ISBN 3-03910-804-2 · US-ISBN 0-8204-7574-2

Vol. 30 Nicholas Brownlees (ed.)
News Discourse in Early Modern Britain. Selected Papers of CHINED 2004.
300 pages. 2006. ISBN 3-03910-805-0 · US-ISBN 0-8204-8025-8

Vol. 31 Roberta Facchinetti & Matti Rissanen (eds)
Corpus-based Studies of Diachronic English.
300 pages. 2006. ISBN 3-03910-851-4 · US-ISBN 0-8204-8040-1

Vol. 32 Marina Dossena & Susan M. Fitzmaurice (eds)
Business and Official Correspondence. Historical Investigations.
209 pages. 2006. ISBN 3-03910-880-8 · US-ISBN 0-8204-8352-4

Vol. 33 Giuliana Garzone & Srikant Sarangi (eds)
Discourse, Ideology and Specialized Communication.
494 pages. 2007. ISBN 978-3-03910-888-6

Vol. 34 Giuliana Garzone & Cornelia Ilie (eds)
The Use of English in Institutional and Business Settings.
An Intercultural Perspective.
372 pages. 2007. ISBN 978-3-03910-889-3

Vol. 35 Vijay K. Bhatia & Maurizio Gotti (eds)
Explorations in Specialized Genres.
316 pages. 2006. ISBN 3-03910-995-2 · US-ISBN 0-8204-8372-9

Vol. 36 Heribert Picht (ed.)
Modern Approaches to Terminological Theories and Applications.
432 pages. 2006. ISBN 3-03911-156-6 · US-ISBN 0-8204-8380-X

Vol. 37 Anne Wagner & Sophie Cacciaguidi-Fahy (eds)
Legal Language and the Search for Clarity / Le langage juridique et la quête de clarté.
Practice and Tools / Pratiques et instruments.
487 pages. 2006. ISBN 3-03911-169-8 · US-ISBN 0-8204-8388-5

Vol. 38 Juan Carlos Palmer-Silveira, Miguel F. Ruiz-Garrido &
Inmaculada Fortanet-Gómez (eds)
Intercultural and International Business Communication.
Theory, Research and Teaching.
2nd edition. 343 pages. 2006, 2008. ISBN 978-3-03911-680-5

Vol. 39 Christiane Dalton-Puffer, Dieter Kastovsky, Nikolaus Ritt &
Herbert Schendl (eds)
Syntax, Style and Grammatical Norms. English from 1500–2000.
250 pages. 2006. ISBN 3-03911-181-7 · US-ISBN 0-8204-8394-X

Vol. 40 Marina Dossena & Irma Taavitsainen (eds)
Diachronic Perspectives on Domain-Specific English.
280 pages. 2006. ISBN 3-03910-176-0 · US-ISBN 0-8204-8391-5

Vol. 41 John Flowerdew & Maurizio Gotti (eds)
Studies in Specialized Discourse.
293 pages. 2006. ISBN 3-03911-178-7

Vol. 42 Ken Hyland & Marina Bondi (eds)
Academic Discourse Across Disciplines.
320 pages. 2006. ISBN 3-03911-183-3 · US-ISBN 0-8204-8396-6

Vol. 43 Paul Gillaerts & Philip Shaw (eds)
The Map and the Landscape. Norms and Practices in Genre.
256 pages. 2006. ISBN 3-03911-182-5 · US-ISBN 0-8204-8395-4

Vol. 44 Maurizio Gotti & Davide Giannoni (eds)
New Trends in Specialized Discourse Analysis.
301 pages. 2006. ISBN 3-03911-184-1 · US-ISBN 0-8204-8381-8

Vol. 45 Maurizio Gotti & Françoise Salager-Meyer (eds)
Advances in Medical Discourse Analysis. Oral and Written Contexts.
492 pages. 2006. ISBN 3-03911-185-X · US-ISBN 0-8204-8382-6

Vol. 46 Maurizio Gotti & Susan Šarcević (eds)
Insights into Specialized Translation.
396 pages. 2006. ISBN 3-03911-186-8 · US-ISBN 0-8204-8383-4

Vol. 47 Khurshid Ahmad & Margaret Rogers (eds)
Evidence-based LSP. Translation, Text and Terminology.
584 pages. 2007. ISBN 978-3-03911-187-9

Vol. 48 Hao Sun & Dániel Z. Kádár (eds)
It's the Dragon's Turn. Chinese Institutional Discourses.
262 pages. 2008. ISBN 978-3-03911-175-6

Vol. 49 Cristina Suárez-Gómez
Relativization in Early English (950-1250). the Position of Relative Clauses.
149 pages. 2006. ISBN 3-03911-203-1 · US-ISBN 0-8204-8904-2

Vol. 50 Maria Vittoria Calvi & Luisa Chierichetti (eds)
Nuevas tendencias en el discurso de especialidad.
319 pages. 2006. ISBN 978-3-03911-261-6

Vol. 51 Mari Carmen Campoy & María José Luzón (eds)
Spoken Corpora in Applied Linguistics.
274 pages. 2008. ISBN 978-3-03911-275-3

Vol. 52 Konrad Ehlich & Dorothee Heller (Hrsg.)
Die Wissenschaft und ihre Sprachen.
323 pages. 2006. ISBN 978-3-03911-272-2

Vol. 53 Jingyu Zhang
The Semantic Salience Hierarchy Model. The L2 Acquisition of Psych Predicates
273 pages. 2007. ISBN 978-3-03911-300-2

Vol. 54 Norman Fairclough, Giuseppina Cortese & Patrizia Ardizzone (eds)
Discourse and Contemporary Social Change.
555 pages. 2007. ISBN 978-3-03911-276-0

Vol. 55 Jan Engberg, Marianne Grove Ditlevsen, Peter Kastberg & Martin Stegu (eds)
New Directions in LSP Teaching.
331 pages. 2007. ISBN 978-3-03911-433-7

Vol. 56 Dorothee Heller & Konrad Ehlich (Hrsg.)
Studien zur Rechtskommunikation.
322 pages. 2007. ISBN 978-3-03911-436-8

Vol. 57 Teruhiro Ishiguro & Kang-kwong Luke (eds)
Grammar in Cross-Linguistic Perspective.
The Syntax, Semantics, and Pragmatics of Japanese and Chinese.
304 pages. 2012. ISBN 978-3-03911-445-0

Vol. 58 Carmen Frehner
Email – SMS – MMS
294 pages. 2008. ISBN 978-3-03911-451-1

Vol. 59 Isabel Balteiro
The Directionality of Conversion in English. A Dia-Synchronic Study.
276 pages. 2007. ISBN 978-3-03911-241-8

Vol. 60 Maria Milagros Del Saz Rubio
English Discourse Markers of Reformulation.
237 pages. 2007. ISBN 978-3-03911-196-1

Vol. 61 Sally Burgess & Pedro Martín-Martín (eds)
English as an Additional Language in Research Publication and Communication.
259 pages. 2008. ISBN 978-3-03911-462-7

Vol. 62 Sandrine Onillon
Pratiques et représentations de l'écrit.
458 pages. 2008. ISBN 978-3-03911-464-1

Vol. 63 Hugo Bowles & Paul Seedhouse (eds)
Conversation Analysis and Language for Specific Purposes.
2nd edition. 337 pages. 2007, 2009. ISBN 978-3-0343-0045-2

Vol. 64 Vijay K. Bhatia, Christopher N. Candlin & Paola Evangelisti Allori (eds)
Language, Culture and the Law.
The Formulation of Legal Concepts across Systems and Cultures.
342 pages. 2008. ISBN 978-3-03911-470-2

Vol. 65 Jonathan Culpeper & Dániel Z. Kádár (eds)
Historical (Im)politeness.
300 pages. 2010. ISBN 978-3-03911-496-2

Vol. 66 Linda Lombardo (ed.)
Using Corpora to Learn about Language and Discourse.
237 pages. 2009. ISBN 978-3-03911-522-8

Vol. 67 Natsumi Wakamoto
Extroversion/Introversion in Foreign Language Learning.
Interactions with Learner Strategy Use.
159 pages. 2009. ISBN 978-3-03911-596-9

Vol. 68 Eva Alcón-Soler (ed.)
Learning How to Request in an Instructed Language Learning Context.
260 pages. 2008. ISBN 978-3-03911-601-0

Vol. 69 Domenico Pezzini
The Translation of Religious Texts in the Middle Ages.
428 pages. 2008. ISBN 978-3-03911-600-3

Vol. 70 Tomoko Tode
Effects of Frequency in Classroom Second Language Learning.
Quasi-experiment and stimulated-recall analysis.
195 pages. 2008. ISBN 978-3-03911-602-7

Vol. 71 Egor Tsedryk
Fusion symétrique et alternances ditransitives.
211 pages. 2009. ISBN 978-3-03911-609-6

Vol. 72 Cynthia J. Kellett Bidoli & Elana Ochse (eds)
English in International Deaf Communication.
444 pages. 2008. ISBN 978-3-03911-610-2

Vol. 73 Joan C. Beal, Carmela Nocera & Massimo Sturiale (eds)
Perspectives on Prescriptivism.
269 pages. 2008. ISBN 978-3-03911-632-4

Vol. 74 Carol Taylor Torsello, Katherine Ackerley & Erik Castello (eds)
Corpora for University Language Teachers.
308 pages. 2008. ISBN 978-3-03911-639-3

Vol. 75 María Luisa Pérez Cañado (ed.)
English Language Teaching in the European Credit Transfer System. Facing the Challenge.
251 pages. 2009. ISBN 978-3-03911-654-6

Vol. 76 Marina Dossena & Ingrid Tieken-Boon van Ostade (eds)
Studies in Late Modern English Correspondence. Methodology and Data.
291 pages. 2008. ISBN 978-3-03911-658-4

Vol. 77 Ingrid Tieken-Boon van Ostade & Wim van der Wurff (eds)
Current Issues in Late Modern English.
436 pages. 2009. ISBN 978-3-03911-660-7

Vol. 78 Marta Navarro Coy (ed.)
Practical Approaches to Foreign Language Teaching and Learning.
297 pages. 2009. ISBN 978-3-03911-661-4

Vol. 79 Qing Ma
Second Language Vocabulary Acquisition.
333 pages. 2009. ISBN 978-3-03911-666-9

Vol. 80 Martin Solly, Michelangelo Conoscenti & Sandra Campagna (eds)
Verbal/Visual Narrative Texts in Higher Education.
384 pages. 2008. ISBN 978-3-03911-672-0

Vol. 81 Meiko Matsumoto
From Simple Verbs to Periphrastic Expressions: The Historical Development of Composite Predicates, Phrasal Verbs, and Related Constructions in English.
235 pages. 2008. ISBN 978-3-03911-675-1

Vol. 82 Melinda Dooly
Doing Diversity. Teachers' Construction of Their Classroom Reality.
180 pages. 2009. ISBN 978-3-03911-687-4

Vol. 83 Victoria Guillén-Nieto, Carmen Marimón-Llorca & Chelo Vargas-Sierra (eds)
Intercultural Business Communication and Simulation and Gaming Methodology.
392 pages. 2009. ISBN 978-3-03911-688-1

Vol. 84 Maria Grazia Guido
English as a Lingua Franca in Cross-cultural Immigration Domains.
285 pages. 2008. ISBN 978-3-03911-689-8

Vol. 85 Erik Castello
Text Complexity and Reading Comprehension Tests.
352 pages. 2008. ISBN 978-3-03911-717-8

Vol. 86 Maria-Lluisa Gea-Valor, Isabel García-Izquierdo & Maria-José Esteve (eds)
Linguistic and Translation Studies in Scientific Communication.
317 pages. 2010. ISBN 978-3-0343-0069-8

Vol. 87 Carmen Navarro, Rosa Mª Rodríguez Abella, Francesca Dalle Pezze & Renzo Miotti (eds)
La comunicación especializada.
355 pages. 2008. ISBN 978-3-03911-733-8

Vol. 88 Kiriko Sato
The Development from Case-Forms to Prepositional Constructions in Old English Prose.
231 pages. 2009. ISBN 978-3-03911-763-5

Vol. 89 Dorothee Heller (Hrsg.)
Formulierungsmuster in deutscher und italienischer Fachkommunikation. Intra- und interlinguale Perspektiven.
315 pages. 2008. ISBN 978-3-03911-778-9

Vol. 90 Henning Bergenholtz, Sandro Nielsen & Sven Tarp (eds)
Lexicography at a Crossroads. Dictionaries and Encyclopedias Today, Lexicographical Tools Tomorrow.
372 pages. 2009. ISBN 978-3-03911-799-4

Vol. 91 Manouchehr Moshtagh Khorasani
The Development of Controversies. From the Early Modern Period to Online Discussion Forums.
317 pages. 2009. ISBN 978-3-3911-711-6

Vol. 92 María Luisa Carrió-Pastor (ed.)
Content and Language Integrated Learning. Cultural Diversity.
178 pages. 2009. ISBN 978-3-3911-818-2

Vol. 93 Roger Berry
Terminology in English Language Teaching. Nature and Use.
262 pages. 2010. ISBN 978-3-0343-0013-1

Vol. 94 Roberto Cagliero & Jennifer Jenkins (eds)
Discourses, Communities, and Global Englishes
240 pages. 2010. ISBN 978-3-0343-0012-4

Vol. 95 Facchinetti Roberta, Crystal David, Seidlhofer Barbara (eds)
From International to Local English – And Back Again.
268 pages. 2010. ISBN 978-3-0343-0011-7

Vol. 96 Cesare Gagliardi & Alan Maley (eds)
EIL, ELF, Global English. Teaching and Learning Issues
376 pages. 2010. ISBN 978-3-0343-0010-0

Vol. 97 Sylvie Hancil (ed.)
The Role of Prosody in Affective Speech.
403 pages. 2009. ISBN 978-3-03911-696-6

Vol. 98 Marina Dossena & Roger Lass (eds)
Studies in English and European Historical Dialectology.
257 pages. 2009. ISBN 978-3-0343-0024-7

Vol. 99 Christine Béal
Les interactions quotidiennes en français et en anglais. De l'approche comparative à l'analyse des situations interculturelles.
424 pages. 2010. ISBN 978-3-0343-0027-8

Vol. 100 Maurizio Gotti (ed.)
Commonality and Individuality in Academic Discourse.
398 pages. 2009. ISBN 978-3-0343-0023-0

Vol. 101 Javier E. Díaz Vera & Rosario Caballero (eds)
Textual Healing. Studies in Medieval English Medical, Scientific and Technical Texts.
213 pages. 2009. ISBN 978-3-03911-822-9

Vol. 102 Nuria Edo Marzá
The Specialised Lexicographical Approach. A Step further in Dictionary-making.
316 pages. 2009. ISBN 978-3-0343-0043-8

Vol. 103 Carlos Prado-Alonso, Lidia Gómez-García, Iria Pastor-Gómez & David Tizón-Couto (eds)
New Trends and Methodologies in Applied English Language Research. Diachronic, Diatopic and Contrastive Studies.
348 pages. 2009. ISBN 978-3-0343-0046-9

Vol. 104 Françoise Salager-Meyer & Beverly A. Lewin
Crossed Words. Criticism in Scholarly Writing?
371 pages. 2011. ISBN 978-3-0343-0049-0.

Vol. 105 Javier Ruano-García
Early Modern Northern English Lexis. A Literary Corpus-Based Study.
611 pages. 2010. ISBN 978-3-0343-0058-2

Vol. 106 Rafael Monroy-Casas
Systems for the Phonetic Transcription of English. Theory and Texts.
280 pages. 2011. ISBN 978-3-0343-0059-9

Vol. 107 Nicola T. Owtram
The Pragmatics of Academic Writing.
A Relevance Approach to the Analysis of Research Article Introductions.
311 pages. 2009. ISBN 978-3-0343-0060-5

Vol. 108 Yolanda Ruiz de Zarobe, Juan Manuel Sierra & Francisco Gallardo del Puerto (eds)
Content and Foreign Language Integrated Learning.
Contributions to Multilingualism in European Contexts
343 pages. 2011. ISBN 978-3-0343-0074-2

Vol. 109 Ángeles Linde López & Rosalía Crespo Jiménez (eds)
Professional English in the European context. The EHEA challenge.
374 pages. 2010. ISBN 978-3-0343-0088-9

Vol. 110 Rosalía Rodríguez-Vázquez
The Rhythm of Speech, Verse and Vocal Music. A New Theory.
394 pages. 2010. ISBN 978-3-0343-0309-5

Vol. 111 Anastasios Tsangalidis & Roberta Facchinetti (eds)
Studies on English Modality. In Honour of Frank Palmer.
392 pages. 2009. ISBN 978-3-0343-0310-1

Vol. 112 Jing Huang
Autonomy, Agency and Identity in Foreign Language Learning and Teaching.
400 pages. 2013. ISBN 978-3-0343-0370-5

Vol. 113 Mihhail Lotman & Maria-Kristiina Lotman (eds)
Frontiers in Comparative Prosody. In memoriam: Mikhail Gasparov.
426 pages. 2011. ISBN 978-3-0343-0373-6

Vol. 114 Merja Kytö, John Scahill & Harumi Tanabe (eds)
Language Change and Variation from Old English to Late Modern English.
A Festschrift for Minoji Akimoto
422 pages. 2010. ISBN 978-3-0343-0372-9

Vol. 115 Giuliana Garzone & Paola Catenaccio (eds)
Identities across Media and Modes. Discursive Perspectives.
379 pages. 2009. ISBN 978-3-0343-0386-6

Vol. 116 Elena Landone
Los marcadores del discurso y cortesía verbal en español.
390 pages. 2010. ISBN 978-3-0343-0413-9

Vol. 117 Maurizio Gotti & Christopher Williams (eds)
Legal Discourse across Languages and Cultures.
339 pages. 2010. ISBN 978-3-0343-0425-2

Vol. 118 David Hirsh
Academic Vocabulary in Context.
217 pages. 2010. ISBN 978-3-0343-0426-9

Vol. 119 Yvonne Dröschel
Lingua Franca English. The Role of Simplification and Transfer.
358 pages. 2011. ISBN 978-3-0343-0432-0

Vol. 120 Tengku Sepora Tengku Mahadi, Helia Vaezian & Mahmoud Akbari
Corpora in Translation. A Practical Guide.
135 pages. 2010. ISBN 978-3-0343-0434-4

Vol. 121 Davide Simone Giannoni & Celina Frade (eds)
Researching Language and the Law. Textual Features and Translation Issues.
278 pages. 2010. ISBN 978-3-0343-0443-6

Vol. 122 Daniel Madrid & Stephen Hughes (eds)
Studies in Bilingual Education.
472 pages. 2011. ISBN 978-3-0343-0474-0

Vol. 123 Vijay K. Bhatia, Christopher N. Candlin & Maurizio Gotti (eds)
The Discourses of Dispute Resolution.
290 pages. 2010. ISBN 978-3-0343-0476-4

Vol. 124 Davide Simone Giannoni
Mapping Academic Values in the Disciplines. A Corpus-Based Approach.
288 pages. 2010. ISBN 978-3-0343-0488-7

Vol. 125 Giuliana Garzone & James Archibald (eds)
Discourse, Identities and Roles in Specialized Communication.
419 pages. 2010. ISBN 978-3-0343-0494-8

Vol. 126 Iria Pastor-Gómez
The Status and Development of N+N Sequences in
Contemporary English Noun Phrases.
216 pages. 2011. ISBN 978-3-0343-0534-1

Vol. 127 Carlos Prado-Alonso
Full-verb Inversion in Written and Spoken English.
261 pages. 2011. ISBN 978-3-0343-0535-8

Vol. 128 Tony Harris & María Moreno Jaén (eds)
Corpus Linguistics in Language Teaching.
214 pages. 2010. ISBN 978-3-0343-0524-2

Vol. 129 Tetsuji Oda & Hiroyuki Eto (eds)
Multiple Perspectives on English Philology and History of Linguistics.
A Festschrift for Shoichi Watanabe on his 80th Birthday.
378 pages. 2010. ISBN 978-3-0343-0480-1

Vol. 130 Luisa Chierichetti & Giovanni Garofalo (eds)
Lengua y Derecho. líneas de investigación interdisciplinaria.
283 pages. 2010. 978-3-0343-0463-4

Vol. 131 Paola Evangelisti Allori & Giuliana Garzone (eds)
Discourse, Identities and Genres in Corporate Communication.
Sponsorship, Advertising and Organizational Communication.
324 pages. 2011. 978-3-0343-0591-4

Vol. 132 Leyre Ruiz de Zarobe & Yolanda Ruiz de Zarobe (eds)
Speech Acts and Politeness across Languages and Cultures.
402 pages. 2012. 978-3-0343-0611-9

Vol. 133 Thomas Christiansen
Cohesion. A Discourse Perspective.
387 pages. 2011. 978-3-0343-0619-5

Vol. 134 Giuliana Garzone & Maurizio Gotti
Discourse, Communication and the Enterprise. Genres and Trends.
451 pages. 2011. ISBN 978-3-0343-0620-1

Vol. 135 Zsuzsa Hoffmann
Ways of the World's Words.
Language Contact in the Age of Globalization.
334 pages 2011. ISBN 978-3-0343-0673-7

Vol. 136 Cecilia Varcasia (ed.)
Becoming Multilingual.
Language Learning and Language Policy between Attitudes and Identities.
213 pages. 2011. ISBN 978-3-0343-0687-5

Vol. 137 Susy Macqueen
The Emergence of Patterns in Second Language Writing.
A Sociocognitive Exploration of Lexical Trails.
325 pages. 2012. ISBN 978-3-0343-1010-9

Vol. 138 Maria Vittoria Calvi & Giovanna Mapelli (eds)
La lengua del turismo. Géneros discursivos y terminología.
365 pages. 2011. ISBN 978-3-0343-1011-6

Vol. 139 Ken Lau
Learning to Become a Professional in a Textually-Mediated World.
A Text-Oriented Study of Placement Practices.
261 pages. 2012. ISBN 978-3-0343-1016-1

Vol. 140 Sandra Campagna, Giuliana Garzone, Cornelia Ilie & Elizabeth Rowley-Jolivet (eds)
Evolving Genres in Web-mediated Communication.
337 pages. 2012. ISBN 978-3-0343-1013-0

Vol. 141 Edith Esch & Martin Solly (eds)
The Sociolinguistics of Language Education in International Contexts.
263 pages. 2012. ISBN 978-3-0343-1009-3

Vol. 142 Forthcoming.

Vol. 143 David Tizón-Couto
Left Dislocation in English. A Functional-Discoursal Approach.
416 pages. 2012. ISBN 978-3-0343-1037-6

Vol. 144 Margrethe Petersen & Jan Engberg (eds)
Current Trends in LSP Research. Aims and Methods.
323 pages. 2011. ISBN 978-3-0343-1054-3

Vol. 145 David Tizón-Couto, Beatriz Tizón-Couto, Iria Pastor-Gómez & Paula Rodríguez-Puente (eds)
New Trends and Methodologies in Applied English Language Research II.
Studies in Language Variation, Meaning and Learning.
283 pages. 2012. ISBN 978-3-0343-1061-1

Vol. 146 Rita Salvi & Hiromasa Tanaka (eds)
Intercultural Interactions in Business and Management.
306 pages. 2011. ISBN 978-3-0343-1039-0

Vol. 147 Francesco Straniero Sergio & Caterina Falbo (eds)
Breaking Ground in Corpus-based Interpreting Studies.
254 pages. 2012. ISBN 978-3-0343-1071-0

Vol. 148 Forthcoming.

Vol. 149 Vijay K. Bhatia & Paola Evangelisti Allori (eds)
Discourse and Identity in the Professions. Legal, Corporate and Institutional Citizenship.
352 pages. 2011. ISBN 978-3-0343-1079-6

Vol. 150 Maurizio Gotti (ed.)
Academic Identity Traits. A Corpus-Based Investigation.
363 pages. 2012. ISBN 978-3-0343-1141-0

Vol. 151 Priscilla Heynderickx, Sylvain Dieltjens, Geert Jacobs, Paul Gillaerts &
Elizabeth de Groot (eds)
The Language Factor in International Business.
New Perspectives on Research, Teaching and Practice.
320 pages. 2012. ISBN 978-3-0343-1090-1

Vol. 152 Paul Gillaerts, Elizabeth de Groot, Sylvain Dieltjens, Priscilla Heynderickx &
Geert Jacobs (eds)
Researching Discourse in Business Genres. Cases and Corpora.
215 pages. 2012. ISBN 978-3-0343-1092-5

Vol. 153 Yongyan Zheng
Dynamic Vocabulary Development in a Foreign Language.
262 pages. 2012. ISBN 978-3-0343-1106-9

Vol. 154 Carmen Argondizzo (ed.)
Creativity and Innovation in Language Education.
357 pages. 2012. ISBN 978-3-0343-1080-2

Vol. 155 David Hirsh (ed.)
Current Perspectives in Second Language Vocabulary Research.
180 pages. 2012. ISBN 978-3-0343-1108-3

Vol. 156 Seiji Shinkawa
Unhistorical Gender Assignment in Laȝamon's *Brut*. A Case Study of a Late Stage
in the Development of Grammatical Gender toward its Ultimate Loss.
186 pages. 2012. ISBN 978-3-0343-1124-3

Vol. 157 Yeonkwon Jung
Basics of Organizational Writing: A Critical Reading Approach.
151 pages. 2014. ISBN 978-3-0343-1137-3.

Vol. 158 Bárbara Eizaga Rebollar (ed.)
Studies in Linguistics and Cognition.
301 pages. 2012. ISBN 978-3-0343-1138-0

Vol. 159 Giuliana Garzone, Paola Catenaccio, Chiara Degano (eds)
Genre Change in the Contemporary World. Short-term Diachronic Perspectives.
329 pages. 2012. ISBN 978-3-0343-1214-1

Vol. 160 Carol Berkenkotter, Vijay K. Bhatia & Maurizio Gotti (eds)
Insights into Academic Genres.
468 pages. 2012. ISBN 978-3-0343-1211-0

Vol. 161 Beatriz Tizón-Couto
Clausal Complements in Native and Learner Spoken English. A corpus-based study with Lindsei and Vicolse. 357 pages. 2013. ISBN 978-3-0343-1184-7

Vol. 162 Patrizia Anesa
Jury Trials and the Popularization of Legal Language. A Discourse Analytical Approach.
247 pages. 2012. ISBN 978-3-0343-1231-8

Vol. 163 David Hirsh
Endangered Languages, Knowledge Systems and Belief Systems.
153 pages. 2013. ISBN 978-3-0343-1232-5

Vol. 164 Eugenia Sainz (ed.)
De la estructura de la frase al tejido del discurso. Estudios contrastivos español/italiano.
305 pages. 2014. ISBN 978-3-0343-1253-0

Vol. 165 Julia Bamford, Franca Poppi & Davide Mazzi (eds)
Space, Place and the Discursive Construction of Identity.
367 pages. 2014. ISBN 978-3-0343-1249-3

Vol. 166 Rita Salvi & Janet Bowker (eds)
Space, Time and the Construction of Identity.
Discursive Indexicality in Cultural, Institutional and Professional Fields.
324 pages. 2013. ISBN 978-3-0343-1254-7

Vol. 167 Shunji Yamazaki & Robert Sigley (eds)
Approaching Language Variation through Corpora. A Festschrift in Honour of Toshio Saito.
421 pages. 2013. ISBN 978-3-0343-1264-6

Vol. 168 Franca Poppi
Global Interactions in English as a Lingua Franca. How written communication is changing under the influence of electronic media and new contexts of use.
249 pages. 2012. ISBN 978-3-0343-1276-9

Vol. 169 Miguel A. Aijón Oliva & María José Serrano
Style in syntax. Investigating variation in Spanish pronoun subjects.
239 pages. 2013. ISBN 978-3-0343-1244-8

Vol. 170 Inés Olza, Óscar Loureda & Manuel Casado-Velarde (eds)
Language Use in the Public Sphere. Methodological Perspectives and Empirical Applications
564 pages. 2014. ISBN 978-3-0343-1286-8

Vol. 171 Aleksandra Matulewska
Legilinguistic Translatology. A Parametric Approach to Legal Translation.
279 pages. 2013. ISBN 978-3-0343-1287-5

Vol. 172 Maurizio Gotti & Carmen Sancho Guinda (eds)
Narratives in Academic and Professional Genres.
513 pages. 2013. ISBN 978-3-0343-1371-1

Vol. 173 Madalina Chitez
Learner corpus profiles. The case of Romanian Learner English.
244 pages. 2014. ISBN 978-3-0343-1410-7

Vol. 174 Chihiro Inoue
Task Equivalence in Speaking Tests.
251 pages. 2013. ISBN 978-3-0343-1417-6

Vol. 175 Gabriel Quiroz & Pedro Patiño (eds.)
LSP in Colombia: advances and challenges.
339 pages. 2014. ISBN 978-3-0343-1434-3

Vol. 176 Catherine Resche
Economic Terms and Beyond: Capitalising on the Wealth of Notions.
How Researchers in Specialised Varieties of English Can Benefit from Focusing on Terms.
332 pages. 2013. ISBN 978-3-0343-1435-0

Vol. 177 Forthcoming.

Vol. 178 Cécile Desoutter & Caroline Mellet (dir.)
Le discours rapporté: approches linguistiques et perspectives didactiques.
270 pages. 2013. ISBN 978-3-0343-1292-9

Vol. 179 Ana Díaz-Negrillo & Francisco Javier Díaz-Pérez (eds)
Specialisation and Variation in Language Corpora.
341 pages. 2014. ISBN 978-3-0343-1316-2

Vol. 180 Pilar Alonso
A Multi-dimensional Approach to Discourse Coherence. From Standardness to Creativity.
247 pages. 2014. ISBN 978-3-0343-1325-4

Vol. 181 Alejandro Alcaraz-Sintes & Salvador Valera-Hernández (eds)
Diachrony and Synchrony in English Corpus Linguistics.
393 pages. 2014. ISBN 978-3-0343-1326-1

Vol. 182 Runhan Zhang
Investigating Linguistic Knowledge of a Second Language.
207 pages. 2015. ISBN 978-3-0343-1330-8

Vol. 183 Hajar Abdul Rahim & Shakila Abdul Manan (eds.)
English in Malaysia. Postcolonial and Beyond.
267 pages. 2014. ISBN 978-3-0343-1341-4

Vol. 184 Virginie Fasel Lauzon
Comprendre et apprendre dans l'interaction. Les séquences d'explication en classe de français langue seconde.
292 pages. 2014. ISBN 978-3-0343-1451-0

Vol. 185 Forthcoming.

Vol. 186 Wei Ren
L2 Pragmatic Development in Study Abroad Contexts
256 pages. 2015. ISBN 978-3-0343-1358-2

Vol. 187 Marina Bondi & Rosa Lorés Sanz (eds)
Abstracts in Academic Discourse. Variation and Change.
361 pages. 2014. ISBN 978-3-0343-1483-1

Vol. 188 Forthcoming.

Vol. 189 Paola Evangelisti Allori (ed.)
Identities in and across Cultures.
315 pages. 2014. ISBN 978-3-0343-1458-9

Vol. 190 Forthcoming.

Vol. 191 Ruth Breeze, Maurizio Gotti & Carmen Sancho Guinda (eds)
Interpersonality in Legal Genres.
389 pages. 2014. ISBN 978-3-0343-1524-1

Vol. 192 Paola Evangelisti Allori, John Bateman & Vijay K. Bhatia (eds)
Evolution in Genre. Emergence, Variation, Multimodality.
364 pages. 2014. ISBN 978-3-0343-1533-3

Vol. 193 Jiyeon Kook
Agency in Arzt-Patient-Gesprächen. Zur interaktionistischen Konzeptualisierung von Agency
271 pages. 2015. ISBN 978-3-0343-1666-8

Vol. 194 Susana Nicolás Román & Juan José Torres Núñez (eds)
Drama and CLIL. A new challenge for the teaching approaches in bilingual education.
170 pages. 2015. ISBN 978-3-0343-1629-3

Vol. 195 Alessandra Molino & Serenella Zanotti (eds)
Observing Norm, Observing Usage. Lexis in Dictionaries and in the Media.
430 pages. 2015. ISBN 978-3-0343-1584-5

Vol. 196 Begoña Soneira
A Lexical Description of English for Architecture. A Corpus-based Approach.
267 pages. 2015. ISBN 978-3-0343-1602-6

Vol. 197-198 Forthcoming.

Vol. 199 Rita Salvi & Janet Bowker (eds)
The Dissemination of Contemporary Knowledge in English. Genres, discourse strategies and professional practices.
171 pages. 2015. ISBN 978-3-0343-1679-8

Vol. 200 Maurizio Gotti & Davide S. Giannoni (eds)
Corpus Analysis for Descriptive and Pedagogical Purposes. ESP Perspectives.
432 pages. 2014. ISBN 978-3-0343-1516-6

Vol. 201 Ida Ruffolo
The Perception of Nature in Travel Promotion Texts. A Corpus-based Discourse Analysis.
148 pages. 2015. ISBN 978-3-0343-1521-0

Vol. 202 Ives Trevian
English suffixes. Stress-assignment properties, productivity, selection and combinatorial processes.
471 pages. 2015. ISBN 978-3-0343-1576-0

Vol. 203 Maurizio Gotti, Stefania Maci & Michele Sala (eds)
Insights into Medical Communication.
422 pages. 2015. ISBN 978-3-0343-1694-1

Vol. 204-205 Forthcoming.

Vol. 206 Maria Pavesi, Maicol Formentelli & Elisa Ghia (eds)
The Languages of Dubbing. Mainstream Audiovisual Translation in Italy.
275 pages. 2014. ISBN 978-3-0343-1646-0

www.ingramcontent.com/pod-product-compliance
Ingram Content Group UK Ltd.
Pitfield, Milton Keynes, MK11 3LW, UK
UKHW020721041026
15590UKWH00002B/794

9 783034 316941